Sigurd P. Ramfjord, L.D.S., M.S., Ph.D.

PROFESSOR OF DENTISTRY, THE UNIVERSITY OF MICHIGAN

Major M. Ash, Jr., B.S., D.D.S., M.S.

PROFESSOR OF DENTISTRY, THE UNIVERSITY OF MICHIGAN

OCCLUSION

SECOND EDITION

W. B. Saunders Company—Philadelphia—London—Toronto

W. B. Saunders Company: West Washington Square
                          Philadelphia, PA 19105

                          1 St. Anne's Road
                          Eastbourne, East Sussex BN21 3UN, England

                          1 Goldthorne Avenue
                          Toronto, Ontario M8Z 5T9, Canada

Listed here is the latest translated edition of this book together with the language of the translation and the publisher.

German (1st Edition) — Die Quintessenz Verlag, Berlin, Germany

Italian (1st Edition) — Piccin Editore, Padova, Italy

Japanese (2nd Edition) — Ishiyaku, Tokyo, Japan

Spanish (2nd Edition) — Nueva Editorial Interamericana, S.A., deC.V.,
                        Mexico

French (2nd Edition) — Julien Prelat, Paris, France

Occlusion   ISBN   0-7216-7441-0

Print No.:   9   8

Preface to the Second Edition

The expanded research and ever-growing interest in occlusion in dental practice and education has stimulated the preparation of a second edition of *Occlusion.* The guiding principles for this edition continue to be an emphasis on knowledge of the physiology of occlusion as the scientific basis for the diagnosis and treatment of dysfunctional disturbances of the masticatory system. The physiologic principles for functional harmony among the various components of the masticatory system have been substantiated further by the inclusion of recent research findings. Therefore, it was necessary to place further emphasis on neuromuscular physiology and the interplay of environmental or emotional frustration and stress with dysfunctional disturbances of the masticatory system.

The concept of an "ideal" occlusion, relating neuromuscular harmony to definite relationships between occlusal and temporomandibular joint guidance, has been defined in details applicable to clinical dentistry.

In keeping with present trends in teaching, a discussion of the relationship between occlusal anatomy and mandibular movements has been included in the chapter on the physiology of occlusion. Also, because of an increased interest in the use of more sophisticated instruments, a review of the use of a "fully adjustable articulator" has been added.

Many new illustrations, photographs, and radiographs have been added to improve understanding of the written text. Some of the photographs and radiographs from the first edition have been replaced with improved illustrations.

An attempt has been made to keep terminology consistent throughout the text; however, this goal was not attainable in all instances because of potential conceptual discrepancies.

The present edition, like the first, was written for practitioners, teachers, students, and investigators, all of whom have a common interest in physiology and dysfunctional disturbances of the masticatory system.

ANN ARBOR, MICHIGAN

SIGURD P. RAMFJORD

MAJOR M. ASH, JR.

Preface to the First Edition

The subject of occlusion is one of the most controversial and challenging aspects of dentistry, and conflicting theories regarding occlusal function and dysfunction have led to a labyrinth of fact and philosophy. However, recent technical advances have made it possible to test the validity of many theories, and we are currently in a period of transition from empirical to scientific concepts of occlusion. Even so, there is still much to be learned about occlusion. Although extensive basic and clinical research may be expected to continue to shed light on occlusal problems in the future, clinical procedures always should be based on the best scientific principles available. These principles are the basis of this book.

The concepts of occlusion presented reflect the extensive legacy of facts and hypotheses now available, and have been acknowledged, at least in part, by the citation of references. In addition to our own interpretation of this legacy, the book contains many concepts of occlusion not previously published. While we may disagree with certain concepts of occlusion or their rationale, to disagree with them is not to deny their place in the process of progressive insight into the problems of occlusion. A number of references attesting to this consideration are presented.

The purpose of this book is to present to students, teachers, and practitioners of dentistry the present status of the science and art of occlusion. Of necessity such a book has to deal more with applicable principles than with specific technical procedures. Principles of physiology, pathology, and the therapy of occlusion form the basis for clinical practice in almost every branch of dentistry, as the function of the masticatory system depends on the occlusion. However, it was not our purpose to generalize about occlusion, for to have done so would be to invite the criticism of being superficial or the hazard of oversimplification. The only clinical procedure that has been covered in detail is occlusal adjustment because of the importance of proper procedures for this basic technique in the correction of occlusal disharmony. The technical principles related to function and stability which are germane to occlusal adjustment should also govern all other phases of occlusal therapy.

It will be noted that the development of occlusion has not been included and that the emphasis has been on the adult occlusion. It was felt that growth and development were not entirely relevant to the objectives of a book of this type. The development of occlusion more logically belongs in textbooks on anatomy and orthodontics. Also, the inclusion of material on detailed techniques for reconstruction of occlusion were not considered to be within the scope of the book. The stress on normal versus ideal occlusion and on the adaptability of the masticatory system, however, does not minimize the importance of restorative dentistry, and a review of the relationship between occlusion and restorative dentistry appears in Section III.

Some concern has been expressed about the tendency for fragmentation of dental subject matters, and even for possible disunity in dental education or the practice of dentistry. Since occlusion involves everyone in dentistry, we have attempted to present the subject in such a way as to bring together the biological, technical, and clinical aspects of dentistry for teachers, students, and practitioners. Occlusion is a complex field in which knowledge of physiology, psychology and psychiatry is often as important for successful diagnosis and therapy as technical skill in clinical practice; it is a field in which basic science training directly supports clinical practice.

The first part of the book is concerned with the anatomy and physiology of the masticatory structures and their relationship to occlusion. Since there already are excellent textbooks available on the anatomy of the masticatory system, the main emphasis has been on advances in the neural and muscle physiology related to occlusal function. The second part of the book is concerned with the etiology of functional disturbances. The third section covers treatment and is based upon the principles of anatomy and physiology outlined in the first part of the book. It is hoped that such a division of the material will enable the reader to establish a progressive foundation in the functional and dysfunctional aspects of the masticatory system, and to insure that the diagnosis and treatment of functional disturbances are cast in a suitable clinical frame of reference for practical use. Although it was inviting to present an entirely pragmatic approach in Section III, to have done so would have been contrary to the goal that the basic sciences and clinical practice should be integrated insofar as possible. It will be apparent to the reader that this goal has not been sacrificed in an attempt to make Section III of practical clinical value.

In keeping with the intent to document the concepts of occlusion presented in the book, an attempt has been made to include as many pertinent publications as possible, even though many of these references have not been translated into the English language. Being cognizant of the importance of the many publications related to the development of present concepts of occlusion, we could not be completely impartial and include all such publications, for to do so would involve a distractingly long list of references.

We wish to acknowledge the constructive criticism provided by Dr. Edward W. Lauer of the Department of Anatomy, and Dr. Arthur T. Storey of the Department of Physiology, The University of Michigan, School of Medicine. Their assistance in neuroanatomy and neurophysiology was most helpful.

Dr. Robert Moyers, Chairman of the Department of Orthodontics, reviewed the chapter on orthodontic therapy and made a number of valuable suggestions.

For the use of histopathologic material and photomicrographs we owe gratitude to Dr. Donald A. Kerr, Chairman of the Department of Oral Pathology.

Our appreciation for their willing assistance is also extended to Mr. Edward Crandell, senior photographer, and to Mrs. Ellen T. Hall and Miss Susan Seger, librarians, The University of Michigan, School of Dentistry.

We also wish to acknowledge the assistance of Mr. William Brudon, medical illustrator for the Department of Anatomy, The University of Michigan, School of Medicine. It was through his artistic ability that our rough sketches were transformed into meaningful illustrations.

Ann Arbor, Michigan

Sigurd P. Ramfjord
Major M. Ash, Jr.

Contents

CHAPTER 4

Physiology of Occlusion 67

SECTION TWO

FUNCTIONAL DISTURBANCES OF THE MASTICATORY SYSTEM

CHAPTER 5

Etiology of Bruxism 115

CHAPTER 6

Etiology of Traumatic Occlusion and Trauma from Occlusion 125

CHAPTER 7

Periodontal Response in Trauma from Occlusion.. 158

SECTION ONE

Anatomy and Physiology
of the Masticatory System

The masticatory system is a functional unit composed of the teeth, their surrounding and supporting structures, the jaws, the temporomandibular joints, the muscles which are attached to the mandible, lip and tongue muscles, and the vascular and nervous systems for these tissues.

The functional activity of this system is performed by the muscles guided by nerve impulses, whereas the jaws, the temporomandibular joints and associated ligaments, and the teeth with their supporting structures are utilized as passive tools.

A harmonious correlation between the component parts is of utmost importance for the functional capacity and maintenance of health within the masticatory system. Adaptations to functional wear and tear (compensatory eruption of teeth, mesial drift, changes in occlusal pattern) signify the unceasing effort to maintain proper physiologic balance of the system throughout the lifetime. The masticatory system or apparatus has been developed as a response to particular demands for function, and it is constituted in such a manner that it is dependent on the frequency and magnitude of functional stimuli for the development and maintenance of a proper physiologic state with a maximum of resistance to possible injury. Any discussion about what part of this system should be considered the most important or dominating is futile because of the close interdependence of stimuli, functional movements, morphology, and state of health in the various closely integrated parts of the system. It also anatomically and physiologically represents a part of the body as a whole and,

1

consequently, it cannot be considered, analyzed, and treated as an autonomous unit without due regard to the complete status of the individual's health.

The integration of the many components and the functioning of the masticatory system are made possible by the complex pathways and mechanisms of the peripheral and central nervous systems. For this reason a brief review of the neuroanatomy and neurophysiology basic to an understanding of the function of the masticatory system is necessary even though somewhat hazardous in view of the fact that many aspects of the neuromuscular mechanisms associated with the masticatory system are still not clearly understood.

Many of the concepts of the neuromuscular aspects of the masticatory system have been based on studies of spinal reflexes, muscles, and receptor systems in areas other than the masticatory system. In general, the neuroanatomy and neuromuscular physiology of systems in other areas provide considerable insight into the mechanisms of the masticatory system.

The coverage here is primarily concerned with the anatomy and physiology of the masticatory muscles; no attempt will be made to cover the autonomic nervous system or the facial muscles and nerves. The components and functions of the various parts of the masticatory system that are of importance in providing the basis for evaluating disturbances of the masticatory system are given in the outline which follows.

OUTLINE FOR CONSIDERING THE FUNCTIONAL RELATIONSHIP OF THE COMPONENTS OF THE MASTICATORY SYSTEM

Anatomy and Physiology of Masticatory Muscles and Temporomandibular Joints
FUNCTIONS OF MASTICATORY MUSCLES
MANDIBULAR MOVEMENTS
REST POSITION
TEMPOROMANDIBULAR JOINTS

Components of the Nervous System
NEURONS
RECEPTORS
NERVE FIBERS
CENTRAL NERVOUS SYSTEM
NERVE PATHWAYS
TRIGEMINAL NERVE
HYPOGLOSSAL NERVE

Neuromuscular Physiology
REFLEXES
MUSCLE SPINDLE
INFLUENCES ON ALPHA MOTONEURONS
OTHER INFLUENCES ON MUSCLE FUNCTION
MUSCLE TONE
REFLEXES AND MANDIBULAR MOVEMENTS

Physiology of Occlusion

CHAPTER 1

ANATOMY AND PHYSIOLOGY OF MASTICATORY MUSCLES AND TEMPOROMANDIBULAR JOINTS

In the past the most common method for studying muscle function has been by dissection and, from that, a reconstruction of known functional patterns. By such a method the interpretation of functional relations was based on the origin and insertion of the muscles. Muscle function has also been studied by direct electrical stimulation of muscles or nerves and clinical observations of muscles during and following surgical intervention or accidents.

Although older methods of studying muscle function have provided valuable information,[22, 36, 57] more recent use of electromyographic methods has produced interesting and promising studies of muscle and temporomandibular joint function in various degrees of rest and movement.[12, 20, 39, 45] Electromyographic methods have made the shortcomings of the previous methods very obvious, especially with reference to neuromuscular relations and synergistic interplay of muscles. However, electromyographic methods indicate only muscle activity, and accurate quantitation of the activity is still not possible at the present time. Even so, electromyographic studies have provided an insight into unexplained relationships between occlusion, muscle tension, and psychic stress.[38, 41, 46] Furthermore, reports of electromyographic and other studies indicate that more muscles are involved and that various masticatory movements are more complex than was generally believed previously.[11, 21, 40, 42, 43] Kinematic studies have benefited from improved cinefluoroscopic, radiographic, laminographic, mechanical, and photographic methods.[5, 16, 26, 34, 44, 58]

It is not possible on the basis of present knowledge to provide a complete analysis of the functions of the various masticatory and related muscles for all movements of the mandible because of the very complex interplay of a large number of muscles, directly and indirectly related to the masticatory system. The clinical observation of muscle function cannot account for the complex

4

synergistic and antagonistic activities nor the magnitude of the activities occurring even in simple mandibular movements. Electromyographic analysis, the technique of single unit recording of the mesencephalic nucleus, and other techniques have made possible more precise evaluation of muscle function than was previously possible by clinical observation. Even so, an account of muscle function in mandibular movements can only be considered to be an incomplete picture. Although certain muscles in the head, neck and shoulders are involved in some aspects of mastication, especially in heavy function or tearing off fibrous food held by the hand, the activities of these muscles will not be discussed.

Although it cannot be concluded that a particular muscle has a primary or single function because of its insertion or origin, important aspects of its functional limitations can be deduced on this basis because of simple mechanics. The location of muscles is important also to the diagnosis of temporomandibular joint disturbances and myalgias.

FUNCTIONS OF MASTICATORY MUSCLES

It is not realistic to attribute a specific function to each jaw muscle in view of the complex nature of functional and nonfunctional jaw movements, but it is necessary to describe the essential anatomic features and major functions of each muscle in order to explain the basic biomechanics involved in moving and positioning the mandible.

Temporal Muscle

The temporal muscle (Fig. 1–1, *A*) has a broad origin on the lateral surface of the skull and extends as far forward as the lateral border of the supraorbital ridge. The insertion is on the coronoid process and along the anterior border of the ascending ramus of the mandible. The temporal muscle has three independent functional components that parallel the direction of the fibers of the muscle. The anterior fibers are almost vertical, the fibers in the middle portion run an oblique course, and the most posterior fibers are almost horizontal before bending downward to meet the mandible. The innervation of the temporal muscle is provided usually by three branches of the temporal nerve, which is a branch of the mandibular division of the trigeminal nerve. Thus, the anatomic features and innervation of the temporal muscle are compatible with the observation that in certain movements the muscle acts as if it consisted of three distinct parts (Fig. 1–1, *B*).

The temporal muscle is the principal positioner of the mandible during elevation and this muscle is more sensitive to occlusal interferences than any other masticatory muscle. Normally, the anterior fibers may contract shortly before the rest of the fibers contract when elevation of the mandible is begun. The posterior fibers of one side are active in abductive mandibular movements of the same side, but bilateral retraction of the mandible from a protruded

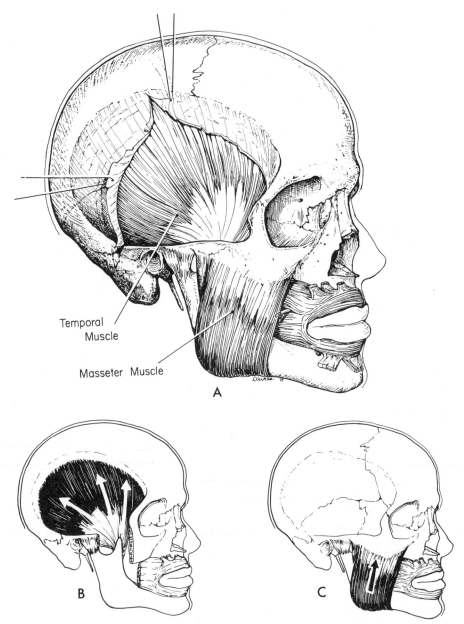

Temporal
Muscle

Masseter Muscle

A

B   C

Figure 1-1. Anatomical features of the temporal and masseter muscles. *A,* The temporal fascia
has been cut and drawn back to show the broad origin of the temporal muscle. The deeper portion of the
masseter muscle can be seen at the posterior superior border of the superficial portion of the masseter
muscle. *B,* The direction of the muscle fibers and the innervation of the temporal muscle provides
for positioning of the mandible during elevation. *C,* The origin and insertion of the masseter muscle
provides principally for elevation of the mandible but may assist in simple mandibular protraction. The
complex integrated function of the temporal, masseter, and other muscles of mastication does not
permit attributing a single or principal function to any muscle.

position involves all fibers of the temporal muscles. There is equal tonus in all parts of the muscle in the resting range of the mandible in the absence of functional disturbances. The activities of the different parts of the muscle are similar during isometric contraction (p. 45) in light centric occlusal closure, provided no functional disturbances or occlusal interferences are present. Heavy occlusal closure will elicit even isometric contraction of all fibers regardless of the presence or absence of occlusal interferences.

Masseter Muscle

The masseter muscle is approximately rectangular and is made up of two main muscle bundles that extend from the zygomatic arch to the ramus and body of the mandible. The insertion on the mandible extends from the region of the second molar on the lateral surface of the mandible to the lower one-third of the posterior lateral surface of the ramus (Fig. 1–1, C).

The principal function of the masseter muscle is mandibular elevation, although it may assist in simple protraction and plays a dominant role in elevation if the mandible is being protracted. It is also active in extreme lateral movements of the mandible. In contrast to the temporal muscle, which is considered to be a positioner of the mandible, the masseter is considered to act mainly in power comminution. As pointed out previously, it is hazardous and unrealistic to attribute a single or principal function to any muscle except for expediency.

Medial (Internal) Pterygoid Muscle

The medial pterygoid muscle is a rectangular muscle with its main origin in the pterygoid fossa and its insertion on the medial surface of the angle of the mandible. The muscle, from its origin, runs downward, posteriorly and laterally to its insertion (Figs. 1–2 and 1–3).

The principal functions of the medial pterygoid are elevation and lateral positioning of the mandible. The pterygoid muscles are very active during simple protraction but somewhat less so if opening and protraction occur together. In combined protrusive and lateral movements, the activity of the medial pterygoid dominates over that of the temporal muscle.

Lateral (External) Pterygoid Muscle

The lateral pterygoid muscle has two origins: one head of the muscle originates on the outer surface of the lateral pterygoid plate while a smaller and upper head originates from the greater sphenoid wing. Both divisions of the muscle join in front of the temporomandibular joint near the condyle of the mandible (Figs. 1–2 and 1–3). The main insertion of the lateral pterygoid muscle is to the anterior surface of the neck of the condyle. There also is an insertion of some muscle fibers to the capsule of the joint and to the anterior

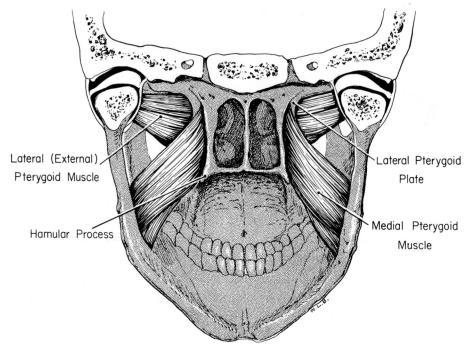

Lateral (External)
Pterygoid Muscle

Hamular Process

Lateral Pterygoid
Plate

Medial Pterygoid
Muscle

Figure 1–2. Schematic representation of the medial and lateral pterygoid muscles. The principal function of the medial pterygoid muscle is elevation of the mandible but it may participate in lateral movements during mastication. The lateral pterygoid muscle is active in protraction of the condyle and anterior movement of the articular disc.

aspect of the articular disc. The direction of the fibers of the upper head is posteriorly and laterally in the horizontal path, while the lower head runs upward and outward to the condyle.

The principal function of the lateral pterygoid muscle is protracting the condyle and at the same time drawing the disc forward. The disc is attached to the neck of the condyle medially and laterally and remains in the glenoid fossa for small movements, but follows the condyle in greater movements.[27] The lateral pterygoid muscles reach their greatest activity sooner than other muscles in a normal unstrained opening or mandibular depression. Thus, the pterygoid muscle appears to be concerned with all degrees of protraction and opening movements of the mandible. The pterygoid muscle also is active during lateral movements but is assisted by the masseter, the medial pterygoid, and the anterior and posterior parts of the temporal muscles.

Digastric Muscle (Anterior Portion)

The attachment of the anterior portion of the digastric muscle is found near the lower border of the mandible and near the midline. The intermediate tendon between the anterior and posterior parts of the muscle is attached to the hyoid bone through fibers of the external cervical fascia. Innervation of the

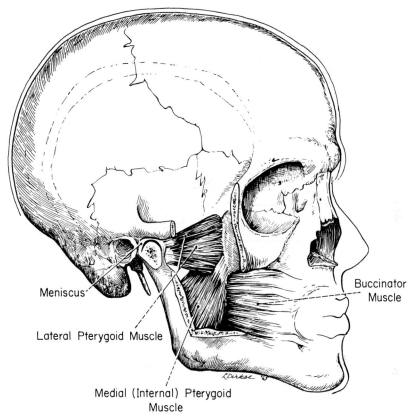

Figure 1–3. The insertion of the lateral pterygoid to the anterior surface of the condyle and some fibers inserting into the articular disc. The main origin of the medial pterygoid muscle is in the pterygoid fossa. As shown in Figure 1–2, the insertion is on the medial surface of the angle of the mandible. As shown here and in Figure 1–2, the lateral pterygoid muscle has one origin on the outer surface of the lateral pterygoid plate and another on the greater sphenoid wing.

anterior portion of the digastric muscle is by a branch of the mylohyoid nerve of the mandibular division of the trigeminal nerve.

The anterior portion of the digastric is concerned with the depression of the mandible along with other suprahyoid muscles and the lateral pterygoid muscle. However, the activity of the digastric is most prominent at the end of mandibular depression, and thus it cannot be considered to be important in initiating opening movements. The lateral pterygoid muscle is most important in initiation of mandibular depression and the anterior digastric in completion of mandibular depression.

MANDIBULAR MOVEMENTS

Many efforts have been made to describe accurately muscle function during movements and postural positions of the mandible; however, more research is needed before a unified concept can be reached. Most descriptions of mandibular movements have been based on the relationship of the mandible to the maxilla in terms of protrusion, retrusion, opening and closing, and lateral movements of the mandible. Other descriptions have been related to the contact patterns of teeth during mastication of various types of food and swallowing, patterns of muscular activity during mastication, swallowing and nonfunctional movements of the mandible, and the relationship of jaw positions to movements of the joint structures. There can be no question that functional movements differ from nonfunctional patterns of jaw movements such as those associated with bruxism or those observed under command, empty articulation or laboratory conditions. Any type of occlusal interference may lead to abnormal muscle activity when the mandible is at rest or between functional occlusal contacts. The contraction patterns of the muscles are more often asynchronous in persons with malocclusion than in those with normal occlusion, and such abnormal muscle activities are reflected in mandibular movements.

Mandibular Opening

During opening movements the lateral pterygoid muscles show initial and sustained activity. The activity of the anterior digastric follows that of the lateral pterygoid muscles when approaching the completion of the opening movement. However, in isometric contraction associated with forced depression, the digastric is activated almost as soon as the lateral pterygoid muscle.

During combined protraction and opening there is activity in the medial and lateral pterygoid muscles, the masseter muscles, and sometimes the anterior fibers of the temporal muscles. The supra- and infrahyoid muscles may function to stabilize the hyoid bone during swallowing, speech, and certain mandibular movements. The participation of passive muscles must also be considered although they are not responsible for active movement in opening. The temporal and masseter muscles, for example, become very active during the final stage of wide opening of the mandible, stopping the opening. Since the passive muscles are not at rest, they are probably important in synergistic and guiding activities. The control of interacting muscles for accurate movements is a function of the central nervous system.

Mandibular Closing

The medial pterygoid, temporal, and masseter muscles are all active during elevation of the mandible. The coordinated activities of these three muscles are under reflex control, and closure patterns may be modified to avoid occlusal interferences. During combined protrusion and elevation of the mandible, the activities of first the medial pterygoid and then the masseter muscles are increased. The lateral pterygoid also is active during combined movements. In forced heavy closure, many of the facial and neck muscles contract, as well as all of the contracting masticatory muscles.

Lateral Mandibular Movements

Krol says No!

Lateral movements of the mandible are brought about by ipsilateral contraction of the posterior and middle fibers of the temporal muscle and contralateral contractions of the lateral and medial pterygoid muscles and the anterior fibers of the temporal muscle. During horizontal movements with minimal separation of the teeth, either the masseter or temporal muscles are active. In this respect, these muscles act as antagonists although they act as synergistic muscles during vertical opening. Thus, parts of the masseter and temporal muscles of the same side may act as antagonists or synergists during horizontal movements and minimum separation of the teeth.[24] Lateral movements are initiated by the lateral and medial pterygoid muscles. The action of the masseter anterior temporal and suprahyoid muscles is considered to be secondary. The temporal muscle is less active during protrusive lateral movements than when lateral movements are made with the jaw retruded.

Protraction and Retraction

The protrusion of the mandible is initiated by the lateral and medial pterygoid muscles acting simultaneously. Retraction of the mandible is accomplished by contraction of the middle and posterior parts of the temporal muscles and the suprahyoid muscles.

Summary

In summary, it has been found electromyographically that mandibular depression is brought about by contraction of the lateral pterygoid[12, 39] and digastric muscles, and other suprahyoid muscles probably to a lesser extent. Elevation of the mandible is due to contraction of the internal pterygoid, masseter, and temporal muscles, and lateral movement is executed by ipsilateral contraction of the temporal muscle and contralateral contractions of the lateral pterygoid and medial pterygoid muscles. Retraction is affected by the contraction of the middle and posterior fibers in the temporal muscle. The suprahyoid muscles are also active in retraction, and they play a definite role in adjusting all of the other movements. Furthermore, it is known that in mastication the tongue, cheek, and lip muscles also participate actively. Electromyography has provided an opportunity to observe the complex activity of the muscles of the jaw, face, and neck as coordinators of mandibular movements, and it has become increasingly evident that a number of muscles participate even in simple jaw movements. However, a shortcoming of electromyographic recordings is that they reveal only when and, to a certain extent, how strongly a muscle acts, but they do not show whether the muscle acts as a stabilizer (isometric contraction) or as a mover (isotonic contraction, p. 45).

Recently, an effort has been made to evaluate the question of whether opening movements are restricted to movements of the lower jaw.[3, 15] The results of the investigation indicate that the upper jaw takes part in opening movements; i.e., the head is slightly tipped backward.[3]

REST POSITION

Concepts regarding the rest position of the mandible should be re-evaluated and revised as the related neuromuscular mechanisms become understood. The complexity of the problem is reflected not only in the many definitions and methods for obtaining it, but in the various significances attached to the rest position in the clinical practice of dentistry.

Postural Rest Position

Rest position has often been described as the postural position of the mandible determined by the resting length of the muscles which elevate or depress the mandible when the person is sitting or standing in an upright position. Also, the term "physiologic" rest position has been used to indicate that the mandibular musculature is in a state of minimal tonic contraction to maintain posture and to overcome the force of gravity. Postural positions of the body, however, are not simply the result of optimal length of the postural muscles and myotatic or antigravity reflexes; such positions and muscle function are complexly related also to other influences, including the gamma efferent (fusimotor) system and related functions of the reticular formation (pp. 31 and 49).

The term "rest position" as used in dentistry implies only one of many postural positions of the mandible, e.g., with the person sitting or standing upright and looking straight forward at eye level.

Clinically Determined Rest Position; Resting Range

Except for minor changes with age, malocclusion[49] and loss of teeth,[54] the relative stability of the clinically determined rest position is generally accepted. However, the rest position is not always indicative of muscle harmony,[17] although most definitions of rest position as they relate to vertical dimensions imply a balance in the tonicity of the elevator and depressor muscles. It has been found that the interocclusal distance averaged 1.7 mm. in the clinically determined rest position, whereas the average distance was 3.29 mm. with an additional resting range of 11 mm. when determined electromyographically on the basis of minimal muscle activity.[17] Thus, at least for the temporal, masseter and digastric muscles, there is a resting range rather than a definite mandibular rest position of minimal muscle activity. The observation that the clinically determined rest position often does not coincide with the range of minimal muscle activity suggests that the neuromuscular mechanisms underlying clinical rest position are more complex than were formerly thought.

In view of the findings that the clinically determined rest position is often situated outside the field of minimum muscle activity, it is possible that different neuromuscular principles are operant in the rest position determined clinically and in the position of the mandible with minimum muscle activity. In reality, the muscles are not at complete rest but are contracting to a limited degree as part of their postural tonicity even in the resting range of the mandible. It may be that the clinically determined rest position is dependent more on the basic myotatic reflexes of the involved muscles than on muscle tonus, which changes readily. The rest position determined electromyographically by a range of minimal muscle activity appears to be influenced to a much greater degree by psychic tension, pain, and occlusal interferences. However, the process of determining the clinical rest position also involves the influences of emotion and exteroceptive and proprioceptive inputs to the neuromuscular system (p. 25). Such inputs from the joints, muscles, lips, cheeks, periodontal membrane (occlusion), and tongue undoubtedly contribute to the learning of rest position, or conditioning of reflexes.

Electromyographic Rest Position. It has been shown that the removal of occlusal interferences can lead to the relative coincidence of vertical dimensions of clinically determined rest position and of minimal muscle activity as determined electromyographically. Also pain associated with temporomandibular joint disturbances or myalgias associated with face and jaw muscles may influence the basic muscle activity associated with electromyographic rest position without appreciably altering the clinical rest position.

It has been shown electromyographically that in order to obtain balanced resting muscle activity in persons with occlusal interferences it is often necessary to open the jaw beyond the rest position determined clinically.[17] Also, it has been observed clinically that occlusal interferences have an increasing tendency to trigger abnormal muscle activity if the interocclusal space is decreased in a given individual. An increase in interocclusal space beyond the previous distance seems to increase the muscle tolerance to occlusal interferences and, in extreme cases, to alter the clinical rest position without change in resting muscle activity.[53] Furthermore, it is sometimes impossible to record electromyographically a harmonious resting activity until an occlusal adjustment has been performed. These observations suggest that pontine brainstem mechanisms and exteroceptive and proprioceptive influences are more nearly in a state of equilibrium at the rest position or resting range (as determined electromyographically with harmonious minimal muscle activity) and exert more influence upon this range than on the clinically determined rest position. Furthermore, such observations suggest that exteroceptive and proprioceptive influences play a minimal role in the determination of clinical rest position.

Fusimotor Activity. The afferent discharge of a muscle spindle depends both on stretch and on impulses from the fusimotor fibers (p. 48). Hunt[24] showed that fusimotor activity increases the afferent response of the spindle to external stretch. Stimulation of areas of the reticular formation in the brainstem also has been found to augment the response to stimulation of peripheral motor areas. Apparently, the reticular system acts mainly through the fusimotor system to influence the activity of the alpha motor neuron and the postural tonus.[50] The threshold for excitation of some fusimotor neurons also has been found to be lower than that required to cause excitation of motor neurons,[25] and fusimotor fibers may initiate a discharge of impulses from the muscle spindle in the absence of external stretch, thereby increasing the sensitivity of the spindle sufficiently to promote a marked increase in the frequency of afferent discharge.

A variation in muscle activity in the rest position may therefore be unrelated to the actual stretch of the jaw muscles within the "resting range," since the cause of such activity may be central nervous system influence through the fusimotor system or impulses created by peripheral stimulation from occlusal interferences or pain. These activities may be unrelated to the myotatic reflex and, possibly, unrelated to the clinical rest position of the mandible.

Such tentative explanations for mechanisms underlying the clinical rest position and the electromyographically recorded "resting range" of the jaw muscles serve only to point out the complex nature of the neurophysiology of mandibular positions and the interacting relationship between the various parts of the masticatory system and the central nervous system relative to the rest position of the mandible.

Interocclusal Space in Clinical Rest Position

An important aspect of clinical rest position of the mandible is the "interocclusal" or "freeway" space which usually is present between the occlusal surfaces of the maxillary and mandibular teeth when antigravity tonus is maintained. The width of this space varies somewhat with the type of occlusion, and probably also with hypo- or hypertonicity of the masticatory muscles. In the anterior part of the mouth it commonly is found to be 1 to 3 mm.; however, it may be much wider (8 to 10 mm. or more) without any indication of a disturbance of the function and health of the masticatory system and therefore may qualify as biologically normal. Both rest position and interocclusal space can be changed by raising[13] or lowering[55] the occlusal vertical dimension. It is easy to conceive that a "bite raising," which encroaches upon the normal interocclusal space for the individual, will act as a constant undue stimulus to the stretch reflex of the masseter, temporal and internal pterygoid muscles and thereby will promote muscle contractions far in excess of the normal antigravity tonus. A strong warning should be made against the application of average values (for example, 2 mm. of interocclusal space) to individual persons. A deviation from this average norm may not be a valid indication of an alteration of a person's occlusion. "Loss of vertical dimension" on the basis of a wider than average interocclusal space has often been used as an unjustified and faulty premise to justify extensive dental procedures that ended by being harmful to the patient.

TEMPOROMANDIBULAR JOINTS

Some of the earliest studies of the function of the temporomandibular joints utilized mechanical devices such as tracing stylus, face bow, intraoral wax, plaster, and other occlusal indices. Radiographic registration of the condyles as well as photographic methods is also found in very early reports of the function of the joints. Later improvements in radiographic techniques include image-intensification cinefluorography, cephalometry, tomography, kymography, laminagraphy, and other special techniques.[6, 32, 34] Numerous descriptions of the functions of the temporomandibular joints have evolved from these methods and anatomic studies, yet many aspects of the function of the joints are still not clearly understood. At least a part of the difficulty lies in attempting to evaluate the joints as entities without simultaneous evaluation of other factors or components of the masticatory system that influence the function of the joints. It is not possible in the present discussion to attempt to correlate all of the factors influencing the functions. The description will be limited to basic positions and movements of the joints.

Anatomy of the Temporomandibular Joints

A temporomandibular joint is a complex ginglymo-arthrodial (hinge and glide) articulation with an articular disc or meniscus interposed between the condyle of the mandible and the glenoid fossa of the temporal bone (Fig. 1–4). The articulating surface of the temporal bone consists of a posterior concave part and an anterior convex part. The concave portion of the temporal bone is the mandibular fossa (glenoid fossa) and the convex part is the articular eminence. The medial and lateral borders of the joint follow the squamotympanic and petrosquamous or petrotympanic fissures.[34, 51]

In adults the articulating surfaces have a well defined cortical layer of bone which is covered by avascular dense fibrous connective tissue containing various amounts of cartilage cells, depending on age and functional stress. No definite synovial membrane is observable on the smooth articulating surfaces of a normal joint, but a synovial capsule is attached to the disc around its circumference and it forms small folds and villi at the distal and lateral borders of the disc, peripherally to its functional borders. Anteriorly, these folds are much larger,

Figure 1–4. Schematic representation of the anatomical features of the temporomandibular joint. The synovial cavities (upper and lower) are greatly enlarged for illustrative purposes. Note the attachment of the pterygoid muscle (cut) to the condyle and to the meniscus (articular disc).

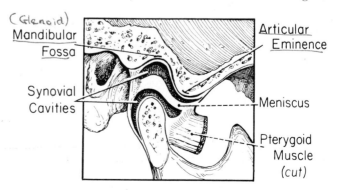

forming bursal sacs to provide space for the condyle in opening movements of the jaw. A small amount of synovial fluid is normally present.

The articular disc consists of dense collagenous connective tissue, which in the central areas is avascular,[2] hyaline, and without nerve tissue. It has a smooth surface but lacks a definite synovial lining. In the peripheral areas small blood vessels and nerve fibers can be seen. The posterior aspect of the disc fits into the glenoid fossa and extends for a short distance down on the distal surface of the condyle,[37] separated from the condyle by the joint space. Behind this extension of the disc, toward the postglenoid spine, there is soft vascular connective tissue with abundant nerve endings. Thus the condyle cannot be moved up and back, but can be moved down and back, as often happens in dysfunctional disturbances of the masticatory system. The disc blends with the connective tissue of the joint capsule and, anteriorly in some areas, rather fine tendons connect the disc to the external pterygoid muscle; however, in other areas this muscle does not appear to be attached to the poorly defined joint capsule. The external pterygoid muscle also has a broad, strong attachment to the neck of the condyle. Anteriorly, the joint capsule is indefinite and loosely arranged. Distally, it is much thicker but without a definite functional capsular arrangement of the fibrous connective tissue. Only in the lateral wall are the fibers arranged in parallel bundles, constituting the temporomandibular ligament.

The fibrous capsule of the joint is attached to the temporal bone along the edge of the articular tissues of the eminence and mandibular fossa, to the neck of the mandible, and to the articular disc. The lateral portion of the capsule is strengthened by the temporomandibular ligament. That part of the capsule from the disc to the temporal bone is considered to be more lax than the inferior portion, which extends from the disc to the neck of the mandible, both medially and laterally.[31] Such looseness of the capsule forming the upper compartment is thought to allow for gliding movements during articulation.

Ligaments. The ligaments of the temporomandibular joint include the temporomandibular ligament and so-called accessory ligaments, and the sphenomandibular and stylomandibular ligaments (Fig. 1–5). The temporomandibular ligament extends from the base of the zygomatic process of the temporal bone downward and obliquely to the neck of the condyle. The sphenomandibular ligament extends from the spine of the sphenoid bone downward and laterally to the region of the lingula of the mandible. The stylomandibular ligament extends from the styloid process to the posterior border of the ramus and angle of the mandible.

The temporomandibular ligament is the ligament most directly related to mandibular articulation and is of importance in limiting mandibular movement. It would be incorrect, however, to assume that the mandible is suspended only by ligaments and that the masticatory muscles are not involved in every phase of jaw positions and movements. The direction of the fibers of the lateral and medial temporomandibular ligaments suggests that these ligaments are of significance in limiting posterior movements of the mandible.[1, 42] The fibrous capsule as well as portions of the temporomandibular ligament is probably of

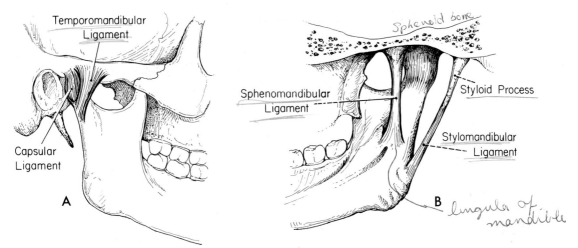

Figure 1–5. Illustration of the ligaments of the temporomandibular joint. *A,* Lateral view showing temporomandibular and capsular ligaments. *B,* Medial view showing position of the sphenomandibular and stylomandibular ligaments.

importance in determining the border of extreme lateral movements in extreme opening. However, in moderate opening, lateral movements are limited, especially with protrusion of the mandible, by the contact of the medial anterior border of the ramus with the posterior maxillary teeth. Even in bilateral condylectomy, where the limiting influence of the capsule and ligament would not be effective, lateral movements are limited. What role receptors in the joint and muscles have in the limitation of lateral movements is not known.

Recent evidence suggests that sensory receptors present in the joint capsule could influence the motor nucleus of the trigeminal nerve and may be important in the control of the activity of muscles of mastication (p. -28).[28, 29, 30] Increasing emphasis is currently being placed upon the role of the ligaments with their nerve receptors as sources of impulses for guidance of muscle function; therefore, it is doubtful that the ligaments alone restrict lateral mandibular movements mechanically. However, it has been established that the posterior functional range of the mandible or centric relation in a normal masticatory system is limited by the ligaments of the temporomandibular joint and meniscus; thus, centric relation may be considered to be a "ligamentous position."[11]

Condylar Positions and Movements

Normally, when the jaws are closed, the condyle contacts the disc and the disc contacts the glenoid fossa. If the contact is maintained between the upper and lower teeth and gliding movements are performed, the contact relationship between the condyle, the disc and the glenoid fossa should be maintained. This basic physiologic relationship depends on harmony among Hanau's well known five factors of occlusion and articulation (condyle guidance, incisal guidance, cusp height, plane of occlusion and compensating curve). During opening movements, a smooth gliding relationship between the parts of the joint also should be maintained. The movements in the lower (condyle-disc) compartment are mainly hinge-like, with only a limited variable amount of slide present. In the upper (glenoid fossa–disc) compartment the disc glides with the condyle during the opening cycle, and the disc seemingly follows the condyle head all the way anteriorly in wide opening movements. (Fig. 1–6 *A*, 1–6 *B*). In extremely wide opening, the functional joint contact is on the distal aspect of the condyle (Fig. 1–6 *C*), and the anterior lateral aspect of the condyle contacts the posterior part of the masseter muscle.[47]

When hard food is masticated the condylar head on the working side may lose its contact with the anterior slope of the glenoid fossa, but, guided by the well integrated neuromuscular system, it is again brought into contact with the disc and the temporal bone. Some observers believe that such contact is always present.[51]

Actually, a combination of three basic movement patterns is found within the temporomandibular joint during mastication: hinge movement, gliding movement with contact between the guiding parts of the joint, and "bodily" or translatory movements of the mandible with light contact between the functioning parts (such a movement also occurs from rest position to centric occlusion, especially in Class II cases with deep overbite). It has been shown that closure from rest position to occlusal contact is not usually a hinge closure with

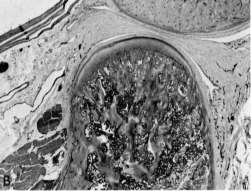

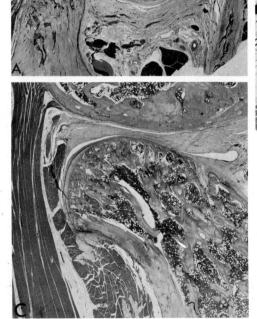

Figure 1–6. *A, B,* In the upper compartment (glenoid fossa-disc) of the temporomandibular joint the disc glides with the condyle during the opening cycle during which the disc seemingly follows the condyle all the way anteriorly in wide opening movements. *C,* In extremely wide opening the functional contact is on the distal aspect of the condyle, and the lateral aspect of the condyle contacts the posterior part of the masseter muscle (adult rhesus monkey).

the axis in the temporomandibular joint, as previously believed.[40] Recent observations of the movement pattern of the condyle by cinefluoroscopic recordings have suggested that there is a zigzagging, up-and-down and back-and-forth movement of the working condyle.[6] If such observations are borne out by further studies, the classic concept of rotation and glide will require revision.

A hinge axis movement in the temporomandibular joint may occur theoretically in various degrees of protrusion; but reference is usually made to the stationary hinge axis movement with the mandible in centric relation. This retrusive opening movement around the terminal hinge axis can be performed only to 20 to 25 mm. of anterior opening. The posterior part of the temporal muscle holds the jaw back during such terminal hinge axis movement, but the movement pattern may also be duplicated by proper manipulation of the jaw by a clinician, provided all the jaw, face and neck muscles are relaxed and muscular dysfunction or pain is not present.

In lateral movements from centric closure, the condyle on the working side appears to rotate with a slight lateral shift in the direction of the movement. The lateral shift or bodily lateral movement of the mandible during lateral jaw movement is called the *Bennett movement* and has immediate and progressive components. The angle formed by the sagittal plane and the path of the advancing condyle during lateral movements (viewed in the horizontal plane) is called the *Bennett angle*[7] (p. 76).

The basic movements described above, however, include only part of the complex functional and nonfunctional movements of the mandible. It should be recognized that the various types of positions and movements, including contact movements, are influenced by the condylar guidance, tooth contacts, ligaments and muscles through complex neuromuscular mechanisms.

In a normal masticatory system with harmony among the guiding factors of occlusion and with a physiologic muscular tonus, the temporomandibular joint is subject to a minimal amount of stress in "empty movements" (such as occlusal contact during swallowing or when the teeth are brought together without food interposed between them). Even in mastication of hard food, the joint normally is protected from injurious stresses by a delicate neuromuscular mechanism of control and coordination of the functional forces. The greatest stress in function is upon the joint on the balancing side. As soon as the normal muscle tonus has been altered either by local disharmony among the guiding factors of occlusion or by nervous tension or pain, a vicious cycle is started consisting of potential traumatic damage to parts of the masticatory system and an increasing muscle tension which will aggravate the tissue damage. Basically, the function of the temporomandibular joint can be compared with that of a bearing in an engine. The joint functions well as long as the moving parts are properly aligned, balanced and lubricated (synovial fluid). Imbalance or improper alignment of the functioning parts will have a disturbing effect upon the bearing of an engine; similarly, dysfunctional movements of the jaw guided by improperly aligned teeth and hypertonic muscles will have an injurious effect on the temporomandibular joint.

Adaptability of the Temporomandibular Joints

Whether the temporomandibular joints can adapt functionally and morphologically to disharmony between occlusal relationships and the joints has been for some time a controversial question. The controversy might be expected in view of the few experimental investigations of the adaptability of the temporomandibular joint that have been made.[4, 10, 14, 18, 19, 56] Since Breitner's report[9] on the effects of anterior displacement of the mandible in young rhesus monkeys, most investigators have indicated that the temporomandibular joint could be changed by orthodontic or other occlusal appliances. Since such studies have been limited to growing animals and one child[19] and to relatively short periods of time, the results of the studies are not conclusive. Only recently have the possible end results of adaptive changes after termination of traumatic effects been studied in both young and adult rhesus monkeys. In these studies no significant changes of the osseous glenoid fossa have been observed.[23, 33]

Reports of limited studies of orthodontic bite-jumping indicate that the ramus and the condyle do not change position in relation to the facial skeleton and the cranial base.[35] In addition, it has been found that changes associated with the orthodontic correction of Class II cases are mainly due to growth in the alveolar processes.[8] Furthermore, there appears to be no acceptable evidence to show that there is adaptability of the temporomandibular joint in adults or even in children more than 10 years of age[35] beyond the physiologic internal remodeling that occurs in all living bone.

In studies of adult rhesus monkeys, when occlusally induced anterior and posterior displacement of the mandible was accomplished, it was found that there were insignificant adaptive changes in the temporomandibular joints compared to the severe trauma and compensatory movement of involved teeth.[23, 48] Although the joints were changed temporarily because of the trauma from occlusally induced displacement, adaptive repositioning of the teeth continued until the temporomandibular joints returned to their previous relationships. In the study of distal displacement of the mandible there were no adaptive or traumatic changes in the base of the glenoid fossa or in the top of the condyle.[48] In the anterior displacement study no traumatic injury occurred to the functioning surfaces of the temporomandibular joints, but there was a slight forward positioning of the condyles that appeared to be nonprogressive and was probably reversible without treatment.[23] The main accommodation for the occlusally induced anterior displacement of the mandible involved movement of the teeth rather than the joints. The results of these studies indicate the need for adapting the occlusion to the joints rather than hoping for the joints to adapt to the occlusion, at least when considering the adult temporomandibular joint. These studies confirm the observations in humans made by Stallard,[52] who observed in all his cases of malocclusion in which the jaws were forced into protrusion by interfering cusps that the joints never become adapted to the forward forced closure.

occlusion adapts to joint

Lindblom[34] found that the condylar path became slightly less steep with age in a large number of patients with functional disturbances of the occlusion. Such changes in the condylar path were not significant for the control patients without functional disturbances. Also, there was no correlation between the type of occlusion and the shape of the temporomandibular joints. It appears that changes which occasionally take place in the temporomandibular joint are the result of pathologic processes rather than physiologic adaptation.

REFERENCES

1. Aarstad, T.: The Capsular Ligaments of the Temporomandibular Joint and Retrusion Facets of the Dentition in Relationship to Mandibular Movements. Oslo, Acad. Forlag., 1954.
2. Agerberg, G., Carlson, G. E., and Hassler, O.: Vascularization of the temporomandibular disk. Odont. Tidsk., 77:451, 1968.
3. Bauer, F.: Are opening movements restricted to movements performed by the lower jaw? Tandlaegebladet, 9:423, 1964.
4. Baume, L. J., and Derichsweiler, H.: Is the condylar growth center responsive to orthodontic therapy? An experimental study in Macaca mulatta. Oral Surg., 14:347, 1961.
5. Berry, H. M., Jr., and Hofmann, F. A.: Cineradiographic observations of the temporomandibular joint function. J. Prosth. Dent., 9:21, 1959.
6. Berry, H. M., Jr., and Hofmann, F. A.: Cineradiographic analysis of temporomandibular joint physiology. J. Prosth. Dent., 14:174, 1964.
7. Boucher, C. O. (Ed.): Current Dental Terminology. St. Louis, C. V. Mosby Co., 1963.
8. Björk, A.: The principle of the Andresen method of orthodontic treatment. Am. J. Orthodont., 37:437, 1951.
9. Breitner, C.: Experimentelle Veränderungen der mesiodistalen Beziehungen der oberen und unteren Zahnreihen I and II. Ztschr. f. Stomatol., 28:134, 620, Heft 2 & 7, 1930.
10. Breitner, C.: Further investigations of bone changes resulting from experimental orthodontic treatment. Am. J. Orthodont., 27:605, 1941.
11. Brill, N., Lammie, G. A., Osborne, J., and Perry, H. T.: Mandibular positions and mandibular movements. Brit. Dent. J., 106:391, 1959.
12. Carlsöö S.: Nervous coordination and mechanical function of the mandibular elevators. Acta Odont. Scandinav., 10:Suppl. 11, 1952.
13. Christensen, J.: Effect of occlusion-raising procedures on the chewing system. Dent. Pract., 20:233, 1970.
14. Derichsweiler, H.: Experimentelle Tieruntersuchunger über Veränderungen des Kiefergelenkes bei Bisslageneränderungen. Fortschr. d. Kieferorth., 19:30, 1958.
15. Ferrein, M.: Sur le mouvement des deux machoires pour l'ouverture de la bouche; et sur les causes de leurs mouvement. Mem. Acad. Roy. Sci., Paris, 509–552, 1748.
16. Granger, E. R.: Functional relations of the stomatognathic system. J. Am. Dent. A., 48:638, 1954.
17. Garnick, J. J., and Ramfjord, S. P.: Rest Position. J. Prosth. Dent., 12:895, 1962.
18. Häupl, K., and Psansky, R.: Experimentelle untersuchungen über Gelenktransformation bei Verwendung der Methoden der Funktionskieferorthopädie. Deutsche Zahn-, Mund-, u. Kieferh., 6:439, 1939.
19. Häupl, K., and Stellmach, R.: Mikroskopische Befunde bei einem Fall von Transformation der Kiefergelenke und allgemeine einschlägige Erlauterungen. Deutsche Zahn-, Mund-, u. Kieferh., 30:324, 1959.
20. Hickey, J. C., Stacy, R. W., and Rinear, L. L.: Electromyographic studies of mandibular muscles in basic jaw movements. J. Prosth. Dent., 7:565, 1957.
21. Hickey, J. C., Allison, M. L., Woelfel, J. B., Boucher, C. O., and Stacy, R. W.: Mandibular movements in three dimensions. J. Prosth. Dent., 13:72, 1963.

22. Hildebrand, G. Y.: Studies in the masticatory movements of the human lower jaw. Skandinav. Arch. Physiol., *61*:Suppl., 1937.

23. Hiniker, J. J., and Ramfjord, S. P.: Anterior displacement of the mandible in adult Rhesus monkeys. J. Pros. Dent., *16*:503, 1966.

24. Hunt, C. C.: The reflex activity of mammalian small-nerve fibers. J. Physiol., *115*:456, 1951.

25. Hunt, C. C., and Paintal, A. S.: Spinal reflex regulation of fusimotor neurons. J. Physiol., *143*:195, 1958.

26. Jankelson, B., Hoffman, G. M., and Hendron, J. A.: The physiology of the stomatognathic system. J. Am. Dent. A., *45*:375, 1953.

27. Jerge, C. R.: The neurologic mechanism underlying cyclic jaw movements. J. Prosth. Dent., *14*:667, 1964.

28. Kawamura, Y., and Majima, T.: Temporomandibular joint's sensory mechanisms controlling activities of the jaw muscles. J. Dent. Res., *43*:150, 1964.

29. Kawamura, Y.: Recent concepts of the physiology of mastication. *In* Staple, P. H. (ed.): Advances in Oral Biology. New York, Academic Press, 1964, pp. 77–109.

30. Kawamura, Y.: Neurophysiologic background of occlusion. J. Am. Soc. Periodont., *5*:175, 1967.

31. Krogh-Poulsen, W., and Mölhave, A.: Om discus articularis temporomandibularis. Tandlaegebladet, *61*:265, 1957.

32. Kydd, W. L.: Rapid serial roentgenographic cephalometry for observing mandibular movements. J. Prosth. Dent., *8*:880, 1958.

33. Lieb, G.: Application of the activator in Rhesus monkeys. Europ. Orth. Soc., 1969, p. 141.

34. Lindblom, G.: On the anatomy and function of the temporomandibular joint. Acta Odont. Scandinav., *17*:Suppl. 28, 1960.

35. Lipke, D. P., and Posselt, U.: Functional anatomy of the temporomandibular joint. J. West. Soc. Periodont. *8*:48, 1960.

36. Lord, F. P.: Movements of the jaw and how they are affected. Internat. J. Orthodont., *23*:557, 1937.

37. Orban, B. (Ed.): Oral Histology and Embryology. St. Louis, C. V. Mosby Co., 1949.

38. Moyers, R.: Some physiologic considerations of centric and other jaw relations. J. Prosth. Dent., *6*:183, 1956.

39. Moyers, R. E.: An electromyographic analysis of certain muscles involved in temporomandibular movement. Am. J. Orthodont., *36*:481, 1950.

40. Nevakari, K.: An analysis of mandibular movement from rest to occlusal position. Acta odont. scandinav., *14*:Suppl. 19, 1956.

41. Perry, H. T., Lammie, G. A., Main, J., and Teuscher, G. W.: Occlusion in a stress situation. J. Am. Dent. A., *60*:626, 1960.

42. Posselt, U.: Studies in the mobility of the human mandible. Acta odont. scandinav., *10*:Suppl. 10, 1952.

43. Posselt, U.: Movement areas of the mandible. J. Prosth. Dent., *7*:375, 1957.

44. Posselt, U.: An analyzer for mandibular positions. J. Prosth. Dent., *7*:368, 1957.

45. Pruzansky, S., Pesek, M., and Osborn, L. F.: Quantitative analysis of the electromyogram in masticating chewing gums of varying toughness (Abstract). Am. J. Orthodont., *44*:149, 1958.

46. Ramfjord, S. P.: Bruxism: A clinical and electromyographic study. J. Am. Dent. A., *62*:21, 1961.

47. Ramfjord, S. P., and Blankenship, J. R.: The interarticular disc in wide mandibular opening in Rhesus monkeys. J. Pros. Dent. (In Press).

48. Ramfjord, S. P., and Hiniker, J. J.: Posterior displacement of the mandible in adult rhesus monkeys J. Pros. Dent., *16*:491, 1966.

49. Ricketts, R. M.: A study of changes in temporomandibular relations associated with the treatment of class II malocclusion (Angle). Am. J. Orthodont., *38*:918, 1952.

50. Ruch, T. C., and Fulton, J. F.: Medical Physiology and Biophysics. Philadelphia, W. B. Saunders Co., 1960.

51. Sicher, H.: Functional anatomy of the temporomandibular joint. *In* Sarnat, B. (ed.): The Temporomandibular Joint. Springfield, Ill., Charles C Thomas, 1951, pp. 3–40.

52. Stallard, H.: Dental articulation as an orthodontic aim. J. Am. Dent. A., *24*:347, 1937.

53. Tallgren, A.: An electromyographic study of the behavior of certain facial and jaw muscles in long-term complete denture wearers. Odont. Tskr., 71:425, 1963.
54. Tallgren, A.: Changes in adult face height due to ageing, wear and loss of teeth and prosthetic treatment. Acta Odont. Scandinav., 15:Suppl. 24, 1957.
55. Tallgren, A.: Positional changes of complete dentures. A 7-year longitudinal study. Acta Odont. Scand., 27:539, 1969.
56. Tiegelkamp, K. H.: Changes in the region of the mandible and the temporomandibular joint during orthodontic treatment. European Orthodont. Soc., 36th Congress Report, July, 1960, pp. 204–223.
57. Ulrich, J.: The human temporomandibular joint: Kinematics and actions of the masticatory muscles. J. Prosth. Dent., 9:399, 1959.
58. Updegrave, W. J.: Roentgenographic observations of functioning temporomandibular joints. J. Am. Dent. A., 54:488, 1957.

CHAPTER 2

COMPONENTS OF THE NERVOUS SYSTEM

NEURONS

The basic unit of the nervous system is the neuron, which consists of a nerve cell body (perikaryon) and its processes. The processes consist of (1) short branching fibers called dendrites that act as the receptor zone of the neuron and conduct impulses toward the cell body, and (2) a single long fiber (axon) for conducting impulses away from the cell body. However, the basic unit is usually more complex because axons generally give off branches or collaterals. Although some neurons have dendrites and others do not, most neurons in the central nervous system have dendrites and are multipolar. Those without dendrites may give off one or two processes (axons) and be bipolar, having a process extending from each end of the cell, e.g., cells of the retina and the vestibular ganglion of the eighth cranial nerve. Most of the neurons of the cerebrospinal ganglia are unipolar neurons, which have a single process that divides into two parts a short distance from the cell body of the neuron. One part, the peripheral process, extends to sensory receptors; and the other part, the central process, extends to the brain stem or spinal cord. The single process of the unipolar neuron that divides and the peripheral and central processes have the features of axons.

Neurons may be grouped according to their function into three general classes: (1) *sensory* neurons, which transmit impulses to the spinal cord and brain, (2) *motor* neurons, which transmit impulses from the brain and spinal cord, and (3) *connecting* neurons (interneurons), which provide for alternate, reciprocal, or distant connections with many of the cells of the nervous system. In general, motor neurons are termed efferent neurons, and sensory neurons are called afferent neurons. Neurons may be classified also according to their location: central neurons are confined to the central nervous system (brain and

24

spinal cord); the neurons remaining on the same side of the central nervous system are the association or ipsilateral neurons; those which cross in the central nervous system are known as contralateral or commissural neurons; and internuncial neurons are those interposed between an initial and a terminal neuron. Neurons vary from a fraction of an inch to more than 3 feet in length. The transmission of signals from one part of the body to another may involve a single neuron or a chain of neurons.

When nerve cell bodies are located in groups outside the brain and spinal cord, they are called ganglia; groups located within the brain or spinal cord are known as nuclei. The nervous tissue of certain portions of the brain and cord is often described as gray matter or white matter. The gray matter consists of aggregations of nerve cell bodies and the white matter consists primarily of nerve fibers or axons. Thus, axons essentially form the nerve fibers of the peripheral nerves (spinal and cranial) and the white matter of the brain and spinal cord.

The transmission of nervous impulses from one neuron to another occurs at a synapse. A simple synapse consists of the junction of the terminal end of the axon of one neuron with the dendritic zone or cell body of another neuron. One neuron may synapse with several neurons whereby an impulse may be propagated to a number of other regions. Most of the synaptic junctions or relays in the brain and spinal cord have interneurons and synaptic activity is more complex than with a simple synapse. For example, the impulses from stretched skeletal muscles not only excite the spinal motor neurons supplying the muscles which were stretched, but also inhibit those supplying the antagonists through an inhibitory interneuron (Fig. 3–5). Synaptic activity is also complicated by the presynaptic and postsynaptic elements, of which there may be a large number within the central nervous system. In addition, synaptic activity is complicated by either inhibitory or excitatory action of the presynaptic impulse upon the postsynaptic cell.

RECEPTORS

Sensory nerve terminations or receptors are specialized organs scattered throughout the body for the transformation of internal and external stimuli to nerve impulses and their relay to the central nervous system. Such receptors have been divided into three classes: (1) *exteroceptors*, which respond to such stimuli as touch, temperature, tactile discrimination, vision, and hearing; (2) *interoceptors*, which are concerned with the viscera and are related to the perception of hunger, visceral pain, and thirst; and (3) *proprioceptors*, which are concerned with the sensibilities of position and pressure and with the sense of movement.[26]

Epicritic sensibility is the term usually applied to discriminatory types of tactile sensation and slight differences in temperature.[11, 12] *Protopathic* sensibility refers to the perception of pain and gross tactile and temperature sensations. *Deep sensibility* refers to the recognition of position of parts of the body by means of impulses from muscles, tendons, and joints. According to this terminology, epicritic and protopathic sensibilities are mediated over the exteroceptive fibers and deep sensibility over the proprioceptive fibers.

A specific receptor is considered to be sensitive to a much lower energy level for a specific stimulus than for any other type of stimulus. Although receptors are specific in that each exhibits a particular sensitivity, the sensation of pain may be related to all types of stimuli (energy) that produce injury. If receptors sensitive to a particular stimulus are stimulated by an abnormal but high intensity stimulus, the usual sensation is aroused. For example, when the eyeball is struck, a flash of light may be seen.

The specificity of receptors is inversely proportional to the size of the area covered by the receptor and the number of endings attached to a fiber. Thus, the most specific tactile sensibility is associated with a single Meissner's corpuscle for a single fiber.[6] Receptors may be classified from an anatomic standpoint as being nonencapsulated or encapsulated.[6, 32]

Nonencapsulated Endings.   The simplest type of receptor is called a free nerve ending and is concerned principally with superficial pain sensibility. However, free nerve endings probably are activiated by gross tactile and other gross stimuli. Some fibers may end as more specialized endings known as the tactile discs of Merkel. Merkel's discs are considered to be receptors for gross tactile stimuli.

Encapsulated Endings.   Included in this category are nerve terminations with thin capsules, such as Meissner's tactile corpuscles, the spherical end-bulbs of Krause, and Golgi-Mazzoni corpuscles.

Meissner's tactile corpuscles are found in dermal papillae, most often in the hairless portion of the skin. However, they are also found in the lips and at the tip of the tongue. These corpuscles serve as receptors of the most discriminatory type of tactile stimulation.

The spherical end-bulbs of Krause have various forms and are found in the mouth, tongue, tendons and ligaments. Although their function is unknown it has been suggested that they distinguish between cool and cold stimulation. Golgi-Mazzoni corpuscles are found on the surface of tendons and in the subcutaneous tissues of the fingers. These corpuscles have been said to be pressoreceptors.

Still another ending with a thin capsule is the Ruffini corpuscle. Large endings of this type have been described in joints and are considered to be pressure receptors. Smaller endings of this type in subcutaneous connective tissue have been considered to be receptors for warmth.

Encapsulated endings with thick capsules include the pacinian (Vater-Pacini) corpuscle, and the cylindrical end-bulbs of Krause. The pacinian corpuscles are pressure receptors located in the subcutaneous connective tissues, periosteum, ligaments and joint capsules. The cylindrical end-bulbs of Krause are found in the skin and mucous membranes and to some extent in striated muscle.

Neurotendinous endings are also encapsulated and are called Golgi tendon organs. They have been found in the tendons of most muscles and respond to tendon stretch and muscle contraction. Impulses from the Golgi tendon organs are inhibitory in that a strong contraction of a muscle activates the tendon organ which inhibits that contraction and thus protects the muscle from disruption or detachment. The threshold of the Golgi tendon organ is much higher than that of the muscle spindle.

Neuromuscular endings (muscle spindles) are found most often in the gross muscle but sometimes lie in the region of transition into tendon. The spindle has its own sensory and motor innervation (p. 48). In this respect muscle spindles are unique, since spindle afferent discharges are produced and modulated by changes in muscle tension and by impulses from the central nervous system.

Although there are a large number of muscle spindles in the masticatory muscles, the lateral pterygoid and the anterior part of the digastric muscles have been considered to be devoid of muscle spindles, or if any are present, they are few in number.[1, 7, 10, 16, 19, 31] However, recently muscle spindles have been found definitely in small numbers in the lateral pterygoid muscle, in both man and monkeys.[13, 17] It has been suggested that the lack of neuromuscular endings or the number of such endings is related to the extensor stress to which the muscle is subjected. Thus, muscles which are not weight-bearing might be expected to contain few, if any, neuromuscular endings. It is generally considered that spindles predominate in extensors and muscles subserving postural functions. Furthermore, a monosynaptic reflex arc has not been established for the digastric muscle.[4] However, one must keep in mind past difficulties in locating muscle spindles in some muscles which later were found to contain neuromuscular endings. The function and details of the muscle spindle will be discussed later (p. 48).

In contrast to tendon organs which are in series, muscle spindles are arranged parallel with the extrafusal fibers of the muscle. Thus, muscle spindles (which have a low threshold to stretch) are excited when the muscle fibers are elongated. It appears that impulses from muscle spindles are excitatory in contrast to tendon organs, which have an inhibitory function (p. 52).

Proprioceptors

The term proprioception, in view of Sherrington's definition, refers to information provided about the movements and positions of the body and its parts by receptors in muscles (spindles), tendons and joints. Such receptors are not generally considered to produce conscious sensations or to be related to conscious control. Since the mesencephalic root and nucleus serve a proprioceptive function, and since some of the sensory information from pressoreceptors of the periodontal membrane go to the mesencephalic nucleus, these pressoreceptors have been termed proprioceptors. In addition, it is common to see proprioception divided into conscious and subconscious proprioception, the former term indicating that certain receptors and fibers mediate sensations relative to positions and movements that reach the sensory cortex.

The proprioceptive or kinesthetic sense (muscle sense) is mediated by such proprioceptors as muscle spindles, tendon organs of Golgi, pacinian corpuscles, and some free nerve endings. Although there are receptors in the periodontal membrane and adjacent soft tissues, their features and characteristics are not well defined; however, their presence has been documented histologically and electrophysically.[2, 3, 16, 19, 21, 22] The joint receptors are primarily pacinian and Golgi type receptors and are situated in the ligaments of the joint; however, sensory fibers also arise from Ruffini end-organs and free nerve endings located in the joint capsule. In general, muscle spindles provide information about the lengths of muscles; joint receptors to some extent indicate position; and tendon receptors provide information relative to the tension of the muscles.

Receptors and Innervation of the Temporomandibular Joints

It is generally accepted that there are nervous receptors in the temporo-mandibular joints that are related to the control of the position and movements of the mandible. Although such acceptance has been based on the innervation of joints other than the temporomandibular joints, recent studies of the in-nervation of the joint capsule indicate that the perception of mandibular posi-tion may be partly related to receptors in the joint capsule.[18, 25, 29]

The innervation of the temporomandibular joints is usually considered to be from the auriculotemporal, masseteric, and posterior deep temporal nerves. However, the location, entrance, and branching of the nerves have not been agreed upon. For example, Costen's syndrome (temporal neuralgia) was attri-buted to the passing of the auriculotemporal nerve between the head of the condyle and the pars tympanica. It is now generally agreed that the auriculo-temporal nerve passes beneath the capsule at its attachment on the ramus of the mandible.

The posterior part of the joint capsule is innervated by a branch of the auriculotemporal nerve which enters the capsule below the articulating part of the condyle. After entry into the capsule the branch divides into a number of twigs. The anterior part of the capsule of the joint may or may not be innervated by branches from either the masseteric or the posterior deep temporal nerve. Present evidence does not support the view that the joint is innervated by branches of the anterior deep temporal nerve, the facial nerve, or other nerves. The distribution of the nerves in the capsule shows some quantitative variation in that the posterior part is more richly innervated than the medial part of the capsule. Branches of the auriculotemporal nerve supply the posterior medial and lateral portions of the capsule and the masseteric nerve innervates the anterior part of the capsule. The anterior lateral aspect of the capsule is supplied by the posterior deep temporal nerve.

Although free nerve endings are numerous in all areas of the capsule, such complicated nerve endings as corpuscles of Ruffini, Golgi tendon organs, and modified corpuscles of Vater-Pacini are relatively few and are primarily localized to the lateral portion of the capsule and the temporomandibular ligament.[29]

Innervation of the temporomandibular joint disc has been observed by special staining of tissues in fetuses, children, and adults.[30] In the fetal disc the nerves from the auriculotemporal, masseteric and posterior deep temporal penetrate the posterior and anterior parts of the disc, giving off branches to the blood vessels and terminating as free nerve endings. In the adult temporomandibular joint the nerve fibers appear to enter only the peripheral parts of the disc in the posterior portion at the border between the disc and capsule, giving off branches to vessels and terminating as free nerve endings.

NERVE FIBERS

Nerve fibers are generally classed according to their size, diameter, and physiological characteristics. In general, large nerve fibers conduct more rapidly than nerve fibers of smaller diameter. Nerve fibers are classified according to several systems. In one system nerve fibers are classified from I through IV, I being the fastest conductor and IV the slowest conductor. Such a classification is not rigid and there are subdivisions. For example, gamma fibers represent a subdivision of Group I fibers. Group Ia nerve fibers have their origin in the primary endings of the muscle spindles and Ib have their origin in the Golgi tendon organ receptors. Group II nerve fibers have their origin in the secondary endings of the muscle spindles and in the receptors for touch and pressure. Group III nerve fibers have their origin in temperature and pain receptors and fibers of Group IV are considered to conduct impulses of poorly localized pain. Thus, large fibers are related to proprioceptive sensations and somatic motor function while the smaller nerve fibers are concerned with pain sensation and autonomic function.

CENTRAL NERVOUS SYSTEM

The central nervous system consists of the spinal cord and brain, whereas the peripheral nervous system consists of the cranial and spinal nerves with their ganglia. Anatomically the brain is described as consisting of three main masses: the cerebrum, the cerebellum, and the brain stem. The brain stem includes the midbrain, pons, and medulla, and contains nuclei of the motor cranial nerves and scattered reticular nuclei. The cerebrum, the most prominent part of the brain, is divided into right and left hemispheres. These hemispheres have an outer coating of gray matter which is called the cerebral cortex. Fissures or sulci divide each hemisphere into areas known as the frontal, parietal, temporal, and occipital lobes and insula.

Cerebral Cortex. The cerebral cortex consists of areas concerned with motor, sensory, and associational functions: (1) the motor or pyramidal cortex, concerned with voluntary movements of striated muscle; (2) sensory or somesthetic areas serving deep and cutaneous sensibility, including touch, pressure, and muscle sense; and (3) associational areas concerned with the integration of activities of other areas and related to such functions as reason, memory and judgment.

The fiber tracts of the white matter of the cerebrum may be grouped into three divisions: (1) the association tracts, (2) the commissural tracts and (3) the projection tracts. The association tracts connect adjacent and distant portions of the same hemisphere, the commissural tracts connect the two hemispheres, and the projection tracts include those fibers which connect the cerebral cortex to other parts of the central nervous system.

Although the motor or pyramidal cortex gives rise to efferent tracts which are important for voluntary movement of striated muscle, subcortical motor mechanisms are also important for effective motor function. Also involved in the motor function are: (1) the basal ganglia and nuclei in the midbrain (collectively called the extrapyramidal system), and (2) the cerebellum with related brain stem structures. Thus, the term extrapyramidal system refers to motor systems other than those of the corticospinal and corticobulbar tracts. Fibers of this system may arise in the prefrontal cortex, basal ganglia, and such nuclei as the red nucleus and reticular nuclei, and also in the cerebellum. From these areas fibers descend in short relays to the reticular formation, to the motor nuclei in the anterior horn cells of the spinal cord, and to the motor nuclei of the cranial nerves and other nuclei in the brain stem. The function of the extrapyramidal system is primarily the coordination of muscle movements and body posture.

Basal Ganglia. The basal ganglia consist of several paired nuclei, including the corpus striatum and the globus pallidum. All subcortical motor nuclei of the forebrain are sometimes included in the term basal ganglia. The corpus striatum is related to the coordination of muscle movements, although some of the functions of the basal ganglia are not motor. Apart from cerebral cortex, the basal ganglia are the highest centers for facilitating motor function, and the globus pallidum is sometimes referred to as the motor center of the extrapyramidal system. Such facilitation of motor function is considered to occur via influencing connections with the premotor and motor cortex, the lower motor neurons (p. 32) by way of the subthalamus and with the reticular formation of the midbrain. Other areas of the corpus striatum are presumed to inhibit the activity of the globus pallidum. Insofar as the muscles of mastication are concerned, a connection from the globus pallidum is made with the masticator nucleus, i.e., motor nucleus of the trigeminal nerve.[8]

Cerebellum. The cerebellum has for its main function the coordination and refinement of muscular movements. The influence of the cerebellum occurs through its connections with the motor systems of the brain stem and with the cerebral motor and sensory cortex. Thus, its chief function is concerned with the control of voluntary skilled movements. The cerebellum receives afferent inputs from proprioceptive and many sensory systems and is important in the regulation of posture and muscle tonus. The relationship of the cerebellum to reflex tonus and the muscles will be described later. In general, the cerebellum exerts both inhibitory and facilitory influences on muscle movements initiated by the motor areas of the cerebral cortex.

Medulla.   The medulla is situated between the spinal cord and the pons, and ascending and descending pathways of the spinal cord are represented here. Two posterior eminences, the gracile and cuneate nuclei (p. 35) and two frontal eminences called the pyramids are present here. In addition to the reticular formation, the cardiac, vasomotor, and respiratory centers are also present in the medulla.

Pons.   The pons lies in front of the cerebellum and above the medulla and is an important connecting link in the path by which the cerebral hemispheres and the cerebellum are united. In the pons are the nuclei of the fifth, sixth, seventh, and eighth cranial nerves.

Thalamus.   The thalamus is a sensory relay station in which all sensory tracts (except the olfactory) are interrupted by a synapse. The sensory fibers which synapse here are projected to the primary cortical sensory areas. Thus, conscious sensory information from the receptors passes through the thalamus to the cerebral cortex. In addition, the thalamus has important efferent inputs from the reticular formation that in turn are relayed to many areas of the cerebral cortex.

Reticular Formation.   The term "reticular formation" is used to describe anatomically a portion of the brain stem which contains centers regulating respiration, blood pressure, heart rate, and other functions. The reticular formation is considered to be capable of modifying or integrating impulses from sensory receptors and is known to be related to arousal and wakefulness. One of the first evidences of the influence of the reticular formation on sensory input to the central nervous system was related to proprioception and modification of muscle spindle activity.[9, 20] The reticular formation, through efferent pathways, appears to facilitate or inhibit the response of motor neurons. Through such action a certain degree of control occurs in motor functions and phasic and tonic muscular activity. Thus, the reticular system, through ascending and descending components, is able to modulate sensory inputs and plays an important role in the formation of conditioned reflexes (pp. 46 and 55).

NERVE PATHWAYS

The spinal cord is connected with the various parts of the body by 31 pairs of spinal nerves. Each of the spinal nerves has a dorsal afferent root and a ventral efferent root. Just before entering the spinal cord the dorsal root forms a spinal ganglion which contains the cells of the afferent fibers. Both dorsal and ventral roots form a mixed spinal nerve or common nerve trunk containing afferent and efferent nerve fibers (Fig. 3–4). The cranial nerves (12 pairs) supply the head and neck, except for the vagus nerve, which goes to the region of the chest and abdomen.

The cerebral cortex and brain stem receive sensory information via sensory (afferent) nerves and their *ascending tracts*. Conversely, muscles receive nerve impulses initiated by the cerebral motor cortex and brain stem that are transmitted by *descending tracts*. The neurons whose cell bodies are in the motor cortex and also compose the descending tracts are usually referred to as *upper motor neurons*. The *lower motor neurons* consist of the anterior horn cells and peripheral nerve processes. Because of the pyramidal shape of this tract in the medulla, it has been called the *pyramidal tract*. It has been found that some neurons whose cell bodies lie outside the motor cortex also constitute a portion of the pyramidal system.

The axons from the higher centers may have connections with a single ventral horn cell. The fibers of the motor nerves arise from cells in the ventral horn of gray matter of the cord and pass to the muscles which they supply. The ventral horn cell and its peripheral processes is called the *final common pathway*.

Descending Tracts

The upper motor neurons make synaptic junctions either directly or through internuncial cells on motor neurons of the motor nuclei of the cranial nerves or the ventral horn cells of the spinal cord. Thus, the efferent pathway from the motor cortex to striated muscles traverses the upper motor neurons and the lower motor neurons. Some of the upper motor neurons form the *corticospinal or pyramidal tracts* that extend from the cortex to the spinal cord (Fig. 2–1). Until recently it had been thought that impulses from the cortex for voluntary movements were transmitted directly by pyramidal fibers to the motoneurons of the muscles. However, most pyramidal and dorsal root fibers end elsewhere in the spinal gray matter to produce motor function. Just prior to entering the spinal cord most of the fibers undergo decussation or crossing in the medulla. These crossed fibers and some of the uncrossed fibers form the *lateral corticospinal tracts*. The remaining uncrossed fibers continue as the *ventral corticospinal tracts*. Most of the uncrossed fibers eventually cross in the spinal cord. Fibers from these tracts end on ventral horn cells or through interneurons. The lateral tracts are the motor supply to the muscles of the extremities, whereas the ventral tracts are the motor supply to the trunk muscles.

Other long descending tracts include: (1) the *reticulospinal tracts* originating in the pontine and medullary reticular formation, which are important to the facilitation and inhibition of reflex activity, voluntary movement, muscle tone, and other functions; (2) the *rubrospinal tract* (Fig. 2–4) originating in the red nucleus, which appears to exert a facilitory influence on flexor-muscle tone; (3) the *vestibulospinal tract* originating in the medulla, which is considered to exert a facilitory influence on the reflex activity of the spinal cord and reflex mechanisms controlling muscle tone; and (4) other tracts related to the autonomic system and reflex postural movements associated with visual and auditory

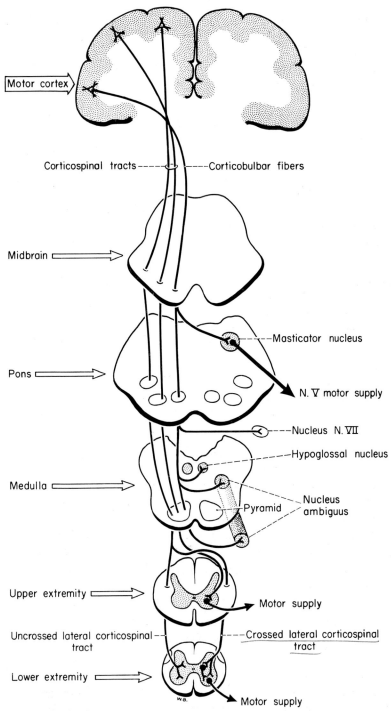

Figure 2-1. Diagrammatic illustration of voluntary motor control showing long descending tracts (corticospinal) to extremities and corticobulbar tracts to region of the head.

stimuli. The nonpyramidal descending fibers, consisting of the reticulospinal, vestibulospinal, rubrospinal, and other tracts, exert control over muscle tone, posture, reflex activity, and automatic movements. In contrast, the corticospinal tracts mediate voluntary, skilled movements.

Other upper motor neurons constitute the *corticobulbar tracts*, whose fibers diverge from the corticospinal tracts at the level of the midbrain and terminate in the brain stem in the reticular formation or on voluntary motor nuclei of the cranial nerves (trigeminal, facial, glossopharyngeal, vagus, accessory, and hypoglossal nuclei [Fig. 2–1]). Although most of these corticofugal fibers which control voluntary movements of muscles innervated by the motor cranial nerves appear to terminate in the reticular formation in lower animals, direct connections to the trigeminal, facial, hypoglossal, and supraspinal nuclei occur in man. The trigeminal and hypoglossal projections are bilateral.

Ascending Tracts

When a sensory receptor is stimulated, an impulse is propagated in an afferent neuron to the central nervous system (brain stem or spinal cord), where the afferent fibers may make synaptic junctions with interneurons and polysynaptic reflex connections with motor neurons in the spinal cord or brain stem, and also with neurons of ascending pathways to the cerebral cortex.

Afferent neurons mediating fine touch and pressure on entering the spinal cord immediately turn upward and ascend on the same side in *dorsal columns* of the spinal cord to the medulla (Fig. 2–2). In the medulla these afferent neurons synapse with second order neurons in the gracile and cuneate nuclei and then cross to the opposite side of the medulla to ascend in a tract called the *medial lemniscus* to the thalamus. The second order neurons make synaptic junction in the thalamus with third order neurons, which then ascend to the cerebral cortex. Thus, information of fine touch, pressure, and proprioception involves three neurons. Some touch and pressure afferent fibers mediating general tactile sensibility synapse on neurons in the dorsal horn of the cord, where they cross the midline and ascend in the *ventral spinothalamic tract*.

Sensory fibers for pain, cold and warmth transmit impulses to the spinal cord through the dorsal roots and end in the dorsal horn of the gray matter of the spinal cord, where they make synaptic junction with axons of second order neurons (Fig. 2–3). The axons of the secondary neurons cross the spinal cord at the same level and turn upward to ascend in the *lateral spinothalamic tracts* to the medulla. In the medulla the second order neurons make synaptic junction with third order neurons, which project to the cerebral cortex.

Proprioceptive pathways leading to the cerebellum from the cord include the *posterior and anterior spinocerebellar tracts* (Fig. 2–4). The posterior spinocerebellar tract contains fibers chiefly from the upper part of the spinal cord and is uncrossed. The anterior spinocerebellar tract contains crossed and

(*Text continued on page 38.*)

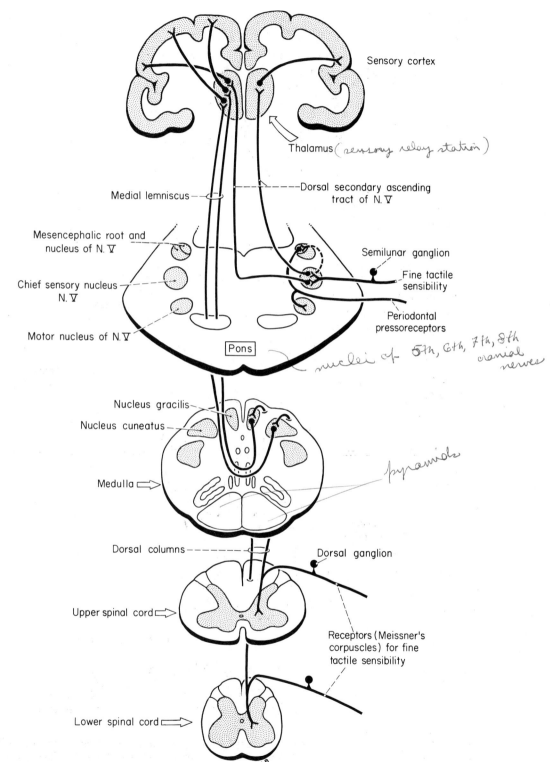

Figure 2–2. The major pathways for fine tactile sensibility and conscious proprioception. Not shown is the ventral spinothalamic tract mediating general tactile sensibility from free nerve endings. Tactile sensibility from the periodontal structures is carried by the mesencephalic root of the trigeminal nerve. The dotted line indicates possible connections to the sensory nucleus of the trigeminal nerve.

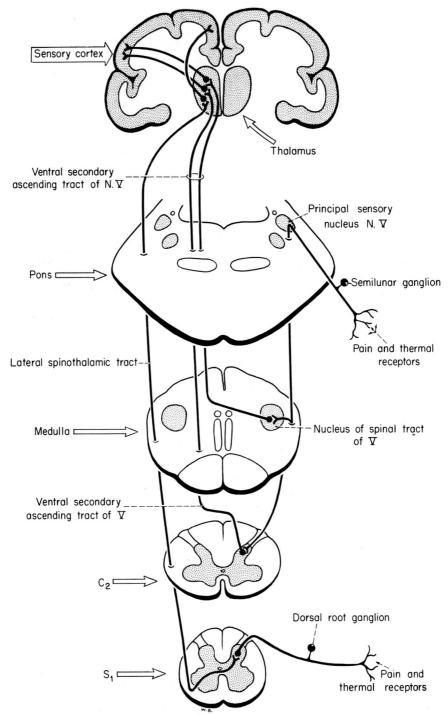

Figure 2-3. Diagram to illustrate major pathways involving pain and thermal stimuli. Impulses set up by gross tactile and temperature as well as pain stimuli travel over the spinal tract of the trigeminal nerve. Deep sensibility, including pain from muscles and around joints, is carried into the brain over the fibers of the mesencephalic root of the trigeminal nerve (Crosby[6]).

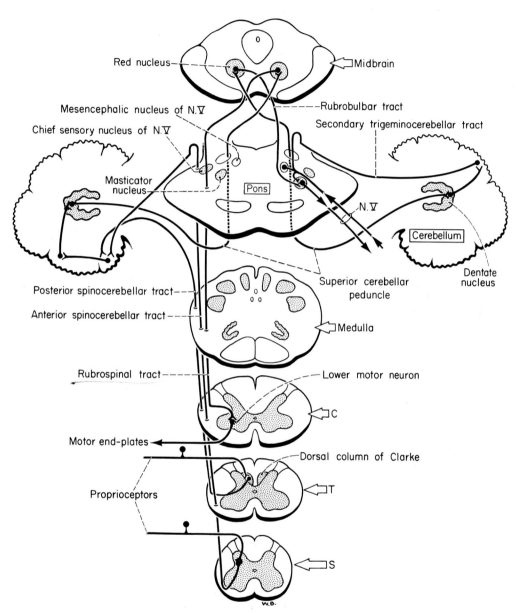

Figure 2-4. Diagram showing some of the connections of the cerebellum with the spinal cord and nuclei of the trigeminal nerve. Efferent cerebellar impulses integrating muscle activity reach the voluntary motor system via the dentatorubrospinal path and the dentatothalamocortical path (Figure 2-5) to the motor area of the frontal lobe.

uncrossed fibers and comes primarily from the lower part of the spinal cord. Until recently, stretch-sensitive muscle spindle and tendon organ receptors were considered to relay signals via the dorsal column-lemniscal system. However, Group I volleys initiated in muscle nerves of the hindlimb in some animals do not ascend in the classical proprioceptive path above the lower thoracic segments but terminate within Clarke's nucleus.[23, 24] Thus, evidence seems to indicate that signals from muscle spindle receptors do not go to cortical levels and in all probability play no part in conscious proprioception. The sense of movement and position is probably mediated by receptors of the joints, ligaments, subcutaneous tissues, and skin.

Secondary trigeminocerebellar fibers (Fig. 2–4) from the mesencephalic nucleus of the trigeminal nerve as well as from the superior sensory and spinal nuclei of nerve V have been found.[14, 32] The fibers from the mesencephalic nucleus of nerve V have been considered to mediate proprioceptive impulses from the muscles of mastication and possibly facial muscles. The cerebellum receives proprioceptive information, and possibly impulses, from the chief sensory nucleus of nerve V. It also projects and receives information from motor and sensory cortical areas and many areas of the brain stem. It thus appears that the cerebellum may modify the activity of most, if not all, neural centers;[27] however, such a concept is not without limitations.[5]

The cortex of the cerebellum receives an account of the program of voluntary motor activities from: (1) the output of the motor cortex and pyramidal tracts by a simultaneous output to corticopontocerebellar pathways (Fig. 2–5); and (2) inputs to the cerebellum from muscles by spinocerebellar and secondary trigeminocerebellar tracts (Fig. 2–4). Modifications of muscular movements may occur over the dentatorubrospinal pathway which leads to lower motor neurons of the spinal cord (Fig. 2–4). Also efferent cerebellar impulses pass over the dentatothalamocortical pathway (Fig. 2–5). The cerebellum influences the activity of the pyramidal system by these pathways.

It has been suggested that the supratrigeminal nucleus, which is dorsal to the masticator nucleus, is important in coordinating or integrating jaw reflexes (p. 60). The neurons of this nucleus appear to function as do the interneurons of the spinal cord.[16]

The facilitory and inhibitory effects of such areas as the cerebellum and cerebral cortex are mediated by descending fibers making contact with either alpha motoneurons or gamma motoneurons or with internuncials. Corticospinal projections, rubrospinal, corticorubral, vestibulospinal, and cerebellovestibular projections present a somatotopical localization which explains how stretch reflexes can be influenced at a local level by supraspinal regions.

TRIGEMINAL NERVE

The trigeminal nerve contains both motor and sensory nerve fibers. Afferent fibers of the trigeminal nerve convey sensory impulses of pain, temper-

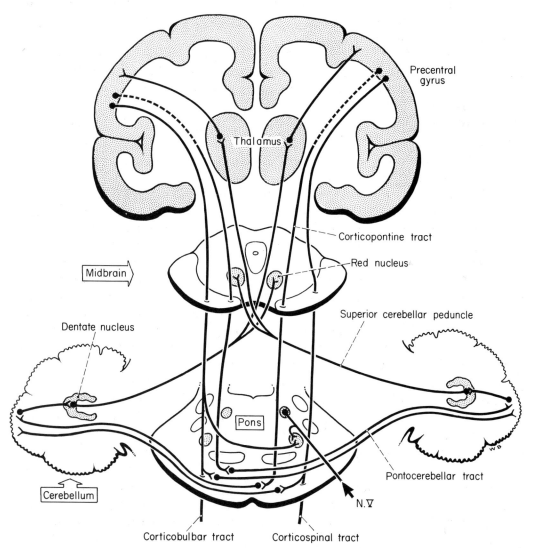

Figure 2–5. Diagram illustrating some of the connections between the cerebellum and the cerebral cortex. Afferent signals of voluntary motor activity from the cerebral cortex are relayed to cortex of the cerebellum via the corticopontocerebellar pathway and from the muscles via spinocerebellar and trigeminocerebellar paths (Figure 2–4).

trigeminal
division; motor
mandibular & sensory
ophthalmic & maxillary
are wholly sensory

ature, and touch from such areas as the face and the oral cavity. Afferent fibers also convey proprioceptive impulses from the masticatory muscles and the periodontal structures. The mandibular division of the trigeminal nerve contains motor as well as sensory nerves, in contrast to the ophthalmic and maxillary divisions, which contain wholly sensory fibers.

Although the cranial nerves appear to be more complex in structure and function than spinal nerves, the two have similar organizational features. Just as spinal afferent fibers have cell bodies in ganglia outside the central nervous system, somatic afferent fibers of the trigeminal nerve have nerve bodies in ganglia outside the brain stem. With the exception of the afferent fibers conveying proprioceptive impulses from the periodontal membrane and muscle spindles, afferent fibers have their cell bodies in the *semilunar ganglion*, which, like a spinal ganglion, contains unipolar neurons. Unlike the spinal nerves supplying proprioceptors, the cell bodies of proprioceptive fibers from the periodontal membrane and muscle spindles lie within the brain stem in the *mesencephalic nucleus* of the trigeminal nerve.

The peripheral processes of the cells of the semilunar ganglion are distributed to exteroceptive endings by way of the three divisions (ophthalmic, maxillary and mandibular) of the trigeminal nerve. Some of the central processes of the ganglion cells bifurcate, one part going to the main sensory nucleus and the other part turning downward to form a part of the descending or *spinal tract of the trigeminal nerve*. This descending tract distributes fibers to the *spinal nucleus of the trigeminal nerve*. Afferent fibers conveying impulses for pain and temperature from the trigeminal sensory areas descend in the spinal tract of the trigeminal nerve (Fig. 2–3). Central processes going directly to the main sensory nuclei are probably related to the most discriminatory type of tactile sensibility (Fig. 2–2). Thus, some trigeminal afferent fibers conveying tactile sense and pressure ascend without bifurcating to the main or superior sensory nucleus; however, gross tactile impulses are conveyed by bifurcating fibers. The most central processes of semilunar ganglion cells concerned with tactile impulses divide into ascending branches, which end in the main sensory nucleus, and descending branches, which terminate in the spinal nucleus.

As already mentioned, a third nucleus in the trigeminal complex, concerned with proprioceptive impulses and associated with the trigeminal nerve, is the *mesencephalic nucleus*. Since the cells of origin for proprioceptive fibers of the trigeminal nerve lie within the brain, the structure of the trigeminal nerve is unique in this respect. The peripheral processes of the cells of the mesencephalic nucleus of the trigeminal nerve travel with the motor root of the trigeminal nerve. The processes collect to form the mesencephalic root of the trigeminal nerve and bypass the motor nucleus of the trigeminal nerve to continue to the mesencephalic nucleus. When bypassing the motor nucleus, axons are given off to the trigeminal motor nucleus,[6] and collaterals from the root fibers are given off to the cerebellum (Figs. 2–2 and 2–4). Since it appears probable that secondary connections may discharge to the main sensory nucleus, the dorsal secondary ascending tract of the trigeminal nerve would then carry deep sensibility impulses from the muscles, tendons, and joints, and tactile sensation from the face.[6]

Whereas the cell bodies of secondary neurons in sensory pathways to the cerebral cortex from spinal levels constitute the tract cells (dorsal gray columns), the cell bodies of secondary neurons that are responsible for transmitting sensory impulses to the thalamus are found in the sensory nuclei of the cranial nerves. The cells in the main sensory and spinal nuclei of the trigeminal nerve, like those constituting the tract cells of the spinal cord, are multipolar. The sensory nuclei of the trigeminal nerve contain internuncial cells which connect through the reticular formation with efferent neurons whose cell bodies are in the motor nuclei of cranial nerves. There is some difference of opinion as to whether corticobulbar fibers discharge in part directly to the motor nucleus or wholly by way of the reticular formation. Monosynaptic connections (two-neuron arc) for proprioceptive control of jaw movements are probably made by mesencephalic root fibers to the motor nucleus (masticator nucleus).[28] Secondary trigeminal fibers also provide reflex control from exteroceptors in the oral mucous membranes, probably via intercalated neurons.

The mesencephalic trigeminal nucleus is related to the transmission of impulses from proprioceptors in certain masticatory muscles, including the medial pterygoid, masseter, and temporal muscles, in the periodontal membrane, and in the hard palate. Deep sensibility, including pain from muscles and around joints, may be relayed to the brain stem in the fibers of the mesencephalic root of the trigeminal nerve. As indicated, there is also the possibility that the axons of cells of the mesencephalic root of the trigeminal nerve end in the chief sensory nucleus of the trigeminal nerve.[6]

Some of the peripheral mesencephalic fibers appear to run in the sensory branches of the trigeminal nerves such as the alveolar nerves and mediate sensations of pressure from the teeth, periodontal membrane, and gingiva. It has been found recently that, in addition to the type of neuron innervating muscle spindles, two other types of neurons are present in the mesencephalic nucleus: (1) a neuron which conveys impulses from pressoreceptors of the periodontal membranes of several teeth as well as the adjacent gingival and oral mucosa, and (2) a neuron which conveys impulses from pressure receptors of the periodontal membrane of single teeth.[15, 16] Although it has been suggested that ganglion cells scattered along the motor root appear to furnish some proprioceptive fibers for the innervation of digastric and mylohyoid muscles, the presence of muscle spindles in these muscles has been questioned (p. 27). Until the recent discovery of muscle spindles in the lateral pterygoid muscle,[13, 17] it was necessary to reconsider the classic concept of reciprocal innervation in cyclic jaw movements (p. 60).[15]

HYPOGLOSSAL NERVE

The hypoglossal nerve is the motor nerve of the tongue and contains proprioceptive fibers and muscle spindles. The nucleus of the twelfth cranial nerve receives fibers and collaterals from reticular neurons and fibers from the corti-cobulbar system. In addition, the nucleus of the hypoglossal nerve receives some secondary trigeminal, glossopharyngeal, and vagal fibers. Such fibers probably enter into the mediation of reflex tongue movements associated with stimulation of the mucous membranes of the tongue (including taste as well as touch, temperature and pain).

REFERENCES

1. Baum, J.: Beiträge zur Kenntnis der Muskelspindeln. Anat. Hefte, *13*:251, 1900.
2. Beaudreau, D. E., and Jerge, C. R.: An electrophysiological study of the gasserian ganglion (abstract). Internat. Ass. Dent. Res., *41*:105, 1963.
3. Bernick, S.: Innervation of teeth and periodontium after enzymatic removal of collagenous elements. Oral Surg., *10*:323, 1957.
4. Blom, S.: Afferent influences on tongue muscle activity. Acta physiol. scandinav., Suppl. 170, *49*:1, 1960.
5. Bremer, F.: Central regulatory mechanisms—Introduction. *In* Handbook of Physiology—Neurophysiology. Washington, D.C., American Physiological Society, 1960.
6. Crosby, E. C., Humphrey, T., and Lauer, E. W.: Correlative Anatomy of the Nervous System. New York, The Macmillan Company, 1962.
7. Freimann, R.: Untersuchungen über Zahl und Anordnung der Muskelspindeln in der Kaumuskeln des Menschen. Anat. Anz., *100*:258, 1954.
8. Fulton, J. E.: Physiology of the Nervous System. London, Oxford University Press, 1949.
9. Granit, R., and Kaada, B. R.: Influence of stimulation of central nervous structures on muscle spindles in cat. Acta physiol. scandinav., *27*:130, 1952.
10. Gregor, A.: Ueber die Vertheilung der Muskelspindeln in der Muskulatur der menschlischen Fötus. Arch. f. Anat. u. Physiol., 112, 1904.
11. Head, H., Rivers, W. H. R., and Sherren, J.: The afferent nervous system from a new aspect. Brain, *28*:99, 1905.
12. Head, H., and Sherren, J.: The consequences of injury to the peripheral nerves in man. Brain, *28*:116, 1905.
13. Honée, G. L. J. M.: An investigation on the presence of muscle spindles in the human lateral pterygoid muscle. Ned. T. and T., *73*:43, 1966.
14. House, E. L., and Pansky, B.: A Functional Approach to Neuroanatomy. New York, McGraw-Hill Book Co., 1960.
15. Jerge, C. R.: The neurologic mechanism underlying cyclic jaw movements. J. Prosth. Dent., *14*:667, 1964.
16. Jerge, C. R.: The organization and function of the trigeminal mesencephalic nucleus. J. Neurophysiol., *26*:379, 1963.
17. Karlsen, K.: Muscle spindles in the lateral pterygoid muscle of a monkey. Arch. Oral Biol., *14*:1111, 1969.
18. Kawamura, Y., and Majima, T.: Temporomandibular joint's sensory mechanisms controlling activities of the jaw muscles. J. Dent. Res., *43*:150, 1964.
19. Kirstine, W. D.: Innervation of the Human Periodontal Membrane and Gingiva. M. S. Thesis, University of Michigan School of Dentistry, 1957.
20. Leksell, L.: The action potential and excitatory effects of the small ventral root fibers to skeletal muscle. Acta physiol. scandinav., Suppl. 10, *31*:1, 1945.
21. Lewinsky, W., and Stewart, D.: The innervation of the periodontal membrane. J. Anat., *71*:98, 1936.
22. Lewinsky, W., and Stewart, D.: The innervation of the periodontal membrane of the cat, with some observations on the function of the end-organs found in that structure. J. Anat., *71*:232, 1957.
23. Lloyd, D. P. C., and McIntyre, A. K.: Dorsal column conduction of group I muscle afferent impulses and their relay through Clarke's column. J. Neurophysiol., *13*:39, 1950.

24. McIntyre, A. K.: Central projections from receptors activated by muscle stretch. *In* Barker, D. (ed.): Symposium on Muscle Receptors. Hong Kong, Hong Kong University Press, 1962, pp. 19–29.
25. Ransjö, K., and Thilander, B.: Perception of mandibular position in cases of temporomandibular joint disorders. Odont. Tskr., *71*:134, 1963.
26. Sherrington, C. S.: The Integrative Action of the Nervous System. New York, C. Scribner's Sons, 1906.
27. Snider, R. S.: Recent contributions to the anatomy and physiology of the cerebellum. A.M.A. Arch. Neurol. & Psychiat., *64*:196, 1950.
28. Szentagothai, J.: Anatomical considerations of monosynaptic reflex arcs. J. Neurophysiol., *11*:445, 1948.
29. Thilander, B.: Innervation of the temporomandibular joint capsule in man. Trans roy. Schools Dent. (Stockh.), No. 7, 1961.
30. Thilander, B.: Innervation of the temporomandibular disc in man. Acta odont. scandinav., *22*:151, 1964.
31. Thilander, B.: Fibre analysis of the lateral pterygoid nerve. Acta odont. scandinav., *22*:157, 1964.
32. Truex, R. C., and Carpenter, M. B.: Strong and Elwyn's Human Neuroanatomy. 5th ed. Baltimore, The Williams & Wilkins Co., 1964.

CHAPTER 3

NEUROMUSCULAR PHYSIOLOGY

The operation of the masticatory system is very complex, and no complete account of the many basic neuromuscular mechanisms underlying its function can be given. However, certain aspects of its general neuromuscular physiology are known to be related specifically to the components of the neuromuscular system of the oral and associated structures. Other aspects of the masticatory system do not appear to be strictly analogous to other aspects of human or animal neuromuscular mechanisms.

When presenting material on neuromuscular mechanisms involving the spinal cord and pointing out *known* dissimilarities of the masticatory mechanism, there is always a tendency to interpret all other neuromuscular mechanisms of the masticatory system and the spinal cord as being similar, if not the same. It must be pointed out that while spinal cord analogies must be drawn upon at the present time because of the difficulty of studying the neuromuscular aspects of the masticatory system, it is to be expected that mechanisms unique to the oral region will continue to be found. In the present brief review of neuromuscular physiology an attempt will be made not to digress into controversial areas except where at least tentative conclusions have been drawn.

The anatomy and the cellular morphology of the masticatory system have been fairly well known for many years, but the physiology of the various parts of this system has always been, and still is, a very controversial subject. It is logical to consider the physiology of the muscles before discussing the other aspects of the system because functional or dysfunctional forces which affect other parts of the system often have their source in these muscles.

The basic unit of muscle is the muscle fiber, which is surrounded by an insulating sheath (sarcolemma); the basic unit of the neuromuscular system is the *motor unit,* which is made up of muscle fibers and one motor neuron. Hundreds to thousands of muscle fibers, with vessels and supporting tissues, make up a muscle. The axon of one motor neuron supplies a variable number of skeletal muscle fibers. It would appear that the more specialized and complex the muscular activity is, the greater the number of motor units for a given number of muscle fibers; i.e., a muscle approximating a one-to-one relation of nerve fibers and muscle fibers would be capable of the most precise movements. For example, the axon of a motor neuron may supply a large number of muscle fibers of large muscles of the back, whereas one nerve fiber may supply only two or three muscle fibers of the eye. It has been estimated that the mean number of muscle fibers per motor unit is 936 for the M. temporalis and 640 for the M. masseter.[11] On the basis of action potentials, these muscles appear to resemble the muscles of the extremities in construction.

Muscle Contraction

The shortening or development of tension in a muscle is the result of contraction. Thus, contracting muscles may produce movement such as elevating the mandible or lifting an arm; or contracting muscles that do not shorten produces tension and may oppose the force of gravity as in standing or holding something between the teeth. Shortening under a constant load is called *isotonic contraction* whereas contraction without shortening is called *isometric contraction.*

The relationship between tension, shortening and length is expressed in terms of equilibrium and resting length. *Equilibrium length* refers to the length of unattached (cut free from bony attachments) relaxed muscle at which tension at rest is zero. *Resting length* refers to the length of muscle at which the developed contraction tension is minimal. The tension developed when a muscle is stimulated in isometric contraction and the tension developed in unstimulated muscle (passive tension) varies with the length of the muscle fiber.

Muscle Sense

Exclusive of pain and deep pressure, deep sensibility (p. 26) may be expressed as muscle, joint and tendon sensibility; proprioception; kinesthesia; and position or movement sense. It has been indicated which receptors are found in the muscles, joints and tendons, i.e., muscle spindle, Golgi tendon organ, pacinian corpuscle and free nerve endings. Prior to discussing the muscle spindle, it is necessary to describe reflexes, which are the basis for automatic movements, posture and muscle tonus.

The functional anatomy of the masticatory system is fairly well understood by most dentists, but for an understanding of the functional disorders of the temporomandibular joint and the periodontium, it is even more important to have a clear concept of the neuromuscular relations within the masticatory system, especially with reference to myotatic reflexes, tonus, flexor reflexes, and influence of the central nervous system upon the conditioned reflex mechanism and the psychosomatic balance of the individual.

REFLEXES

Reflex action may be considered the response that occurs when nervous impulses from a receptor pass through sensory fibers to the central nervous system and out again through motor fibers to muscles which produce the response. This reflex arc in its simplest form consists of a sensory or afferent neuron and the motor or efferent neuron (Fig. 3–1). However, interconnecting neurons between the afferent and efferent fibers are usually present in most reflex arcs. Although afferent impulses may originate at different sites and pass through widely divergent paths to the central nervous system, such impulses may converge on the same motor neurons, called the final common path. The concept of the final common path requires some adjustment when considering organized movements. The simplest reflexes consisting of two neurons are monosynaptic reflexes; reflexes containing one or more interconnecting neurons are called polysynaptic reflexes. Other criteria for defining reflex action include conditioned reflexes or other motor activity acquired from conditioning or training.

Unconditioned reflexes are those in which a stimulus brings about a response without previous training and the response is considered to be specific for the stimulus. However, in the conditioned reflex, the responses elicited require previous training and the formation of new associations. In respect to the associations, the cerebrum is essential for the establishment of conditioned reflexes. Simple unconditioned reflexes include jaw opening and jaw closing reflexes.

Stretch (Myotatic) Reflex

When a muscle is stretched by pulling on it, the muscle contracts; this response is called a stretch reflex. The stretch reflex is initiated by receptors in the muscles being elongated; the receptor or sense organ for the initiation of these impulses is the muscle spindle. Stretch implies increased length, which is related to the muscle spindle, and increased tension, which is related to the Golgi tendon organ. Although it was previously considered that the function of the stretch reflex was primarily related to the opposition of the forces of gravity (for example, standing and the rest position of the mandible), it is now apparent that the stretch reflex is active during reflex and voluntary contraction of muscles, and is present in flexor and in extensor muscles.

The simple spinal cord reflex illustrated in Figure 3–1 provides the underlying mechanism for posture and locomotion and is basic to the concept of reciprocal innervation. In the simple spinal reflex the afferent neuron, whose cell body is in the dorsal root ganglion, is activated by the muscle spindle through lengthening of the muscle. In turn, the alpha motoneuron in the ventral horn is activated, bringing about reflex contraction of the muscle containing the spindle. The components of a simple disynaptic spinal reflex are also illustrated in Figure 3–1. It should be pointed out that the foregoing description is elemen-

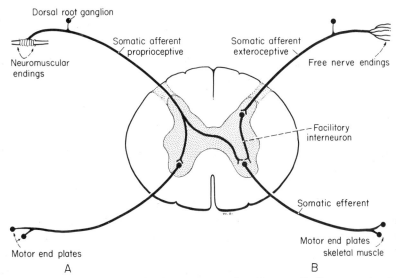

Figure 3–1. *A*, Components of a simple monosynaptic reflex arc. *B*, Components of a disynaptic reflex arc.

tary and does not take into consideration activation of the afferent neuron by the gamma efferent system (p. 49) and facilitation or inhibition of reflexes (p. 54).

Another example of the myotatic (stretch) reflex consists of the reflex contraction of the temporal and masseter muscles in the jaw jerk, which is activated by a downward percussion of the chin, tapping lower incisors, or tapping the tendon of the masseter muscle. In these instances the afferent neuron, whose cell body is in the mesencephalic nucleus (Fig. 3–2), is activated by the stretching of the muscle (the afferent neuron makes synaptic junction with the alpha motoneuron in the masticator nucleus in the pons). In turn, the alpha motor or effector neuron is activated and brings about reflex contraction of elevator muscles of the jaw. Slow as well as rapid stretching of the muscle elicits the reflex and, within rather narrow limits, the strength of the contraction continues to increase with increasing muscle lengthening force (bite raising). As previously indicated, there are several considerations which have not been included in this elementary description but will be taken up later. It has been established that the mesencephalic nucleus pathway is activated by lengthening of the mandibular elevator muscles and stimulation of pressoreceptors in the periodontal membrane. The pathway involves a monosynaptic reflex arc with cells of the mesencephalic and masticator nuclei taking part.[14, 70]

Flexor (Flexion, Nociceptive, Withdrawal) Reflex

Flexor reflexes involve the withdrawal from noxious stimuli. Thus, the primary function of the flexor reflex is protective. In general, it involves more muscle groups than the stretch reflex, and greater integration. It is a polysynap-

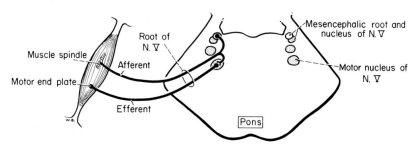

Figure 3–2. Pathways of stretch (myotatic) reflex involving trigeminal nerve. Gamma efferent system has been omitted.

tic reflex in which the response to a noxious stimulus brings about contraction of flexor muscles and inhibition of extensor muscles, and results in withdrawal of the part stimulated. Flexor reflexes are prepotent so that they take precedence over other reflex activity occurring at the same time. Spatial and temporal facilitation occurs in the various synapses of the polysynaptic pathway.

A flexor reflex involving the lower extremity is illustrated by the withdrawal of the entire limb when a strong stimulus such as stepping on a nail occurs. Similarly, during mastication when an encounter is made with a hard object which causes a painful stimulus, the jaw reflexly opens. It can be seen that the stretch and flexor reflexes are essentially antagonistic in that one is related to extension and the other to flexion and one inhibits the other. Such reflexes in which there is inhibition of one muscle group so that another may be activated is basic to the concept of reciprocal innervation (p. 52). Posture and locomotion are dependent upon the principles of reciprocal innervation as well as rhythmic mastication, although the latter may involve somewhat different components from the classical concept of reciprocal innervation (p. 60). The flexor reflex usually involves contraction of several different muscle bundles, whereas stretch reflex may be manifest in only a few muscle fibers. The flexor reflex plays a definite part in the clinical manifestations of traumatic temporomandibular joint arthritis.

MUSCLE SPINDLE

The muscle spindle consists of embryonal-like striated muscle fibers (intrafusal fibers) enclosed in a thin connective tissue capsule (Fig. 3–3). The capsule of the muscle spindle is attached to the tendinous end and the sides of the extrafusal muscle fibers (main contractile muscle fibers). The central portion of the muscle spindle is called the nuclear bag region. Afferent nerve endings in this portion of the spindle are called primary or annulospiral endings and are concerned with stretch reflexes. The afferent nerve fibers from the primary endings are called Group Ia fibers (p. 29). Adjacent to the primary ending is a secondary or flowerspray ending which responds to stretch and may be concerned with increased flexor and decreased extensor motor activity. The afferent nerve

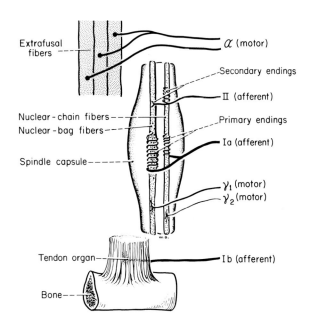

Figure 3-3. Schematic representation of innervation of skeletal muscle. Type III fibers from paciniform corpuscles and free nerve endings, and type IV fibers from vasomotor supply have not been included.

fibers from the secondary endings are called Group II fibers. It has been shown that fibers of the mesencephalic tract of the trigeminal nerve come from the primary and secondary endings of the spindles of the masticatory muscles. It has also been shown[70] that collaterals of the tract neurons pass to the motor nucleus of the infrahyoid muscles (ipsilateral hypoglossal nucleus).

Recently, a second type of intrafusal muscle fiber has been described and called the nuclear chain fiber.[6] Both the nuclear bag and nuclear chain fibers receive motor innervation by gamma fibers. The gamma efferent fibers (γ_1 and γ_2) constitute the fusimotor fibers. Also, as is the case with the nuclear bag fiber, afferent impulses from the primary ending of the nuclear chain fibers are conducted by Group Ia nerve fibers, and impulses from the secondary endings on the nuclear chain fiber are conducted by Group II nerve fibers. Thus, it appears that the motor as well as the sensory supply to the neuromuscular spindle is double.[7, 55]

The fusimotor nerve fibers are sometimes referred to as the small motor nerve system of the muscle spindle. Similarly, the extrafusal muscle fibers (regular contractile units of the muscle) which are innervated by large alpha type fibers are referred to as the large motor nerve system. Functional connections via gamma and alpha fibers with intra- and extrafusal muscle fibers are made at motor end plates.

Afferent sensory fibers (Group Ia) from the primary endings of the muscle spindle end directly on motoneurons supplying the extrafusal fibers of the same muscle containing the muscle spindle. The primary ending of the spindle is sensitive not only to elongation but also to stimulation by the fusimotor nerve fibers. When gross muscle is stretched, the primary endings of the nuclear bag region of the muscle spindle are lengthened and impulses initiated in the ending are transmitted via the spindle afferent Group Ia fibers to the cell body of the motoneuron supplying the muscle that was stretched. The impulses are then transmitted by the motoneuron via alpha type efferent fibers to the muscle (extrafusal fibers), and the muscle contracts. The impulses arriving from primary endings excite monosynaptically the alpha motoneurons supplying the same and protagonistic muscles and inhibit antagonistic muscles. Thus, the monosynaptic reflex is the basis of the stretch reflex (p. 46) and reciprocal innervation (p. 52). Impulses from the secondary ending are thought to excite flexor motoneurons whether located in flexor or extensor muscles.

Stretch Reflex as Servomechanism

As previously stated, excitation of the fusimotor fibers may cause contraction of the contractile portion of the muscle spindle. In effect, the contraction of the intrafusal fibers via the fusimotor fibers elongates the nuclear bag and distorts the primary endings of the muscle spindle, thereby increasing the sensitivity of the spindles to stretch since this sensitivity varies directly with the rate of gamma efferent activity. In one sense, the fusimotor system may serve as a "starter" of the motor activity of the alpha fibers, although contraction of the spindle fibers is not sufficiently strong in itself to cause shortening of the large mass of extrafusal muscle fibers. Thus, the fusimotor system serves as a "biasing" mechanism regulating the sensitivity of the muscle spindle and thereby the sensitivity of the stretch reflex by contributing to the excitation of the alpha motor neurons. It is generally agreed at the present time that the main function of the muscle spindle is the subconscious nervous control of muscular contraction during movement and steady contraction. Muscle spindles are not important to "conscious proprioception" or sense of position.

The stretch reflex has been likened to a servomechanism in which feedback signals from a muscle exert an influence on the length of the muscle.[26, 56] The servomechanism or automatic control mechanism is actuated by an "error signal" occurring in a closed-loop control cycle. The closed-loop cycle consists of: stretch of the muscle–elongation–excitation of primary endings–monosynaptic excitation of the motoneurons–contractions–shortening of the muscle. In this system the loop gives negative feedback from detectors of change in the length of the muscles and thus tends to hold the muscles at a required constant length.[55]

Since the muscle spindles are in parallel with the extrafusal muscle fibers, the spindles provide information about differences in the length of the extrafusal muscle fibers as well as the intrafusal muscle fibers. The discharges from the muscle spindles in turn excite the motor neurons of the extrafusal muscle fibers, which then shorten. The length of the main muscle (extrafusal muscle) is maintained by the length of the intrafusal muscle fibers, which act as error detectors in the servo loop mechanism and feed the information back to the reflex center. Because the delay time for the signals to pass around the reflex arc would not allow for the correction of length of the main muscle instanta-neously, it is apparent that a signal indicating the rate of change of length as well as length itself would be required. It is apparent that the muscle spindles are sensitive to the rate of change of elongation as well as to the elongation of muscle.[54]

Velocity Control

In addition, the concept of velocity control is suggested by the following generalization: When a muscle is being stretched the primary endings signal both instantaneous length and the velocity of stretching, while the secondary endings signal mainly the instantaneous length of the muscle.[9, 38] Primary end-ings give a large response to dynamic components of a stimulus above their response to the static component, whereas secondary endings do not. "Dynamic" response refers to the response of the receptor to being stretched (rate of change of length), whereas "static" response is the maintained contraction (absolute length). Both are independently controlled by the central nervous system. In view of the presence of the two types of intrafusal muscle fibers (nuclear bag and nuclear chain fibers) such independent control appears possible. As was pointed out previously, the primary ending of the muscle spindle has termina-tions on both types of intrafusal fibers. In view of the finding that the two kinds of intrafusal fibers have an independent motor supply, it has been suggested that possibly the dual innervation provides independent control of "bias" and "dampening" of the servo loop.[55] Thus, the central nervous system could adjust the dampening of the stretch reflex or time delay in the reflex arc to different movements.

Each motoneuron is subjected to many influences (Fig. 3–4), some facili-

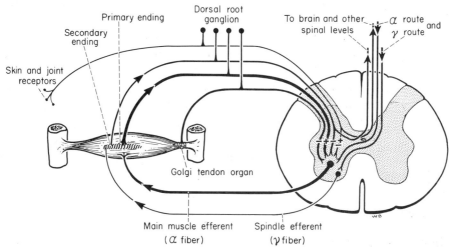

Figure 3–4.   Schema of the innervation of skeletal muscle and connections with the central nervous system.

tory and some inhibitory, and the results of these influences determine the excitation of the motoneuron. These many influences, depending on the location of the motoneuron, consist of numerous pathways of afferent inputs from many types of receptors and higher brain centers terminating directly or indirectly upon the motoneuron.[9, 55] Various stimuli reflexly alter fusimotor discharge, including light touch, pressure and pain. The muscle spindle provides information about mechanical events by means of two outputs (afferent fibers from primary and secondary endings) and is controlled by two inputs (gamma efferent fibers). Regions of the central nervous system which appear to have effects on the fusimotor system include the reticular formation, motor cortex, pyramidal tract, basal ganglia, red nucleus, thalamus, cerebellum, hypothalamus and the amygdala.[2, 3, 21–23, 30, 31, 38, 59, 67, 68]

Other Receptor Functions

The Golgi tendon organs are served by Group Ib fibers, whereas pacinian corpuscles, the vascular bed and free nerve endings are served by Group III fibers. It is possible also that Group IV (C) afferent fibers originate from the vascular bed, free nerve endings, tendon organs and muscle spindles.[4] The tendon organs are generally considered to have a higher threshold than the muscle spindles and are concerned primarily with protection of the muscle against excessive tension.

INFLUENCES ON ALPHA MOTONEURONS

Reciprocal Innervation

When a part is moved, the muscles which ordinarily oppose the movement are caused to relax. This phenomenon is known as *reciprocal innervation* (Fig. 3–5). Since flexors and extensors can be made to contract voluntarily at the same time, it is apparent that reciprocal innervation is not employed in all types of muscle function. When a stretch reflex occurs, impulses from the muscle spindles of a protagonist inhibit directly the motoneuron of the antagonist muscle. Thus, in addition to excitatory fibers to the protagonist muscles, there is a collateral from the Ia fibers which passes to an inhibitory interneuron in the cord that synapses directly with the motoneuron supplying the antagonist muscle. Thus, afferent neurons from the spindles in protagonistic muscles provide for both protagonistic and antagonistic muscle function.

Inverse Stretch Reflex

When a muscle is stretched severely enough, contraction ceases and the muscle relaxes (Fig. 3–5). Such a response to a strong stretch is called the *inverse stretch reflex* (autogenic inhibition).[18, 19] The receptor for this reflex is the

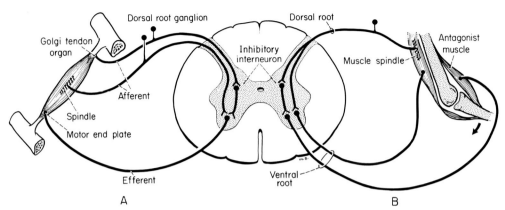

Figure 3–5. *A, Autogenic inhibition* (inverse stretch reflex). Excessive tension stimulates the Golgi tendon organ, which activates the interneuron and inhibits contraction. *B, Reciprocal innervation.* Possible neuromuscular connections for inhibiting antagonist muscle in response to stretch. Impulses from muscle spindle in protagonist are conveyed to same muscle for contraction; at the same time impulses activate interneuron, which inhibits the antagonist muscle. The gamma efferent system has not been included.

Golgi tendon organ. Golgi tendon organs, being in series with the muscle fibers, are stimulated by both passive stretch and active contraction of the muscle. The sudden relaxation in the inverse stretch reflex is thought to protect the muscle from detachment from its origin or insertion or both. However, other than protective functions for the Golgi tendon organs have been suggested. Some Golgi tendon organs appear to have sufficiently low thresholds to play a part in the control of muscle contraction and thus may not be present simply to provide protection against excessive muscle tension. It also appears that autogenic inhibitory effects of extensor muscles can be derived from Group II afferent impulses originating in the secondary endings in the muscle spindles[50] and thus it is suggested that autogenic inhibition can be directly influenced by the central nervous system through the nuclear chain fusimotor system.[15, 39, 52]

Inputs to Spinal Neurons

The spinal motoneuron of an extensor muscle has monosynaptic excitatory inputs from the muscle spindles, polysynaptic inhibitory inputs from spindles that relax antagonists, inhibitory inputs from secondary endings of the muscle spindle, afferent inhibitory inputs from nerves in the skin, muscles and periosteum, and inhibitory inputs from Golgi tendon organs (inverse stretch reflex). Similar central connections excitatory to motoneurons supplying flexor muscles are found with afferent nerve fibers from cutaneous, subcutaneous, muscle and periosteal tissue. It should be pointed out that monosynaptic spinal reflexes originate in Group I afferent fibers found only in muscles.[62] Thus, the input from one muscle facilitates and inhibits motoneurons supplying antagonistic muscles. However, the afferent limbs of polysynaptic reflex arcs have Group II, III and IV fibers.

Excitatory and Inhibitory Inputs

In addition to the inputs to a spinal neuron outlined above, there are excitatory and inhibitory inputs from other levels of the spinal cord and from long descending tracts from the brain (Fig. 3–4). Such inputs to cranial nerve neurons are also present. It has been stated that inhibitory and facilitory nerve relationships exist only in the masticator nucleus and not in the mesencephalic nucleus.[45] Also the collaterals from a muscle's center in the mesencephalic nucleus pass to other muscle centers in the masticator nucleus. Such collateral pathways have been considered to be responsible for inhibition and facilitation.

Although Golgi tendon organs have been inferred for certain jaw muscles[41, 69, 70] and no direct analogy between their functions in cranial and spinal nerve systems can be made,[41] it seems appropriate to point out possible relationships. Of interest here are the common observation that patients cannot comfortably close forcibly against periodontally involved teeth and the observation that there is a fall in amplitude of the electrical activity of the temporal and masseter muscles with a maintained closing force as the vertical dimension is increased.[69] In the former, stimulation of the receptors in the periodontal membrane results in inhibition of the elevator muscles of the mandible. In the fall in electromyographic amplitude with sustained voluntary isometric muscular contraction with increased vertical dimension, the inhibition of alpha and gamma afferent fibers might be mediated by the secondary endings of the muscle spindles on the gamma efferents or by Golgi tendon organs on both alpha and gamma afferent fibers.[35] Like inhibition by interneurons in the spinal cord, inhibition of activity may take place through an inhibitory neuron in the masticator nucleus. However, it is possible that the neurons of the nucleus supratrigeminalis respond the same as the inhibitory neurons of the spinal cord.[40] It is doubtful that Golgi tendon organs are of significance in the inhibition of small closing forces; it is more likely that pressoreceptors in the periodontal membrane and other receptors in the gingiva, palate and other oral mucous membranes are responsible.[69]

OTHER INFLUENCES ON MUSCLE FUNCTION

The emotional influences on the muscles of mastication are well known to clinicians. Superficial emotional reactions such as apprehension of dental procedures increase muscle tone, and positioning of the jaw accurately becomes difficult if not impossible. In deeper emotional conflicts as well as in superficial emotional reactions, changes in cortical and subcortical activity influence other parts of the brain such as the reticular formation and those areas to which the reticular formation projects.[48, 49] Such changes may be excitatory or inhibitory.

The ability to perform all kinds of muscle activity is present in each segment of the spinal cord. However, skilled and voluntary actions are initiated when necessary by highly integrated facilitory and inhibitory influences arising in cerebral structures. It is difficult to divide the brain stem anatomically into facilitory and inhibitory areas; however, such a division exists, at least functionally.[9] Such brain stem areas also are controlled by facilitory and inhibitory inputs from the spinal cord, cerebral cortex, cerebellum and basal ganglia. The reticular formation is capable of modifying sensory inputs to the central nervous system and, as already indicated, the reticular formation influences proprioception through its influence on the fusimotor system.

The role of the reticular formation in the habituation (decreasing awareness of a sensation) of animals to repeated stimuli and arousal with new and strange stimuli may be of importance to understanding the mechanism of habituation to "high" restorations.[24] Furthermore, the habituation associated with monotonously repeated stimuli and conditioning may well be related to the inhibitory influence of the reticular formation.[17, 28] The avoidance patterns of mandibular movement associated with occlusal interferences implies that a higher integrative mechanism, possibly in the reticular formation, may be involved in the avoidance adaptation. It is believed that the conditioned discharge of gamma neurons may significantly facilitate the establishment and maintenance of lateral behavioral responses.[10] There is acceptable evidence that the central nervous system exerts adaptive influence over the postural control system by regulating the neural loop gain and adjusting the muscle spindle time constant.[32, 57]

The general pattern for functional movements of the mandible is determined from a combination of impulses derived from the various receptors in the masticatory organ, later evaluated and guided by nerve centers of the reflex system. A conditioned or acquired reflex pattern is thereby established which, under physiologic conditions, will come as close as possible to satisfying the basic requirement of optimal function without damage to any part of the masticatory organ. The importance of a reflex controlled combination of synergistic and antagonistic activities for the establishment of well balanced and smooth function of the masticatory apparatus cannot be overlooked. A knowledge of the source of influence on the masticatory system is of greatest importance in an analysis of masticatory function or dysfunction.

MUSCLE TONE

Muscle *tone* may be defined in several ways; however, most simply it refers to the clinical sense of firmness of skeletal muscles. Muscle tone is also defined as the clinically assessed passive resistance of muscles to stretch. Increased passive resistance to stretching of the muscle has been called increased tone; such muscles are referred to as hypertonic or spastic. In the presence of a diminished passive resistance, the muscles are said to be hypotonic or flaccid. Somewhere in between these two states is the normal passive resistance, which is termed normal muscular tone.[71] According to Sherrington's terminology[65] muscle *tonus* or reflex tonus is that part of muscle tone based on the myotatic reflex. However, in a general sense, muscle tone is determined by passive mechanisms such as elastic properties of muscle and the investing tissues as well as by myotatic reflexes (stretch reflexes).

Myotatic reflexes and tonus can be influenced and altered (1) by facilitation or inhibition of the gamma motoneurons which influence the alpha motoneuron and (2) by facilitation or inhibition of the alpha motoneurons which innervate the gross muscle (extrafusal fibers). The reticular formation acts mainly through the gamma efferents and affects chiefly myotatic extensor reflexes. The extensor inhibitory reticular system is dependent on impulses from the cortices of the cerebellum and cerebrum. The extensor facilitory reticular system receives impulses from the ascending afferent systems including impulses originating in muscles. In this respect, the ascending afferent systems facilitate myotatic reflexes of extensor muscles and inhibit nociceptive flexor reflexes, whereas cerebral and cerebellar impulses inhibit myotatic reflexes and facilitate flexor reflexes.[62] Such control mechanisms suggest that tonicity may be altered by cerebral and cerebellar impulses.

Mechanism of Muscle Tonus

When muscle fibers are stretched, the proprioceptive organs (muscle spindles) in the stretched muscles are elongated. Afferent impulses from the stretched spindle travel via spindle afferents to the spinal cord or brain stem, where connections are made with alpha motoneurons. Stimulation of motoneurons causes impulses to be carried to the motor end plates of the stretched fibers, resulting in contraction of the muscle fibers. The contractile ends of the muscle spindle are subject to adjustment via the fusimotor nerves whereby the muscle spindles are kept at a level of tension favorable for firing the afferents. The level of adjustment or degree of contraction of the spindle controls the "bias" of the stretch reflex, which is basic to muscle tone. When a muscle contracts, tension on the spindle decreases because the spindle is in parallel with the extrafusal muscle fibers and fusimotor discharge decreases. However, when a muscle is stretched, the tension on the spindle is increased and the discharge increases until the muscle reflexly contracts and the discharge ceases. Increased fusimotor activity increases spindle sensitivity to stretch because the contractile portion of the spindle contracts and the spindle is shorter. Thus, spindle sensitivity varies with fusimotor activity (rate of gamma efferent discharge). In effect, this self-regulatory mechanism influenced by the central nervous system largely determines muscle tone.[34]

Activity of the alpha motoneurons may be influenced by other sensory receptors as well as the muscle spindles. It is a common experience in electromyographic procedures to note the influence produced on muscle activity by touching of the skin of the face. There can be no question that receptors in the skin influence the stretch reflex[20, 36] and thus influence mandibular position and tonicity of the muscles. Such considerations are important in the clinical recording of rest position.

Muscle Splinting

"Splinting" refers to the increased tonus (hypertonicity) of muscles in which there is resistance to passive movement of a joint. Splinting of muscles has been described as a protective mechanism whereby injury to a joint is avoided or reduced.[52] Occlusal interferences often lead to myalgias and pain associated with disturbances of the temporomandibular joints, and splinting of the involved muscles occurs.[61]

Inasmuch as the tonicity of the muscles of mastication can be influenced by impulses from the peripheral and central nervous system, it follows that hypertonicity of the masticatory muscles may be caused by functional disharmony of the components of the masticatory system, and/or to altered activity of the higher centers such as may occur under psychic stress. Hypertonicity of masticatory muscles tends to develop when the adaptability of the components of the masticatory system has been exceeded. For example, occlusal interferences may lead to hypertonicity and "splinting" of the masticatory muscles, in association with injury of the temporomandibular joints and its accompanying discomfort. The limits of adaptability of the supporting structures of the teeth may also be exceeded, but discomfort is not often of the same magnitude or type as pain of the temporomandibular joints. Without treatment of the occlusal disharmony, afferent signals from the receptors of the periodontal membrane and related to protective reflexes tend to further aggravate and perpetuate the problem. Also, muscle and temporomandibular joint dysfunction, as well as discomfort when present, increasingly influences the activity of the higher centers, leading to even further hypertonicity of the masticatory muscles. Such a self-perpetuating mechanism for the increase of muscle tension is a basis for bruxism.

It is often found in bruxism that the patient is unaware of the act of grinding the teeth or of the occlusal disharmony.[60] The only manifestation that the patient may be aware of is muscle discomfort due to increased muscle tonus or temporomandibular joint discomfort or pain. The fact that the subject is not aware of the act or of the local factor (occlusal interference) which is triggering the bruxism might be explained on the basis that the bruxism has become habitual. The contribution of awareness provided by the interplay between the cerebral cortex, reticular formation and the extrapyramidal system (p. 30) is no longer functioning to the same degree since the process of learning to avoid or wear down the occlusal disharmony has been accomplished. Thus, the conscious mind is no longer concerned with the automatic pattern of bruxism, but rather with the discomfort that may be associated with it.

In summary, the steady reflex contraction of muscles, especially of those that are concerned with maintenance of posture and counteraction of gravity, is called muscle tonus. Active fiber groups mingled with inactive groups, according to the "all-or-none principle" of muscle contraction, are scattered throughout the muscle, and alternating periods of rest and activity of the muscle fibers explain the maintenance of tonic contractions over long periods of time without evidence of fatigue. The fundamental basis for tonus of skeletal muscle is the myotatic reflex with pathways from cerebellar, midbrain and cerebral centers conveying impulses which are capable of altering the degree of tonus. Factors such as learning, pain, fear, tiredness, fatigue, mental relaxation and position of the subject will affect muscle tonus. Less distinct are the effects of hormonal or histochemical alterations on muscle tone. The tonus of a given group of muscles may also be influenced through the spinal centers by impulses arising in other muscle groups and in skin receptors. The muscular contractions which cause movements are fundamentally of the same nature as the contractions which maintain tonus. An active muscle contraction is different from tonus only in the respect that more muscle fibers participate. The factors which influence tonus therefore play a role in determining the functional action of the masticating muscles.

REFLEXES AND MANDIBULAR MOVEMENTS

Simple reflex opening and closing jaw movements are part of the suckling and nursing reflexes in infants prior to the eruption of teeth. Such movements are not chewing movements but are well organized movements involving oral and perioral muscles. With the growth of the infant and the eruption of the teeth, afferent stimuli from the receptors in the periodontal membrane influence the central nervous system and reflexly the position of the mandible. With the eruption of the teeth, the process of mastication is learned, and learning depends upon association involving the cerebral cortex, the reticular formation and the extrapyramidal system.

Adaptation to Changes

In the adult, alterations in tooth position, loss of teeth, high fillings, and other influences calling for new learning of masticatory patterns also occur. Of major consideration in such changes is whether the components of the masticatory system are capable of adapting to the changes. Since the higher centers are associated with the active learning process, an awareness of the failure to adapt may occur. For example, a new higher restoration may be so objectionable that normal function is impossible. If, however, a pattern of movement is learned so that the high filling can be avoided, functional movements then become automatic, probably regulated by the fusimotor system. However, in time the avoidance pattern of jaw movements may contribute to dysfunctional states in other components of the masticatory system which cannot adapt or compensate for the avoidance pattern of movement. Although the muscle patterns learned in the act of mastication are rather complex, and to a large extent represent complex conditioned reflexes, the basic opening and closing movements of the mandible represent stable muscle patterns based on the simple reflexes.

Rhythmic Chewing

The question of whether the rhythmicity of chewing is fundamentally related to higher centers or requires for its generation reverberating circuits through participating muscles is not known. It has been suggested[51] that the role of the motor cortex is doubtful in man and that mastication, like walking, may be one of the automatic functions which have become localized in subcortical regions. However, some investigators feel that the cortical motor area for the masticating muscles should be considered as contributing to the elicitation of skillful masticatory movements of the tongue and jaw.[41] The removal of cortical areas implicated in rhythmic chewing does not seem to interfere with such masticatory mechanisms in man.[16]

Although the basic mechanisms of mastication have been attributed to the jaw-closing and jaw-opening reflexes,[66] it is questionable that the rhythm of chewing is determined by a sequence of such reflexes set up by the movement of the mandible. It is quite likely that such reflexes can function to some extent without impulses from sensory receptors in the masticatory organ and that rhythmic chewing does not depend solely upon reflexes from the periphery of the organ.[64] While reflexes are important in the modification of chewing, the organization of rhythmic chewing may be internal and not dependent on a sequence of reflexes.[58] Although the principle of reciprocal innervation plays a large part in inhibitory processes, not all muscular actions involve reciprocal innervation. When the mandible is held stationary, both opening and closing muscles act together. Only during movement does reciprocal innervation operate.

Silent Period (EMG) – Motor Pause

A silent period or pause in electromyographic (EMG) patterns has been observed in association with tooth contacts during chewing and biting, mechanical tapping of the teeth, and abrupt release of tension on a muscle.[1, 5, 8, 25, 27, 53, 63] The term *silent period* was initially used to describe the brief cessation of tonic motor activity following a tendon jerk,[29] but this term has broader meaning now.

The mechanism underlying the motor pause (Fig. 3–6) has been related to

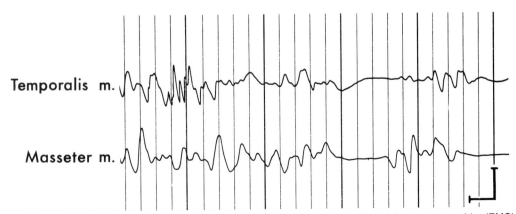

Temporalis m.

Masseter m.

Figure 3–6. Silent period associated with occlusal contact seen in electromyographic (EMG) record. Muscle response to a single voluntary tooth tap. Calibrations represent 10 msec and 1.5 mV.

a response of the receptors in the periodontal membrane (jaw opening reflex) as a protective measure against excessive occlusal forces.[1, 5, 8, 25, 63] The silent period has also been attributed to a decrease in muscle spindle activity during the initial reflex muscle contraction, and to have only a minor role in producing reflex changes in elevator muscle activity as a protective mechanism, except for heavy forces.[27, 53] Although Golgi tendon organs have a much lower threshold for stimulation than previously believed,[33, 37] there is no evidence to conclude it has a role in the silent period of jaw elevator muscles.[1, 5] However, certain receptors in the periodontal membrane have been likened anatomically and functionally to Golgi tendon organs.[46, 47]

It is evident that inhibition of elevator muscle activity as indicated by the silent period is an important component of the complex mechanism of mandibular control. The complex feed-back systems involving receptors in the periodontal membrane and muscles cannot be resolved by assuming that any one explanation that has been proposed is adequate to explain the silent period. Whatever the underlying mechanism may be, the silent period or motor pause appears to be important in some degree for noci-influences on occlusion.

Role of Cerebellum

The role of the cerebellum in masticatory function is not clear. Connections with the cerebellum from the mesencephalic root have been suggested; however, adequate mastication may occur in the presence of disturbances of the cerebellum which produce intention tremor. Tremor also depends on inadequacies of organization of voluntary control mechanisms without the cerebral cortex, and concurrent compensation for cerebellar function may occur.

In addition to the masticator nucleus (motor nucleus of nerve V) and the sensory nuclei within the brain stem, the nucleus supratrigeminalis (an extension of the main sensory nucleus) contains units whose responses are similar to those attributed to spinal interneurons, and thus could be important for coordinating or integrating jaw reflexes.

Cyclic Jaw Motions

When a noxious stimulus is applied to the oral structures there is reflex jaw opening and inhibition of jaw closing muscles.[43, 66] However, until the discovery of muscle spindles in the lateral pterygoid muscle, it did not appear that the classic concept of reciprocal innervation would apply to certain aspects of the neuromuscular mechanisms involving cyclic jaw motions, and a modified reciprocal relationship was suggested.[41, 42] It was proposed that closing movements of the jaw are based on a stretch reflex mechanism involving muscle spindles in the jaw elevators (Fig. 3–7) and that reflex opening occurs as a result of inputs from intraoral pressure receptors of the periodontal membrane and soft tissues such as the palate (Fig. 3–7). However, it has also been reported that most of the signals from the periodontal membrane are transmitted to the sensory nuclei of the trigeminal nerve, and that responses in the mesencephalic

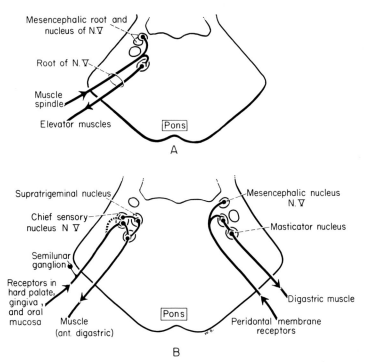

Figure 3–7. Representation of possible reflex paths for cyclic jaw movements. *A,* Jaw closing by activating stretch reflex. *B,* Jaw opening pathways (Jerge [40, 41]) involving interneuron in the sensory nucleus and/or supratrigeminal nucleus.

nucleus are presumably due to impulses from activity of jaw-closing muscles through slight jaw opening rather than impulses passing to the mesencephalic nucleus from pressoreceptors in the periodontal membrane.[55, 56] Even so, sensory impulses from the periodontal structures or oral mucous membranes, or both, have been considered to inhibit the activity of jaw closing muscles once the teeth are occluded and to activate jaw opening muscles. Such a reciprocal reflex relationship has been considered to be in the background of routine chewing movements of the jaw.[42] Recently it has been proposed that the inhibition or silent period in muscle activity following tooth contact may be due to stimulation of muscle spindles, and that periodontal receptors are not involved in any reflex system operating to maintain cyclic jaw movements during chewing.[27] The complex innervation of the masticatory system and the evidence that reciprocal innervation exists do not allow for final conclusions regarding the basis for cyclic movements. However, the evidence presented thus far suggests that both reciprocal innervation in the classical sense and the mechanism of reflex opening involving inputs from pressoreceptors of the periodontal membrane and soft tissues may be present in cyclic jaw movements.

Tongue Movements

As indicated previously (p. 41), the muscles of the tongue are innervated by the hypoglossal nerve. In addition, general sensations and taste are carried by the glossopharyngeal, vagus and facial (chorda tympanic branch) nerves. Sensations involving the tongue are important in the regulation of tongue movements. Although some controversy exists regarding the presence of muscle spindles in the tongue, it is likely that some type of muscle sense is present to account for the high degree of skilled tongue movements.[12, 13] It would appear essential for some type of feedback mechanism to be present, not only as a protective measure in swallowing and mastication, but also to influence masticatory movements. The coordination of tongue and jaw movements during mastication and other functions must be considered on the basis of some type of functional relationship between the mesencephalic nucleus of the trigeminal nerve and the hypoglossal nucleus. Whether this relationship is reciprocal is not clear; however, it has been indicated that there is a reciprocal inhibitory relationship between the tongue muscles and the jaw-closing muscles.[45] There can be no question that certain sensory mechanisms influence not only the masticator nucleus but also the swallowing, respiratory and vomiting centers. The patency of the air passage; the inhibition of respiration during swallowing; the positioning of the tongue during swallowing, jaw-opening and vomiting; and other coordinated activities point out the inhibitory and facilitory influences on the masticator, hypoglossal and other nuclei by sensory mechanisms and the necessity for the coordination and integration of various groups of muscles by some form of reciprocal functional relationship.

Summary

It has been indicated in this chapter that the relationship between the components of the masticatory system (including the neuromuscular components) is complex and to a certain degree unknown. Although Figure 3–8 is an oversimplification of the relationship, such a schematic representation is helpful for an understanding of dysfunctional disturbances of the masticatory system, including trauma from occlusion and bruxism.

Psychic stress can alter the myotatic reflex (stretch reflex) by influencing the function of proprioceptors (muscle spindles). Also, stimulation of exteroceptors in oral and facial structures can alter the stretch reflex. In these ways the tonicity of muscles and mandibular position can be influenced. Adverse alteration with hypertonicity of the masticatory muscles and restricted jaw movements are common features of dysfunctional disturbances of the temporomandibular joints.

The flexor or nociceptive reflex is protective in nature and is elicited by the application of noxious stimuli to exteroceptors in the oral tissues, including those in the periodontal membrane. In the presence of occlusal interferences and psychic stress, avoidance patterns of mandibular movement may occur as a protective response to bypass the interfering occlusal contacts. Such patterns of mandibular movement may not be compatible with harmonious muscle function and consequently lead to dysfunctional disturbances.

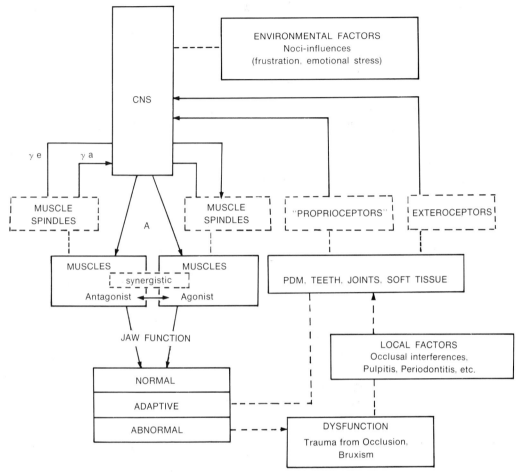

Figure 3–8. Schematic representation of the relationship of local and environmental factors to dysfunctional disturbances of the masticatory system. Normal, adaptive, and abnormal jaw function is represented as a function of the neuromuscular system involving the small motor system (γe, γa), the large motor system (A), proprioceptors and exteroceptors in the oral structures and temporomandibular joints, and the central nervous system (CNS) at all pertinent levels discussed in Chapters 2 and 3 (see text).

Fortunately there is a certain degree of tolerance in the masticatory system for less than an ideal occlusion and optimal psychic states. The tolerance is due in part to the adaptive capacity of several of the components of the system to change. For example, teeth may move as a result of traumatic occlusal forces to a more favorable location when possible; however, there appears to be little or no adaptive capacity of the adult temporomandibular joint for morphologic alteration to avoid trauma from occlusion.

If the adaptive capacity of the masticatory system has been exceeded, noci-influences from local and environmental sources tend to increase and augment the existing disharmony to a point at which the disturbance becomes self-perpetuating. Treatment is directed toward the reestablishment of harmony between the various components of the masticatory system.

REFERENCES

1. Ahlgren, J.: The silent period in the EMG of the jaw muscles during mastication and its relationship to tooth contact. Acta Odont. Scand., *27:*219, 1969.
2. Appelberg, B.: The effect of electrical stimulation of nucleus ruber on the gamma motor system. Acta physiol. scandinav., *55:*50, 1962.
3. Appelberg, B.: The effect of electrical stimulation in nucleus ruber on the response to stretch in primary and secondary muscle spindle afferents. Acta. physiol. scandinav., *56:*140, 1962.
4. Barker, D.: The structure and distribution of muscle receptors. *In* Barker, D. (ed.): Muscle Receptors. Hong Kong, Hong Kong University Press, 1962, pp. 227–240.
5. Beaudreau, D. E., and Daugherty, W. F.: Two types of motor pause in masticatory muscles. Am. J. Physiol., *216:*16, 1969.
6. Boyd, I. A.: The diameter and distribution of the nuclear bag and nuclear chain fibers in the muscle spindles of the cat. J. Physiol., *153:*23, 1960.
7. Boyd, I. A.: The motor innervation of mammalian muscle spindles. J. Physiol., *159:*7, 1961.
8. Brenman, H. S., Black, M. A., and Coslet, J. G.: Interrelationship between the electromyographic silent period and dental occlusion. J. Dent. Res., *47:*502, 1968.
9. Brodal, A.: Spasticity—anatomical aspects. Acta. neurol. scandinav., Suppl. 3, *38:*9, 1962.
10. Buchwald, J. S., and Eldred, E.: Activity in muscle spindle circuits during learning. *In* Barker, D. (ed.): Muscle Receptors. Hong Kong, Hong Kong University Press, 1962, pp. 175–183.
11. Carlsöö, S.: Motor units and action potentials in masticatory muscles. Acta morph. neerl.-scand., *2:*13, 1958.
12. Cooper, S.: Muscle spindles in the intrinsic muscles of the human tongue. J. Physiol. (London), *122:*193, 1953.
13. Cooper, S.: Afferent impulses in the hypoglossal nerve on stretching the cat's tongue. J. Physiol. (London), *126:*32, 1954.
14. Corbin, K. B., and Harrison, F.: Function of the mesencephalic root of the fifth cranial nerve. J. Neurophysiol., *3:*423, 1940.
15. Eccles, R. M., and Lundberg, A.: Synaptic actions of motoneurons by afferents which may evoke the flexon reflex. Arch. ital. biol., *97:*199, 1959.
16. Eliasson, S. G.: Central control of digestive function. *In* Field, J. (ed.): Handbook of Physiology, Section 1: Neurophysiology. Vol. 2. Washington, D. C., American Physiological Society, 1959, pp. 1163–1171.
17. Galambos, R., Sheatz, G., and Vernier, V.: Electrophysiological correlater of a conditioned response in cats. Science, *123:*376, 1956.
18. Granit, R.: Reflex self-regulation of muscle contraction and autogenetic inhibition. J. Neurophysiol., *13:*351, 1950.
19. Granit, R., and Strom, G.: Autogenetic modulation of excitability of single ventral horn cells. J. Neurophysiol., *14:*113, 1951.
20. Granit, R., Job, C., and Kaada, B. R.: Activation of muscle spindles in pinna reflex. Acta physiol. scand., *27:*161, 1952.
21. Granit, R., and Kaada, B. R.: Influence of stimulation of central nervous structures on muscle spindles in cat. Acta physiol. scand., *27:*130, 1952.
22. Granit, R.: Receptors and Sensory Perception. New Haven, Yale University Press, 1955.
23. Granit, R., and Holmgren, B.: Two pathways from brain stem to gamma ventral horn cells. Acta physiol. scandinav., *35:*93, 1955.
24. Green, J. D., and Arduini, A. A.: Hippocampal electrical activity in arousal. J. Neurophysiol., *17:*533, 1954.
25. Griffin, C., and Munro, R.: Electromyography of the jaw closing muscle in the opening-close-clench cycle in man. Archs oral Biol., *14:*141, 1969.
26. Hammond, P. H., Merton, P. A., and Sutton, G. G.: Nervous graduation of muscular contraction. Brit. Med. Bull., *12:*214, 1956.
27. Hannam, A. G., Matthews, B., and Yemm, R.: Receptors involved in the response of the masseter muscle to tooth contact in man. Archs oral Biol., *15:*17, 1970.
28. Hernández-Peón, R., Scherrer, H., and Jouvet, M.: Modification of electric activity in cochlear nucleus during "attention" in unanesthetized cats. Science, *123:*331, 1956.

29. Hoffmann, P.: Untersuchungen über die Eigenreflexe (Sehnenreflexe) Menschlicher Muskeln. Berlin, Springer, 1922.
30. Hongo, T., Shimazu, H., and Kubota, K.: A supraspinal inhibitory action on the gamma motor system. *In* Barker, D. (ed.): Muscle Receptors. Hong Kong, Hong Kong University Press, 1962, pp. 59–65.
31. Hongo, T., Kubota, K., and Shimazu, H.: EEG spindle and depression of gamma motor activity. J. Neurophysiol., *26:*568, 1963.
32. Houk, J. C.: A mathematical model of the stretch reflex in human muscle systems. M.S. thesis, Mass. Inst. Tech., 1963.
33. Houk, J., and Henneman, E.: Responses of Golgi tendon organs to active contractions of the soleus muscle of the cat. J. Neurophysiol: *30:*466, 1967.
34. Hunsperger, R. W.: Postural tonus and cardiac activity during centrally elicited affective reaction in the cat. Ann. N.Y. Acad. Sci., *159:*1013, 1969.
35. Hunt, C. C.: Diameter and function of afferent fibres from muscle. Montreal, Proceedings of the XIXth International Congress of Physiological Sciences, 1953.
36. Hunt, C. C., and Paintal, A. S.: Spinal reflex regulation of fusimotor neurons. J. Physiol., *143:*195, 1958.
37. Jansen, J., and Rudjerd, T.: On the silent period and Golgi tendon organs of the soleus muscle of the cat. Acta physiol. scand., *62:*364, 1964.
38. Jansen, J. K. S., and Matthews, P. B. C.: The central control of the dynamic response of muscle spindle receptors. J. Physiol. (London), *161:*357, 1962.
39. Jansen, J. K. S., and Matthews, P. B. C.: The effects of fusimotor activity on the static responsiveness of primary and secondary endings of muscle spindles in the decerebrate cat. Acta physiol. scand., *55:*376, 1962.
40. Jerge, C. R.: The function of the nucleus supratrigeminalis. J. Neurophysiol., *26:*393, 1963.
41. Jerge, C. R.: The neurologic mechanism underlying cyclic jaw movements. J. Prosth. Dent., *14:*667, 1964.
42. Kawamura, Y.: Neurophysiological background of occlusion. Periodontics, *5:*175, 1967.
43. Kawamura, Y. and Fujimoto, J.: Study of the jaw opening reflex. Med. J. Osaka Univ., *9:*377, 1958.
44. Kawamura, Y., Funakoshi, M., and Takata, M.: Reciprocal relationships in the brain stem among afferent impulses from each jaw muscle in the cat. Jap. J. Physiol., *10:*585, 1960.
45. Kawamura, Y.: Recent concepts of the physiology of mastication. *In* Staple, P. H. (ed.): Advances in Oral Biology. Vol. I. New York, Academic Press, 1964, pp. 77–109.
46. Kizior, J., Cuozzo, J., and Bowman, D.: Functional and histologic assessment of the sensory innervation of the periodontal ligament of the cat. J. Dent. Res., *47:*59, 1968.
47. Lewinsky, W., and Stewart, D.: The innervation of the periodontal membrane of the cat, with some observations on the function of the end organs found in that structure. J. Anat., *71:*232, 1936.
48. Livingston, R. B.: Some brain stem mechanisms relating to psychosomatic functions. Psychosom. Med., *17:*347, 1955.
49. Livingston, R. B., and Hernandez-Peón, R.: Somatic functions of the nervous system. Ann. Rev. Physiol., *17:*269, 1955.
50. Lloyd, D. P. C.: Neuron patterns controlling transmission of ipsilateral hind-limb reflexes in cat. J. Neurophysiol., *6:*293, 1943.
51. Magnus, O., Penfield, W., and Jasper, H.: Mastication and consciousness in epileptic seizures. Acta psychiat. et neurl. scandinav., *27:*91, 1952.
52. Magoun, H. W., and Rhines, R.: Spasticity: The stretch reflex and extrapyramidal systems. *In* Pitts, R. F. (ed.): American Lectures in Physiology. Springfield, Ill., Charles C Thomas, 1947.
53. Matthews, B., and Yemm, R.: A silent period in the masseter electromyogram following tooth contact in subjects wearing full dentures. Archs oral Biol., *15:*531, 1970.
54. Matthews, B. H. C.: Nerve endings in mammalian muscle. J. Physiol., *78:*1, 1933.
55. Matthews, P. B. C.: Muscle spindles and their motor control. Physiol. Rev., *44:*219, 1964.
56. Merton, P. A.: The silent period in a muscle of the human hand. J. Physiol., *114:*183, 1951.
57. Milhorn, H. T.: The Application of Control Theory to Physiological Systems. Philadelphia, W. B. Saunders Co., 1966.
58. Monnier, M.: Physiologie du tronc cérébral. Le rôle du système réticulaire dans l'organization de la motricité extra-pyramidale. Ergebn. Physiol. *45:*321, 1944.

59. Mortimer, E. M., and Akert, K.: Cortical control and representation of fusimotor neurons. Am. J. Phys. Med., *40*:228, 1961.
60. Ramfjord, S. P.: Bruxism, a clinical and electromyographic study. J. Am. Dent. A., *62*:35, 1961.
61. Ramfjord, S. P.: Dysfunctional temporomandibular joint and muscle pain. J. Prosth. Dent., *11*:353, 1961.
62. Ruch, T. C., Patton, H. D., Woodbury, J. W., and Towe, A. L.: Neurophysiology. Philadelphia, W. B. Saunders Co., 1961.
63. Schaerer, P., Stallard, R. E., and Zander, H. A.: Occlusal interferences and mastication: an electromyographic study. J. Prosth. Dent., *17*:438, 1967.
64. Schärer, P., and Pfyffer, G.: Comparison of habitual and cerebrally stimulated jaw movements in the rabbit. Helv. Odont. Acta, *14*:6, 1970.
65. Sherrington, C. S.: The Integrative Action of the Nervous System. New York, Charles Scribner's Sons, 1906.
66. Sherrington, C. S.: Reflexes elicitable in the cat from pinna vibrissae and jaws. J. Physiol. (Lond.), *51*:404, 1917.
67. Shimazu, H., Hongo, T., and Kubota, K.: Two types of central influences on gamma motor system. J. Neurophysiol., *25*:309, 1962.
68. Stern, J., and Ward, A.: Inhibition of muscle spindle discharge by ventrolateral thalamic stimulation. Arch. Neurol., *3*:193, Aug., 1960.
69. Storey, A. T.: Physiology of a changing vertical dimension. J. Prosth. Dent., *12*:912, 1962.
70. Szentagothai, J.: Anatomical considerations of monosynaptic reflex arcs. J. Neurophysiol., *11*:445, 1948.
71. Winton, F. R., and Bayliss, L. E.: Human Physiology. 5th ed. Boston, Little, Brown and Co., 1962.

CHAPTER 4

PHYSIOLOGY OF OCCLUSION

Although there is general consensus concerning the anatomy and cellular morphology of the masticatory system, the physiology and the functional relationships of the various parts are still controversial in spite of recent research with complex tools and new methods.

"Occlusion," by dictionary definition, refers to the act of closure or being closed. In dentistry the word "occlusion" includes both closure of the dental arches and the various functional movements with maxillary and mandibular teeth making contact. Furthermore, "occlusion" is used to designate the anatomic alignment of the teeth and their relationship to the rest of the masticatory system.

Until recently two main concepts of occlusion have been taught in dental schools and used as a basis for the practice of dentistry. One is the prosthetic concept of balanced occlusion for complete dentures whereby functional stability and effectiveness are enhanced by bilateral tooth contacts in lateral and protrusive excursions. The other concept is orthodontically oriented in that certain acceptable static cusp and fossa relationships are emphasized; an occlusion that does not conform to this relationship is designated as malocclusion. Until fairly recently the analysis of the occlusion of the natural dentition has to a great extent been based upon these two concepts and criteria. It is also apparent that a large number of persons have received extensive "oral rehabilitation" and orthodontic treatment for no other reason than that their occlusion did not conform to these standards. During the last 10 to 20 years a third concept of a dynamic individual occlusion has emerged wherein the criteria for diagnosis of occlusion and the need for treatment have been based upon an evaluation of the health and function of each individual's masticatory system.

It has become increasingly evident that the previously alleged close relationship between form and function of the dentition is not dependent upon the common standards such as over-bite and cusp-fossa relationships. The appearance of the occlusion is not much more related to function than the external appearance of the nose is to breathing. Function and esthetic criteria should be considered separately.

GUIDANCE OF OCCLUSION

Certain terms that relate occlusion to the practice of dentistry have to be defined and explained before the function of the masticatory system can be discussed in detail.

Supporting Cusps. These are the lingual cusps of the maxillary molars and bicuspids and the buccal cusps of the mandibular molars and bicuspids (Fig. 4–1). The incisal edges of the mandibular anterior teeth are usually included in this designation. In the normal adult dentition the supporting cusps maintain centric stop contacts with the opposing fossae and interproximal embrasures and determine the occlusal vertical dimension of the face. The areas of contact of the supporting cusps with the opposing teeth in maximal closure should be well established and stable. These contact areas, which are called *centric stops*, have no rigidly set relationships for normal occlusion except occlusal stability. Such stability should be maintained by axially directed forces which are the resultants of the forces applied to the centric stops.

Guiding Inclines. These are the bucco-occlusal inclines (the lingual inclines of the buccal cusps) of the maxillary posterior teeth (Fig. 4–2), the lingual inclines of the maxillary anterior teeth, and the linguo-occlusal inclines (buccal inclines of the lingual cusp) of the mandibular posterior teeth. The guiding inclines are the planes and occlusal ridges that determine the path of the supporting cusp during normal lateral and protrusive working excursions.

Incisal Guidance. This term refers to the influence on mandibular movements of the lingual surfaces of the maxillary anterior teeth. The incisal guidance may be expressed in degrees with the horizontal plane.

Cusp Angle. This is the angle made by the slopes of a cusp with a plane that passes through the tip of the cusp and is perpendicular to a line bisecting the cusp.

Curve of Spee. This term refers to the curvature of the occlusal surfaces of teeth from the tip of the mandibular cuspid and following the buccal cusps of the mandibular posterior teeth (called the compensating curve for dentures).

Plane of Occlusion. This is an imaginary plane that touches the incisal edges of the central mandibular incisors and the tip of the disto-buccal cusps of the second mandibular molars.

Condylar Guidance. This term refers to the path that the horizontal rotation axis of the condyles travels during normal mandibular opening. It can be measured in degrees as related to the Frankfort (orbitale to tragion) plane.

The relationship between these various factors related to occlusion or articulation has been classically expressed in Hanau's quint or Thielemann's formula or principle, which states that balanced occlusion is equal to the product of condylar guidance and incisal guidance divided by the product of the cusp

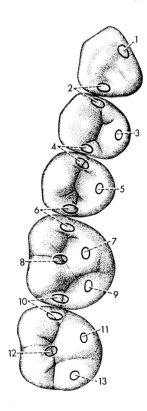

Figure 4-1. Location of centric stops. The supporting cusps include the lingual cusps of the maxillary molars and premolars and the buccal cusps of the mandibular molars and premolars. The relationship of centric stops to the occlusal surfaces is not rigidly set and may vary considerably from one individual to another. The cusp, fossa, and ridge relationship between the maxillary and mandibular teeth is indicated by like numbers. Such relationships are usually considered as pertaining to a "normal" occlusion; however, occlusal stability is of greater importance than rigidly set relationships for normal occlusion.

Very seldom, if ever, will all contact areas conform to this schematic "ideal." The centric stops are often in the central fossa, related to the inner surface of the marginal ridges rather than to the embrasure surfaces of the ridges as indicated in the illustration.

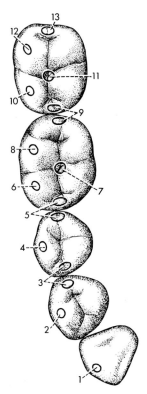

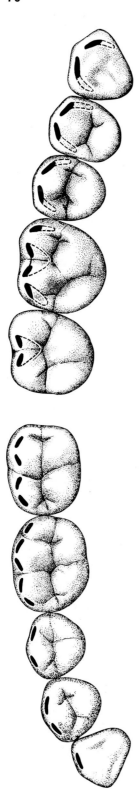

Figure 4–2. Location of occlusal contacts in working relation and guiding inclines. The guiding inclines include the lingual inclines of the buccal cusps of the maxillary posterior teeth and the lingual inclines of the maxillary anterior teeth. Also included, but not illustrated, are the buccal inclines of the lingual cusps of the mandibular posterior teeth.

angle, curve of Spee, and the plane of occlusion. Except for condylar guidance, all these factors may be altered by prosthetic dentistry and orthodontic therapy; however, only cusp angle and incisal guidance can be appreciably changed by occlusal adjustment. There does not seem to be a correlation in the natural dentition between condylar guidance and incisal guidance, and this formula is of limited value for analysis and adjustment of the natural dentition where balanced occlusion is not even an objective.

KINESIOLOGY OF OCCLUSION

Kinesiology describes the movements of body parts on the basis of anatomy, physiology and mechanics. The kinesiology of the mandible related to the maxilla during function is extremely complex since it commonly involves a combination of movements in the sagittal, frontal and horizontal planes.

Many attempts have been made to explain jaw movements in simple terms since the classical works of Bonwill, Bennett, and Gysi on mandibular kinesiology. However, the complexity of the mechanical and neuromuscular principles involved in the various jaw movements defies all attempts at simple descriptions or explanations.

Mandibular movements have been studied by a number of techniques, such as clinical and anatomic observations, engraving and graphic methods, roentgenographic and other photographic methods, check bite registration, recording of facet patterns on the teeth and, in recent times, by electromyography and telemetry (radio transmitters built into bridgework). These studies have been concerned with the movement patterns of both the teeth and the rest of the mandible, including the temporomandibular joints.

In order to simplify the description of mandibular kinesiology it will be discussed relative to the sagittal plane first, then to the horizontal and the frontal planes.

Border Movements and Positions of the Mandible Related to the Sagittal Plane

When the various parts of the mandible are projected perpendicular to the median or sagittal plane during movements a characteristic pattern can be registered, for example, for the incisive point between the incisal edges of the two mandibular central incisors and similarly for the condyles and the other parts of the mandible. Since Posselt[73] showed that border movements of the mandible are reproducible, and all other movements take place within the framework of the border movements, it appears logical to start the description of mandibular movements with border movements. The border movements of the mandible recorded in the sagittal plane are shown in Figure 4–3.

If the mandible is held back either by the patient or by the operator, a hinge movement can be traced for the lower incisors from CR to B (a distance of 3/4 to 1 inch). The axis (point C) for this movement is stationary and usually within

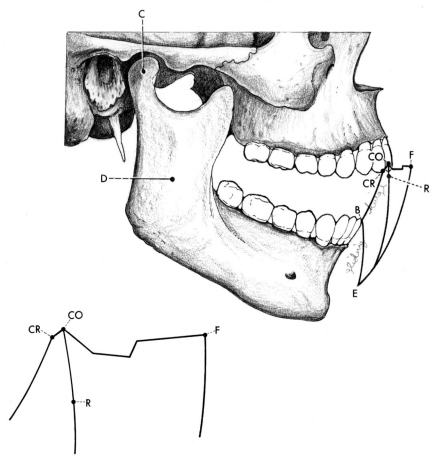

Figure 4–3. Border movements of the mandible recorded in a sagittal plane (see text).

the condyles. In this movement, called the terminal hinge movement of the mandible, the rotation axis through the two temporomandibular joints is stationary. This is also called *centric relation, terminal hinge position* or *retruded contact position*. Since this position or path is determined by the ligaments and structures of the temporomandibular joints it has also been called the *ligamentous position*. This position denotes the posterior functional range of the mandible and has been defined as the most retruded position of the mandible from which opening and lateral movements can be performed comfortably. Under normal physiologic conditions of the masticatory system, this center of rotation and the path of mandibular movements are constant and reproducible. However, in order for these to be constant and reproducible the condyles have to be seated against the meniscus in the bottom of the glenoid fossa; this is predicated upon normal function of the ligaments and the jaw muscles. The functional significance of centric relation will be discussed later (p. 95).

If an attempt is made to open the jaw in a retrusive path below B (Fig. 4–3), the movement changes character and the axis of rotation is then at D (slightly behind the mandibular foramen) and the condyle moves down and forward while the incisive point moves down to E. There is, of course, still rotation around the intercondylar axis combined with the down and forward movement of this axis. Closure with the jaw in a forward or protrusive position will follow the path E to F while the condyle is placed on the articular tuberculum. When the posterior teeth make contact, the protrusive closure stops at F. The path from F to CO (while the teeth are making contact) is determined by the occlusal relationship of the teeth in both arches. *centric occlusion*

The position CO (Fig. 4–3) is determined by maximum intercuspidation of the teeth and is usually called *centric occlusion*. It is also called *intercuspal position, tooth position, acquired centric* and *habitual centric*. This is the vertical and horizontal position of the mandible in which the cusps of the mandibular and maxillary teeth interdigitate maximally. This position is a tooth-to-tooth determined relationship of the jaws guided by the relation of the occlusal surfaces of the teeth. The position is subject to change by alterations of the occlusal surfaces. Ideally, in centric occlusion the lingual cusps of the maxillary bicuspids make contact with the marginal ridges of the mandibular bicuspids and the marginal ridges of the second bicuspid and first molar (Fig. 4–1). The mesial lingual cusps of the maxillary molars occlude in the central fossae of the mandibular molars, while the distal lingual cusps of the maxillary molars occlude on the marginal ridges of the mandibular molars. Similarly, the supporting cusps of the mandibular teeth occlude on the marginal ridges and fossae of the maxillary molars and bicuspids.

Between CR and CO there is a short movement path that can be recorded by bringing the teeth in contact in centric relation (CR) and having the patient squeeze his jaws together into centric occlusion (CO) (Fig. 4–3). This movement is called *slide in centric* or *excentric slide*, dependent on how the word *centric* is applied. The slide is often a combination of forward and lateral movements. Measurements referring to this slide are not directly comparable since different landmarks have been used to obtain the measurements. However, the average distance for the slide in adults[10, 30, 73] and in children[45] seems to be about 1 mm, with greater variance in adults than in children.

If a person sits or stands with his mandible in rest position R (Fig. 4–3) and is asked to open his jaw, the incisor point will follow the path from R to E, and the condyle will move forward and down with a center of rotation close to D. If he is asked to tap his teeth into light initial contact from R, he will hit somewhere close to CO (centric occlusion), but the initial contact will depend on posture. Since this initial contact from rest position is to some extent dependent on muscle balance (but is, of course, also influenced by "muscle memory" of occlusal contacts), it has been called muscular position[22] or *centric position*. It has been assumed incorrectly that this centric position could be recorded by recording of rest position and closure in an articulator around a hinge axis in the temporomandibular joint region. However, cephalometric studies by Nevakari[61] often showed a translatory movement of the mandible in such closure with an imaginary hinge axis in the mastoid region.

A fourth "centric" or *power centric* has been recorded by Boos[14, 15] and

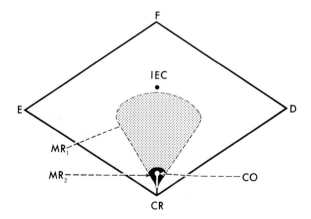

Figure 4–4. Border movements of the mandible recorded in the horizontal plane. The incisal point is at *CR* when the condyles are in centric relation, and at point *CO* when the teeth are in centric occlusion. The small dark area MR$_2$ is the approximate region of function during the latter stages of mastication. The larger stippled area MR$_1$ extending to IEC (incisal edge contact) is the approximate region of function in earlier stages of mastication.

Page [81] by having the patient close against force and determining the position of the mandible in which the patient can bite the hardest. This position again does not necessarily correspond to any of the three previously defined "centrics," since it is based on a different premise.

Border Movements and Positions of the Mandible Recorded in the Horizontal Plane

Similarly to recordings in the sagittal plane, one can project mandibular movement perpendicular to the horizontal plane (Fig. 4–4). The border movements for the incisor point can be traced by a gothic arch or Gysi[37] tracing in the horizontal plane (CR, D, E, F). Such a figure can be recorded at various degrees of opening. With the mandible in the stationary hinge position or centric relation, point CR corresponds to centric relation (also called the arrow point[73] in Gysi's tracing). As the mandible moves in retrusive lateral excursions and the condyle

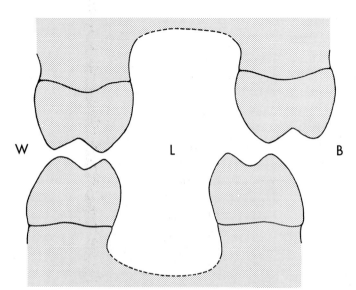

Figure 4–5. Mandible in right lateral excursion showing working (W) side and balancing (B) side as viewed from the frontal plane. The lingual cusp (L) of the left maxillary first molar is opposite the buccal cusp of the left mandibular molar on the balancing side. On the working side the maxillary buccal cusps oppose the mandibular buccal cusps.

moves from C to B, the incisal point records the line from CR to D. From D the mandible can be moved forward and medially to point F. A similar tracing can be done for the other side to point E from point CR.

When the mandible is moved, for example, to the right side so that the mandibular buccal cusps oppose the maxillary buccal cusps and inclines, the right side is called the *"working"* or the *functioning side* (Fig. 4–5). At the same time, the relationship of the mandibular buccal cusps and inclines to the maxillary lingual cusps and inclines on the left side of the arch is called the *"balancing"* or the *nonfunctioning side* (Fig. 4–5). The converse is true when the mandible is moved to the left side. These terms have been transferred from full denture terminology to occlusion of natural teeth and they are used without consideration to actual working and balancing functional contacts.

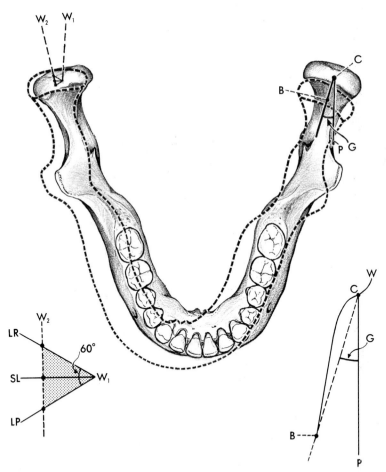

Figure 4–6. Right lateral movement of the mandible viewed from above (horizontal plane). The condyle, during a side shift on the working side, may move straight outward laterally (SL), lateral and protrusively (LP), or lateral and retrusively (LR) from W_1 to W_2. In effect the condyle may move to any point within the borders of the 60° triangle shown in the horizontal plane. On the balancing side the condyle may move from C to point B. The angle (G) made by the sagittal plane and a line drawn from point C to point B is called the Bennett angle. Bilateral straight forward movement of the condyles (C-P) is protrusive. The curved line (C-B) is the type of path made by the balancing condyle as recorded by the pantograph.

The lateral shift of the mandible, called Bennett movement, is measured by the distance that the condyle on the working side moves from W_1 to W_2 (Fig. 4–6). The opposing or balancing condyle (B) moves down, forward and inward and makes an angle (G) with the median plane when projected perpendicularly on the horizontal plane. This angle (G) is called the Bennett angle. The lateral movement may have immediate as well as progressive components. On the working side the rotating condyle (Fig. 4–6) may move from W_1 to W_2 laterally up to approximately 3 mm.[35] The lateral movement may have a retrusive (LR) or protrusive (LP) component or move straight laterally (SL) as shown in Figure 4–6. The movement may end at any point in the 60° triangle. Viewed from the frontal plane the rotating condyle may move laterally or outward only, laterally and superiorly (upward), or laterally and inferiorly (downward). The envelope of these possible movements is analogous to a right circular cone (Fig. 4–7) with the vertex at W_1. Sagittal displacement of the rotating condyle may occur from W_1 to any point within the cone. On the balancing side the orbiting condyle usually does not follow a straight line from C to B, but rather some form of curved path as indicated in the pantographic tracing (Fig. 4–6). Sagittal movements and occlusal morphology are related to the principles of restorative dentistry. These movements influence the placement and height of cusps and the orientation of ridges and grooves in restorations.

The guidance of the teeth is eliminated by the temporary raising of the bite level in Gothic arch tracings of the natural dentition, and the movements represented in the tracing express the temporomandibular joint and muscle potential for border movements rather than a recording of functional movements.

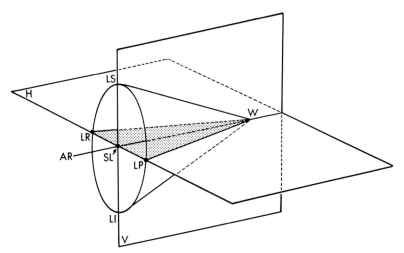

Figure 4-7. Schematic representation of the condylar shift on the working side. Movements up to approximately 3 mm. may occur to any point within the 60° circular cone. Line AR represents the center of rotation of the condyle. Viewed from the horizontal plane (H), the movement from W may be straight lateral (SL), lateral and protrusive (LP), or lateral and retrusive (LR). Viewed in the vertical plane (V), the movement from W may be straight lateral, lateral and inferior (LI), or lateral and superior (LS).

Border Movements and Positions of the Mandible in the Frontal Plane

Although most descriptions of mandibular movements are projected to the median or sagittal and the horizontal planes, projections into the frontal plane have to be considered in order to complete the picture of mandibular movements. Lateral masticatory function and bruxism have patterns that are recorded in a more meaningful way in the frontal than in the other planes. The patterns of jaw movements recorded in the frontal plane vary greatly with the type of occlusal contact relations.[4, 57] With excellent occlusions and with uninhibited masticatory movements, as seen in Australian aborigines, the masticatory cycle has a fairly uniform, wide oval form;[10] the cycle is wider and more regular than that found in subjects of European origin.[4, 41] The mean range of contact gliding from lateral to the intercuspal position during mastication has been found to be 2.8 mm. at the incisors for Australian aborigines,[10] but only half that amount or less for modern man. The return or opening part of the chewing cycle from centric occlusion is very irregular according to most investigators, and may even revert close to the path of the closing stroke. Most common in persons with unrestricted freedom of occlusal contact movements is a smooth, uncrossed path of movements that return very closely to the same closed position for every chewing stroke[10, 56] (Fig. 4–8). Occlusal contact during mastication occurs almost invariably in centric occlusion, but in most cycles there are occlusal contacts for part of the closing movement, and occasionally even in the opening movement.[10]

Mandibular Movements and Occlusal Morphology

For all aspects of dentistry it is necessary to understand the relationship between the patterns of mandibular movements and occlusal form. Although cusps, fossae, grooves, and ridges should be compatible with functional and parafunctional mandibular movements, the concept of an ideal occlusion (p. 104) does not suggest that the absence of a specified relationship in the natural dentition can or must be corrected by the reconstruction of an entire occlusion. However, in required restorative procedures involving one or more teeth one

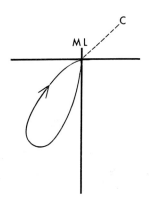

Figure 4–8. Jaw movement in function recorded at the midline (ML) of the mandible. In individuals with unrestricted movements, the incisal point of the mandible makes a record in the frontal plane similar to that shown.

does not knowingly contribute to, predispose to, or treat dysfunctional disturbances by ignoring the relationship between occlusion and mandibular movements. Thus, functional occlusion should be anticipated for indicated restorations on the basis of mandibular movements that have been determined to the degree necessary or possible for an individual patient. At the present time there is no acceptable way to determine functional or parafunctional movements, or both, of the mandible that can relate completely the relationship between these movements and occlusion.

The intercondylar distance influences the position and direction for placement of ridges and grooves (Fig. 4–9). The greater the intercondyle distance, the more distal is the placement of the ridges and balancing (idling) grooves on the mandibular teeth, and the more mesial is the placement on the maxillary teeth. Also, the greater the intercondylar distance, the greater must be the lingual concavity of the maxillary teeth. Related is the influence of the distance of the teeth from the center of rotation and from the midsagittal plane: the greater the distance of the teeth from the midsagittal plane or from the center of rotation, the greater is the angle between the working and balancing grooves.

The relationship between the medial aspect of the glenoid fossa, Bennett movement (side shift), and occlusal morphology is shown in the horizontal plane in Figure 4–10. The greater the Bennett movement, the more mesial

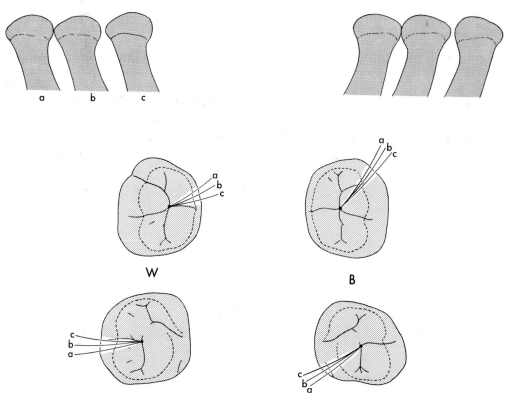

Figure 4–9. Effect of intercondylar distance on position and direction of placement of ridges and grooves.

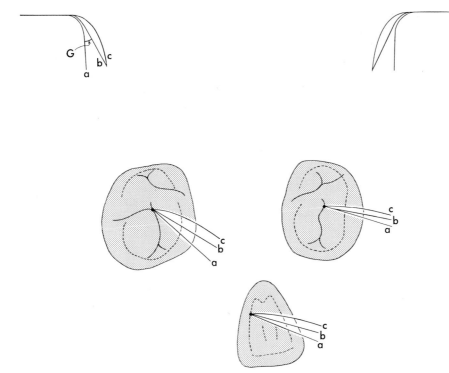

Figure 4–10. Relationship of medial aspect of glenoid fossa, side shift, and occlusal morphology (horizontal plane).

must be the directional placement of the ridges and grooves on the mandibular teeth, and the more distal must be the placement on the maxillary teeth. Also, the greater the side shift, the shorter the cusps must be relative to fossa depth, and the greater the lingual concavity should be of the anterior maxillary teeth.

The influence of the lateral lip of the posterior wall and side shift of the rotating condyle in determining functional occlusion in restorations is shown for the horizontal plane in Figure 4–11. When the condyle on the working side (rotating condyle) moves laterally and posteriorly, the ridge and groove direction must be placed more toward the mesial on the mandibular teeth and more toward the distal on the maxillary teeth than otherwise would be the case if the movement was straight lateral. When the rotating condyle moves laterally and anteriorly, the ridge and groove direction must be placed toward the distal on the mandibular teeth and more toward the mesial on the maxillary teeth. A greater concavity of the lingual aspect of the maxillary anterior teeth is required when the effective movement is both outward and forward than when the movement is outward and backward.

The influence of the superior contour of the glenoid fossa on the rotating condyle and its relationship to occlusal morphology is shown in the vertical plane in Figure 4–12. The condyle may move laterally and superiorly, straight laterally, or laterally and inferiorly. These outward as well as backward or forward movements (viewed in the horizontal plane) can be logically combined,

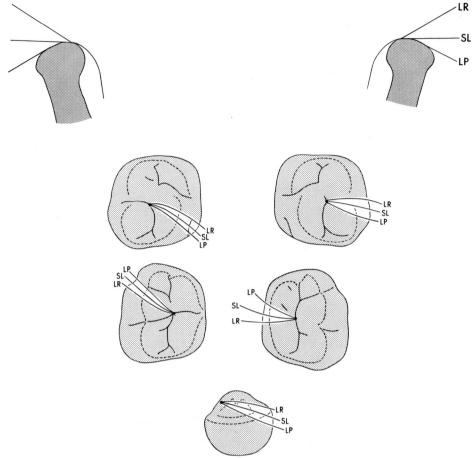

Figure 4–11. Effect of posterior wall of glenoid fossa and side shift on determining occlusal morphology in restorations (horizontal plane).

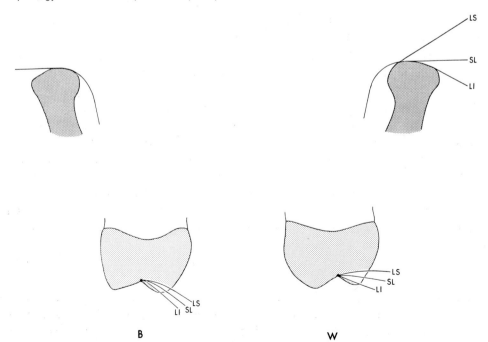

B   W

Figure 4–12. Influence of superior contour of the glenoid fossa on the rotating condyle (working side) in relationship to determining occlusal characteristics (vertical plane).

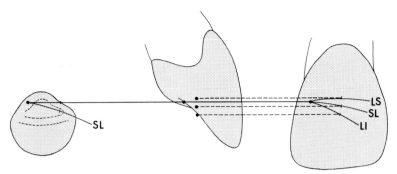

Figure 4–13. Relationship of side shift of the condyle to the lingual concavity of the maxillary anterior teeth. Lateral superior (LS), straight lateral (SL); lateral inferior (LI).

giving rise to a large number of possible movements within the geometric borders of a right circular cone. However, considering only the direction of the rotating condyle in the vertical plane, if the movement is lateral and inferior (outward and downward), the heights of the cusps relative to fossa depth can be made greater than if the movement were straight lateral (outward only). If the movement is outward and upward, the height of the cusps of a restoration have to be less than when the movement of the rotating condyle is outward. The lingual concavity of the maxillary anterior teeth must be greater when the movement is outward and upward (Fig. 4–13) than when the movement is straight lateral (outward only) or lateral and inferior (outward and downward).

Considering occlusal morphology in the vertical plane and Bennett movement only, the importance of the relationship of cusp height and depth of fossa is illustrated in Figure 4–14. The greater the side shift, the shorter the cusps

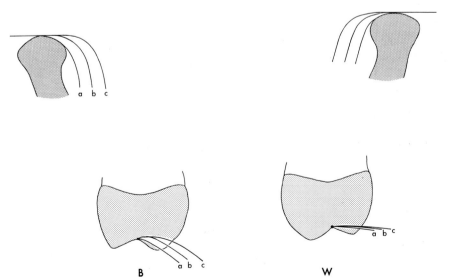

Figure 4–14. Influence of condylar side shift in determining functional occlusion (vertical plane).

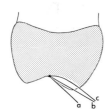

Figure 4–15. Influence of condylar shift in determining functional occlusion. Letter *a* indicates the absence of a side shift; *b* indicates a linear side shift such as is incorporated in a semi-adjustable articulator; *c* indicates immediate and progressive side shift. Failure to anticipate adequately the side shift can result in significant occlusal interferences.

must be made to prevent interferences. Although not readily apparent from Figure 4–14, the greater the side shift, the greater the lingual concavity must be in restorations of the maxillary anterior teeth.

The effect on determining occlusal morphology relative to the side shift as viewed in the vertical plane is shown in Figure 4–15. If an average (line b with no immediate side shift) or no shift (line a) is considered to be present when one in fact is present (line c), significant occlusal interference may be incorporated in the restoration. Other factors to be considered that relate to cusp height are the angle of the eminentia, curve of Spee, occlusal plane, and the overlap of the maxillary anterior teeth. These factors are additional to those involving the direction and magnitude of the side shift of the mandible, or direction of the rotating condyle.

As the angle of the eminentia increases, the posterior part of the mandible moves with increasing rapidity away from the maxillary teeth. Thus, the greater the angle, the longer the cusps of restorations of posterior teeth can be made. With maxillary anterior restorations the lingual concavity needed decreases as the angle of the eminentia increases.

In the natural dentition (excluding complete dentures) an important goal is to make sure that contacts between opposing posterior teeth or restorations are not made in straight protrusive movements of the mandible. In protrusive movements the relationship of the occlusal plane to the angle of the eminentia is important to cusp height relative to the depth of the fossae. The greater the divergence between the angle of the plane of occlusion and the angle of the eminentia, the shorter the cusps should be made in posterior restorations. In effect, the closer the plane of occlusion and the path of the condyle are to being parallel, the shorter the cusps of restorations must be made to prevent posterior contact in protrusive movement.

The relationship between the curve of Spee and the angle of the eminentia (Fig. 4–16) is associated also with posterior contact of the teeth in protrusive movement. Considering that the angle of the eminentia is constant and that the plane of occlusion will be held constant, the shorter the radius of the curve of Spee, the shorter the posterior cusps have to be made to prevent contact in protrusive movement. The relationship between the angle of the plane of occlusion and the radius curve of Spee is clear: the more nearly the plane of occlusion is parallel to the path of the condyle in protrusive movement of the mandible, the greater the effect that the curve of Spee has on cusp height. The greater the divergence anteriorly from a parallel relationship, the less influence a smaller radius of the curve of Spee would have on dictating that the cusp height be shorter.

In a straight protrusive movement of the mandible the degree of horizontal and vertical overlap, as well as the inclination of the maxillary anterior teeth, is related to requirements of cusp height for posterior teeth. The greater the horizontal overlap of the maxillary teeth, the shorter the cusps are required to be to prevent posterior contact. Assuming reasonable coronal morphology of the maxillary incisors, the greater the labial inclination of the maxillary anterior teeth the shorter the heights of the cusps of posterior restoration must be made. In relation to vertical overlap, the smaller the overlap, the shorter the cusps of posterior teeth must be made.

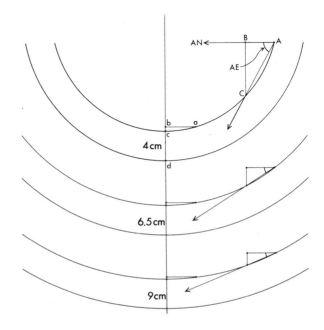

Figure 4–16. Relationship between the curve of Spee and the angle of the eminentia. If the angle of the cusps is not considered and the distance from c to d is considered to be the lower arch, it is necessary for the lower arch with a curve of Spee of radii 4, 6.5, and 9 cm. to move downward the distance B to C in order to move anteriorly (AN) from A to B. Considering the arch to be less of an arc, the lower arch must move downward the distance of b to c in order to move protrusively and avoid posterior contacts. As the radii of the curves of Spee diminish, the greater the angle of the eminentia becomes. Since in reality the angle of the eminentia (AE) is constant, the height of cusps must be made less as the radius of the curve of Spee decreases.

FUNCTIONAL MOVEMENTS OF THE MANDIBLE

Mastication and Occlusion

Patterns for masticatory movements are developed at the time of eruption of the primary teeth. An infant first acquires the sense of position of the teeth as soon as the maxillary and mandibular incisors erupt and contact of the teeth occurs. The mandibular position that is required for the mandibular and maxillary teeth to touch is learned and then contact movements are initiated. The first movements are poorly coordinated, like those of initial walking. Later, conditioned reflex patterns are established guided by the proprioception in the periodontal membrane and temporomandibular joints as well as by sense of touch in tongue and mucosa. As more teeth erupt into functional positions, the movement patterns are modified to conform to the general principle of maximum efficiency with minimum expansion of energy and avoidance of pain or discomfort. A person's individual movement pattern of the mandible is based upon coordination of the previously listed factors governing functional jaw movements (condylar guidance, incisal guidance, plane of occlusion, curve of Spee and cusp angles). This pattern is developed in a way similar to that of the characteristic individual gait of walking.

Movement patterns of the mandible and the tongue as well as the occlusion of the teeth are interdependent. Although the act of mastication is a highly complex neuromuscular activity that is based on conditioned reflexes, the complex organization of mastication cannot be considered as a cascade or chain of reflexes or devoid of guiding influences from the occlusion. It is quite likely that internal motor mechanisms cause the appropriate muscles to contract, and proper guidance near centric occlusion depends upon past and present responses related to tooth contacts and receptors in the periodontal membrane and other areas. With ideal contact relationships there is a well synchronized and integrated contraction pattern of activity of the masticatory muscles.

There has been considerable controversy with regard to actual tooth contacts and movement patterns during mastication of food. Some investigators have on the basis of cinefluoroscopy maintained that few, if any, occlusal contacts occur during chewing,[46] but that occlusal contacts do occur during deglutition. However, recent evidence derived from studies using telemetry systems (radio transmitters)[2] and electric circuits to inlays[5] has established that actual tooth contact takes place regularly in centric occlusion as well as lateral and protrusive to this position in mastication of average foods. Depending upon the type of food being masticated, the duration of occlusal contacts in centric occlusion increases and decreases during the chewing cycle probably in relationship to the power required for comminution and to the size of the particles. The frequency of contacts increases in centric occlusion and lateral positions as the food is broken into progressively smaller particles.

The interdigitation of the teeth in lateral excursion on the working side is guided by the buccal aspects of the supporting buccal cusps of the mandibular teeth contacting the slopes of the lingual aspects of the buccal cusps of the maxillary teeth (Fig. 4–2). Since there are both mesial and distal slopes involving these cusps, the occlusal contacts in working excursions may be between the mesial and distal slopes of the buccal maxillary cusps and the mesial and distal slopes of the buccal surfaces of the supporting buccal mandibular cusps. The lingual maxillary cusps have similar working relationships to the buccal inclines of the mandibular lingual cusps. Such contact relationship may not necessarily be present for all of the teeth on the working side to have a normal function. The extent of lateral functional contacts out from centric occlusion is dependent upon convenience (absence of restrictive occlusal interferences) and type of food to be masticated.

Balancing side contacts may be made along the surfaces of the buccal inclines of the maxillary lingual cusps (including these cusp tips in wide excursion) and the lingual inclines of the buccal mandibular cusps (including these cusps in wide excursions). These contact relationships again involve mesially and distally directed inclines extending to the embrasures and include the ridges and fossae between the cusps of molars (Fig. 4–17).

Recently, extensive studies made of the jaw movements, contact patterns and occlusal facets of aboriginal Australians indicate that after heavy functional wear, the teeth on the balancing side do not make contact during mastication.[10] However, if the wear has been produced mainly by bruxism, the contacting wear facets on the balancing side often interfere with masticatory movements to the other side.

Bilateral Mastication. Multidirectional, alternating bilateral mastication is ideal for stimulation of the entire supporting structures, for stability of occlusion and for cleansing of the teeth.[9] It also has been observed by clinical studies[9] and combined clinical and electromyographic studies[74] that bilateral function is assumed whenever a convenient unrestricted bilateral occlusal relationship has been provided with equal bilateral cuspal guidance and functional capacity. Although mastication may be accomplished satisfactorily with unilateral, or even no lateral movements, this accomplishment does not constitute ideal occlusal function.

Unilateral Mastication. Habitual unilateral or protrusive preference patterns of mastication are often the result of adaptation to occlusal interferences.* Such patterns are commonly seen in persons who have been living on soft nonabrasive foods or whose normal occlusal pattern has been disturbed by dental and periodontal irregularities or disease. In persons with occlusal interferences the initial asynchronous muscle action may indicate inhibited reflex action by the untimely and disorganized excitation of receptors in the periodontal membrane. Later, the nerve centers may succeed in establishing a compromise pattern of masticatory movements which will inflict minimal or no irritation upon the involved tissues. Such patients may then show good muscle coordination and no temporomandibular joint and muscle disturbances, but disturbances may arise when an attempt is made to masticate away from this preference pattern because of the occlusal interferences. Such disturbances,

---

*Occlusal interferences are occlusal contacts hampering or hindering smooth, gliding, harmonious jaw movements with the teeth maintaining contact.

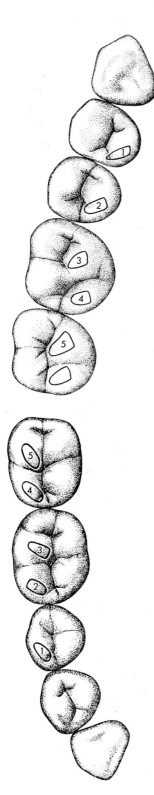

Figure 4–17. Occlusal contacts in balancing relation. The relationship of the mandibular cusps and inclines to the maxillary lingual cusps and inclines on the side of the arches opposite to working relation (Fig. 4–2) is referred to as the "balancing" side. Contact relations are indicated by like numbers. Balancing side contacts are not necessary in the natural dentition. Unless such contacts are light, they frequently are balancing interferences.

however, are usually minimal unless a severe balancing side interference is present.

A unilateral restricted pattern of mastication may also be the result of a splinting or protective action of the jaw muscles in patients with temporomandibular joint disturbances. If a sufficient number of teeth are present, such patients prefer to chew on the side of the painful joint since there is more pressure on the balancing side condyle than on the working side condyle in the process of biting through food.

Masticatory Habits. The sequence and distribution of the activities of the jaw muscles during mastication depend normally upon the type of food being chewed and upon the individual's habitual masticatory pattern. During the chewing of hard foods, such as a carrot, there is heavy masseter action on both sides coinciding with the action of the temporalis. As the carrot is reduced in size, chewing usually alternates bilaterally but may be unilateral, or even bilaterally simultaneous until the act of swallowing has been initiated. During the last phase of chewing a carrot and during chewing of soft food, the masseter muscle on the working side shows more activity than the balancing masseter and the temporal muscle will show a burst of activity prior to the maximal masseter activity—more so the farther the lateral excursions extend out from centric occlusion. In a study[72] of persons with full complements of teeth more than two-thirds were shown to have an alternating bilateral masticatory pattern, about 10 per cent chewed bilaterally simultaneously, and about 12 per cent had unilateral mastication restricted to one side (equal number right and left). According to cineradiographic studies, the bicuspid-molar segments are used most in regular mastication.[93] The presence of food between the teeth eliminates in part the unquestionable influence of occlusal interferences upon the patterns of jaw movements, but there are no comprehensive studies available on the effect of lateral occlusal interferences upon the functional masticatory pattern except that elimination of occlusal interferences may change the masticatory pattern.[9, 74] In some instances, when the occlusal interferences are avoided in empty lateral occlusal movements through established convenience pattern, the patient will strike these interferences in chewing when there is food between the teeth.[74]

It has been shown that if dentures were made to fit only in centric occlusion most patients could adapt to an up-and-down movement pattern,[87] but tracings in the frontal plane have indicated that the patients would make eccentric movements during mastication if the occlusion permitted such movements. In the natural dentition prominent cuspids may restrain normal lateral movements and the patient may develop chewing motions with a steep path of closure into centric occlusion.

The lack of abrasiveness of modern diet is probably conducive to the development of restricted masticatory movements. Although it has been shown recently that the frequency of lateral tooth contacts is not significantly altered by the type of food being eaten at the time of the recording,[2] it is quite likely that hard foods, such as raw fruits and vegetables and fibrous or dry meat, are more effective in eliminating the influence of occlusal interferences and total occlusal guidance than soft foods. It also appears from tests on biting strength that really heavy biting is more comfortably done close to centric occlusion than in lateral or protrusive positions of the jaw,[15] so that the crushing of very hard food probably involves very limited lateral excursions.

Effect of Loss of Teeth. The muscle activity and the chewing pattern may also be radically altered by loss of teeth. It has been shown by taking electro-myographic records before the loss of the posterior teeth, after the loss of the posterior teeth with only anterior teeth present, and finally after insertion of dentures following loss of posterior teeth, that the facial and circumoral muscles become very active in mastication, whereas there is minimal masseter activity. This is reversed again to normal activity following insertion of well fitting dentures.[85]

It is worth noting that besides the "masticatory muscles," a number of head and neck muscles are actively and passively participating in the act of mastication and the muscle activity is always guided towards the optimal functional result with the masticatory "tool" available.[80]

Stages of Mastication. Mastication is often described as occurring in three stages: (1) incision, (2) crushing and diminishing the size of large particles, and (3) "milling" or trituration of the food preparatory to deglutition. There is no clear-cut sequence of stages 2 and 3 since some larger particles may have escaped the crushing before the milling was started and crushing may again be needed.

The registration of the actual jaw movements during normal uninhibited mastication is extremely difficult. Hildebrand's[35] classical work 40 years ago still is the best source of information. He recorded masticatory movements by positional photography, roentgenkymography, kinematography and fluoroscopy from the frontal and sagittal planes. Similar clinical investigations have been done more recently by several other investigators[56, 82] and by Adams and Zander[2] with radio transmitters giving signals from fixed bridge pontics. It appears from practically all of these investigators' findings that small lateral and combined lateral and protrusive strokes ending in centric occlusion constitute the normal pattern of mastication, but the strokes vary considerably from individual to individual. In some instances, instead of ending in centric occlusion the chewing stroke in the milling stage of mastication carries over slightly laterally or retrusively from centric occlusion. It also appears that there may be gliding contact back over the working side in opening from centric occlusion.[2]

Masticatory Adaption. Masticatory performance or effectiveness has been tested and related to occlusal contacts recorded both by size of contact area and number of contacts.[52] It appeared from the study that the masticatory performance was well correlated in a linear manner with food platform areas, less well with molar imprint length, and poorly with tooth units. The food platform area or total occlusal contact is influenced by occlusal interferences, missing teeth, and irregular positions of the teeth. Attrition usually increases the food platform area, and so does occlusal adjustment.

The entire dentition undergoes a continuous adaptation to functional wear. This is manifest as compensatory eruption of teeth, mesial drift to compensate for interproximal wear, and changes in tooth position in an attempt to compensate for pathologic tooth movements or loss of teeth. These changes signify an unceasing effort to maintain a properly balanced physiologic status of the masticatory system throughout a person's lifetime.

Advanced attrition with loss of cusps leads, by uneven wear of enamel and dentition, to the formation of "inverted" cusps and fossae which are wholly as efficient in masticatory function as the original cusps and fossae, thus maintaining the efficiency of the masticatory system.

Deglutition and Occlusion

Stages of Deglutition. Mastication is based on a learned reflex pattern and like the initiation of swallowing is partially under voluntary control; however, when the bolus of food has reached the upper pharynx, the rest of the swallowing function is based on primary unlearned reflexes.[23] Bosma[14] has divided the process of swallowing into four stages: (1) the swallow-preparatory position of the bolus within the mouth, (2) passage from the mouth to the pharynx, (3) passage through the pharynx, (4) passage through the hypopharyngeal sphincter.

The first stage, which is under voluntary control, involves placing the chewed food or liquid between the tongue and the anterior teeth and palate. At this stage the facial and circumoral muscles as well as the tongue muscles are active, but there is minimal activity in the temporal and masseter muscles. The tongue then propels the bolus posteriorly against the palate and into the pharynx with a wave-like motion and the pharynx is opened in advance of the bolus. The hyoid bone is raised by the myohyoid muscles, the soft palate is elevated, the palatopharyngeal muscles constrict to close the passage of the nasal cavity, and the mandible is stabilized in a posterior position. The teeth are pressed together and the larynx is raised, with the glottis closed to interrupt respiration while the bolus passes.

The bolus passes over and around the epiglottis and is forced through the hypopharynx into the upper esophagus. When the bolus reaches the level of the clavicle, the palate relaxes, the larynx descends, the glottis opens, the tongue moves forward, the mandible is moved into rest position, and respiration is resumed.[27] The swallowing action in man is rapid and the bolus reaches the upper end of the esophagus one second after the initiation of the act of swallowing.[72]

The exact position of the trigger for the primary swallowing reflex action is not known, but reflex swallowing can be initiated by stimulation of the mucosa of the anterior and posterior pillars of the fauces, the uvula, the anterior aspect of the soft palate, the posterior and lateral walls of the lower pharynx, and the epiglottis.[71] The center for the complex act of deglutition is situated in the floor of the fourth ventricle, slightly above the respiratory center.

Muscular Action in Deglutition. Swallowing in infancy prior to the establishment of occlusion has been called infantile or *visceral swallowing.*[79, 89] This swallowing seems to be based upon an unconditioned reflex system in which the facial and circumoral muscles initiate the swallowing and the jaw is braced against the tongue, the gum pads being held separated by the tongue. Later, with the eruption of the posterior teeth, the infant assumes a tooth-together swallowing that has been called adult or *somatic swallowing.* It has been assumed by Rix,[79] Tulley[89] and others that these are two different types, infantile swallowing being dominated by the seventh cranial nerve muscles and adult swallowing by the fifth cranial nerve muscles. However, after complete loss of teeth, swallowing is again dominated by muscles innervated by the seventh cranial nerve and very little demarcation action is seen in the masseter muscle during swallowing until dentures are inserted. Some people with teeth also avoid bringing the teeth together during swallowing in that they place the tongue between the teeth to accomplish bracing of the jaw for the act of swallowing. This type of mandibular bracing is seen mainly in persons with severe occlusal prematurities* in centric relation; however, following elimination of these prematurities they may assume a tooth-together swallow.[76]

An electromyogram of a normal tooth-together swallowing of a bolus or mouthful of liquid is shown in Figure 4–18. Note how the action is initiated by

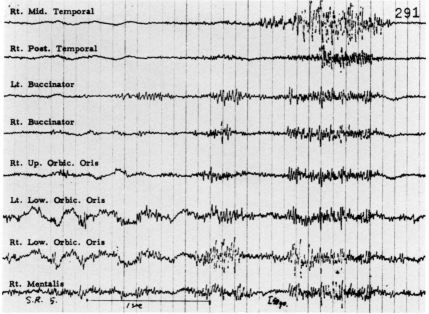

Figure 4–18. Electromyogram of a subject with harmonious occlusion drinking a large mouthful of water (glass separated from the lips). *Left,* Movement of lip muscles. *Middle,* Initiation of the swallow by the circumoral muscles. *Right,* Completion of the swallow with participation of both circumoral and masticatory muscles in the normal "tooth-together" swallow.

---

*A premature contact is an occlusal contact or interference that occurs before a balanced and stable jaw-to-jaw relationship is reached in either centric relation or centric occlusion, or in the area between these two positions.

the facial muscles. The next phase of activity is bringing the teeth together. Then at the time of swallowing both the facial and masticatory muscles are active, with most activity in the masticatory muscles. This burst of activity of the masticatory muscles is partially missing in an edentulous person, but the basic neuromuscular mechanism of swallowing is essentially the same; the differentiation of two types of swallowing may be meaningless and misleading.

A command swallow with the mouth empty may not involve the initial phase of facial and circumoral muscle activity since the person may bite together and force a swallow afterwards instead of going through the normal sequence of bringing the bolus back to the palate. An electromyogram of such a forced empty swallow is seen in Figure 4–19; the subject was the same as shown in Figure 4–18.

It should, of course, be understood that the drinking of liquids is often done with the teeth apart and that any person can brace his jaws with the tongue and lips so that he does not have to bring his teeth together during swallowing.

Tooth contacts in swallowing are of longer duration than in chewing,[33] but there is wide variation in frequency and duration from one subject to another.[74] Until recently there has been considerable controversy about the occlusal relations resulting from the jaw closure in swallowing. Jankelson and co-workers[46] observed by cinefluoroscopy a distal thrust of the mandible during swallowing. Furthermore, it was found that occlusal interferences or prematurities in the retrusive range disturbed the muscle contraction patterns (as seen on electromyograms) during swallowing but did not appreciably affect mastication.[76] Removal of these interferences had to be extended all the way back to centric relation before muscle harmony in swallowing could be estab-

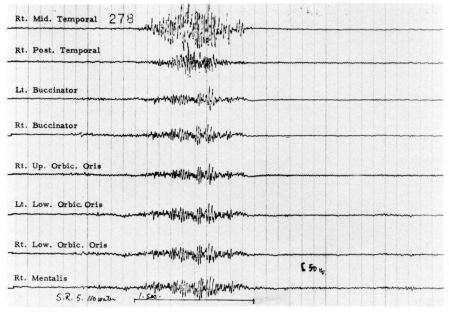

Figure 4–19. Forced "empty" swallow with the mandible in centric occlusion. Note heavy contraction of both circumoral and masticatory muscles.

lished. More recently, Zander and co-workers[31, 32, 34] have shown by means of radio transmitters that occlusal contacts (with the mandible in centric relation) are made regularly during swallowing of food and occasionally during cleaning of the mouth, during assembling of the bolus of food and placing it in position for swallowing, and occasionally during sleep without swallowing. However, telemetry studies by Glickman et al.[33] indicated that centric relation was rarely used during chewing and was used only infrequently during swallowing. The study also reported that elimination of premature contacts in centric relation did not result in an increased use of centric relation. However, Butler and Zander[25] reported tooth contact in the retruded position (centric relation) during chewing and swallowing after occlusal adjustment.

It is commonly believed that the mandible normally slides forward from the initial contact in centric relation and is seated in centric occlusion during swallowing.[31, 32, 34] The applied forces appear to be related to the individual muscle tone, which again is related to psychic tension (fusimotor activity) and occlusal interferences or prematurities.

The posterior thrust of the mandible during swallowing is part of the primary unconditioned reflex pattern of swallowing, and biting together for bracing of the mandible comes as a natural part of swallowing. It appears to be more difficult, if not impossible, to retrain or recondition the muscles so that interfering teeth will not make contact during this act than to retrain or recondition the learned reflexes associated with mastication so that interferences may be avoided (if there are not unavoidable balancing side interferences present).

Although retrusive or distal facets of occlusal wear have been attributed to mandibular excursions during function,[1] it now appears that the mandible does not move into the retruded position or centric relation except during clearing of the mouth of food, swallowing,[2, 34] and possibly bruxism. (At least bruxism is triggered by interferences or prematurities in this retrusive position.[76]) During the waking state occlusal contacts associated with swallowing occur about every two minutes,[49] but are irregular and much less frequent in deep sleep.[74] This frequency of contacts associated with swallowing explains the wear facets seen in the retrusive range between centric relation and centric occlusion. In contrast, the wear facets laterally and protrusively to centric occlusion are probably caused by masticatory function and in some instances by bruxism.

During normal adult swallowing, the distal thrust of the mandible and closure first to centric relation and then to centric occlusion (if there is a "slide in centric") will be evident on an electromyogram as synchronous bilateral muscle contractions (Fig. 4–20), provided that there are no interferences in the retrusive range of the occlusion. However, unbalanced muscle contractions with lack of synchronization often occur when the teeth come into contact during swallowing in the presence of premature contacts between centric relation and centric occlusion (Fig. 4–21). The elimination of such premature contacts in the retrusive range will provide for harmonious muscular contractions in swallowing.

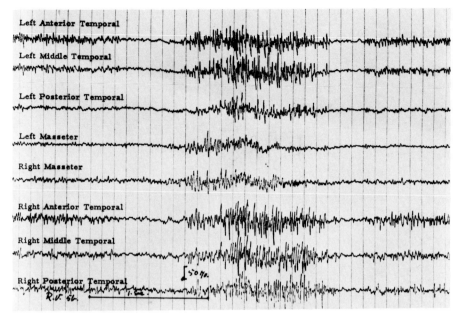

Figure 4–20. Electromyogram of a subject swallowing a large mouthful of water and sliding from centric relation to centric occlusion with even contacts in this retrusive range of the occlusion. An occlusal adjustment had been performed and, although the "slide" has not been completely eliminated, the contacts are even on both sides of the arches.

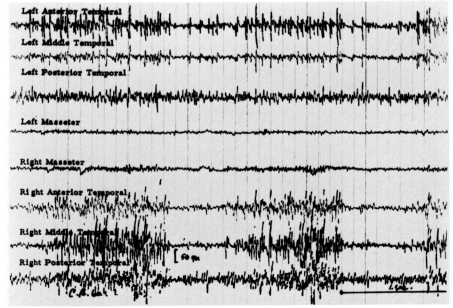

Figure 4–21. Electromyogram of subject with severe occlusal interferences in centric relation with the initial premature contacts being on the right side (swallowing a large mouthful of water). Note unharmonious contractive activity, mainly of the temporal muscles.

In conscious swallowing or swallowing with a small bolus of food, the mandible does not always go back to centric relation, but the initial occlusal contact may be made anywhere between centric relation and centric occlusion. It is therefore important that this area as well as both centric relation and centric occlusion be in harmony with the temporomandibular joint and the muscles. This is the reason for a need for a *freedom of movement in centric* or a *long centric*.[53] If there is an interference in centric relation, a second swallow with the jaw set in centric occlusion will often follow immediately (Fig. 4–22).

A discrepancy between centric relation and centric occlusion that involves a lateral slide is much more likely to be accompanied by unbalanced muscle contractions during swallowing than a straightforward slide, and such a lateral slide is particularly significant for patients with temporomandibular joint disturbances of a dysfunctional nature. Further discussion of the significance of occlusal interferences in the retrusive range can be found in Chapter 5, Bruxism.

From the foregoing it is apparent that occlusal interferences in the path from centric relation to centric occlusion are most significant during swallowing.[83] Such interferences are important in the occurrence of neuromuscular disharmony, and may also be of significance in the development of traumatic occlusion both to teeth with premature contacts and to teeth that receive the impact of the slide into centric occlusion.

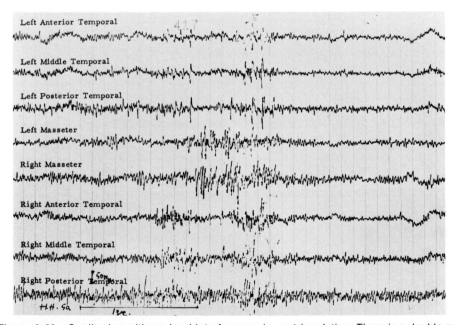

Figure 4–22.　Swallowing with occlusal interferences in centric relation. There is a double swallow present; the first in centric relation with fleeting tooth contact and unharmonious muscle activity, and the second swallow following with heavy tooth contact in centric occlusion and fairly well-balanced muscle activity.

SIGNIFICANCE OF "CENTRIC"

"Centric" is probably the most controversial word in dental terminology. Even when it is used in combination with other words, as in centric relation, centric occlusion, centric position, etc., the meaning of these terms varies to a very great extent both in the literature and among clinicians. The controversy is, in part, semantic, but more significant is the serious difference in concepts. It is questionable whether there ever will be one word that can convey all the meanings that have been attached to this word. An attempt will be made to summarize, without extensive documentation or discussion, the current status of "centric."

Summary of Current Status of "Centric"

The teeth commonly make contact both during chewing and during swallowing in centric occlusion.

Centric relation is a functional border position which is reached chiefly during swallowing, but also occasionally during chewing.

Centric relation and centric occlusion do not coincide in the average healthy human dentition.

Lateral and protrusive excursions are parts of normal masticatory function, and chewing strokes converge to centric occlusion.

Occlusal interferences between centric relation and centric occlusion are more apt to create neuromuscular disharmony associated with swallowing than during mastication.

Occlusal interferences laterally and protrusively to centric occlusion are apt to interfere with the muscle harmony in mastication rather than during swallowing.

Centric relation is stable and reproducible when the temporomandibular joint is normal and in the absence of unbalanced muscle activity.

Recording of a stationary hinge axis or a Gothic arch tracing with a definite arrow point does not prove that this is the normal centric relation, since splinting action of muscles and disturbed guidance from ligaments may lead to a false recording. The stationary hinge axis may then change position following elimination of the joint and muscle dysfunction, and finally settle down as a stable stationary hinge axis (within one or two millimeters of error inherent in the method of recording).

A lateral slide from centric relation to centric occlusion is apt to create much more neuromuscular disharmony than a straight forward slide.

A completely well balanced straight forward slide from centric is tolerated well, but such a slide would be extremely difficult to produce and maintain in stability.

A flat area between centric relation and centric occlusion ("long centric") is compatible with occlusal, temporomandibular joint, and muscle harmony.

Oral rehabilitation carried out according to gnathological principles and in such a way that centric relation and centric occlusion coincide is well tolerated if properly done. However, neuromuscular adaptation is required and there is a tendency for a slide to reoccur as the teeth move. Thus, there are no demonstrated advantages over the much easier to construct "long centric."

Centric position or "muscle centric" and "power centric" seem to fall within or close enough to the "long centric" that these poorly defined positions (which are difficult to record) do not seem to be of practical value as reference positions.

Since it is not known what determines the magnitude of the "slide in centric" there is no way to predetermine the ideal length of a "long centric." However, as long as the centric relation is determined correctly and there is some (0.3 to 0.8 mm.) freedom of movement in the long centric, this seems to be within the adaptive range of the overwhelming majority of patients.

There is no valid reason to institute therapy just because a patient has a "slide in centric" if there are no signs or symptoms to indicate any harmful effect from such a slide and the masticatory system is otherwise normal.

For persons with bruxism and functional temporomandibular joint disturbances the safest therapy is to eliminate the slide in centric completely and to have a horizontal "long" centric or, depending on the direction of the original slide, a "wide" centric.

A centric occlusion that is 2 to 3 mm. in front of centric relation in dentures has proved to be acceptable for mastication, but has resulted in muscle spasms and pain.[22]

It appears that centric relation is extremely important as a functional border position of the mandible in swallowing. Any occlusal interferences within the field of occlusal contacts laterally and protrusively to centric relation may result in occlusal, neuromuscular and temporomandibular joint disorders.

Of extreme clinical significance for "centric" as well as for other occlusal problems is a patient's adaptive capacity or tolerance level to occlusal imperfections.

Centric relation is the only "centric" which is reproducible and stable with or without teeth present, and recent research has confirmed the great clinical significance of this position as the main key for the solution of occlusal problems.

Centric relation is the only reference position that assures simultaneous harmonious alignment of both temporomandibular joints.

OCCLUSAL STABILITY

The modern concept of a dynamic individual occlusion naturally includes an increased interest in stability of the occlusion before, during and after dental and periodontal treatment. A stable occlusion is dependent on the resultant of all forces acting on the teeth, including the ever-present eruptive force. Neither the disturbing forces nor the restraint to such forces can be described accurately, although it is the equilibrium of all such forces that counts for the stability of occlusion. Adjustment of tooth position occurs throughout a person's lifetime in response to naturally induced changes of occlusal forces associated with wear, in response to pathologic changes in the support mechanism or muscle tonicity, and following placement of restorations and other dental procedures. However, within the adaptive capacity of the masticatory system, a balance of forces is maintained. Periodontal disease, increased mobility of teeth, unfavorable alteration of occlusal anatomy and position of the teeth, habits and dysfunctional muscle forces may induce an imbalance of forces which is beyond the adaptive range and which may become manifest as traumatic occlusion.

The patterns of forces that act on the teeth are far more complex than usually conceived. Research in this area has been largely directed toward magnitude of biting forces[3, 5, 12, 90] and the orthodontic aspects of tooth mechanics.[24, 39] Although recent research has explored some of the mechanics of occlusal forces, the equilibrium of a tooth relative to its surrounding,[29, 38, 92] tooth mobility,[59, 68] and tilting movements,[69] few deductions can be made from these studies that are of direct practical value for stabilization of teeth by occlusal adjustment or other dental procedures. It has been observed that teeth move and new interferences develop if the occlusal adjustment does not

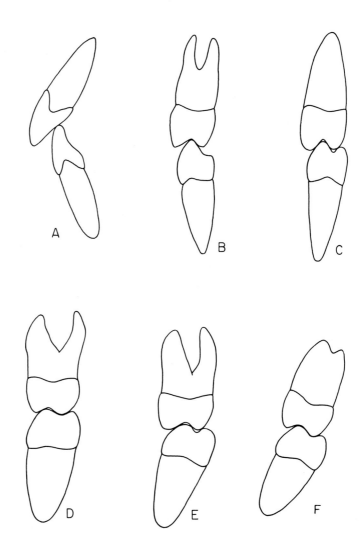

Figure 4-23. Angulation of the axes of teeth. Because of the interdigitation of the teeth, the occlusal relationship of opposing teeth is not necessarily represented in the illustration. The point which is to be emphasized is the direction of the axes of the mandibular and maxillary teeth, and the necessity for directing occlusal forces along the long axes of the teeth during occlusal adjustment and placement of restorations. *A, B, C, D, E* and *F* show incisors, 1st and 2nd premolars, and 1st, 2nd, and 3rd molars, respectively. Forces from lips and tongue also play an important role in occlusal stability, especially for the anterior teeth.

include in principle the establishment and maintenance of occlusal stability. Whether a tooth remains in equilibrium with its environment is dependent on many factors such as occlusal forces, status of supporting structures, size, form and number of roots,[62] and inclination of the teeth.

A practical principle for stabilization of teeth following occlusal adjustment or placement of dental restorations is to make centric stops in centric relation closure on the same horizontal level as the centric stops in centric occlusion and in such a manner that the biting forces in centric will be directed along the long axis of the teeth. Vertical forces have less tendency to create excessive mobility of teeth than lateral forces and less tendency to move teeth into new interferences than unbalanced laterally directed forces.[9, 18, 21] In order to direct the occlusal forces along the long axis of the teeth during occlusal adjustment and placement of restorations it is important to know the general location of the axes of opposing teeth. These axes vary with the arrangement and location of the teeth,[28] and the angulation of the axes is seldom coincident for mesiodistal and the buccolingual directions (Figure 4–23).

Occlusal stability is also intimately related to stable temporomandibular joint relationships, and even to physiologic wear and balanced muscle function.

PERIODONTAL REACTION TO PHYSIOLOGIC FORCES

A functional orientation of the principal periodontal fibers with the teeth in function is evident in histologic sections of jaws. The change from a non-functional to a functional arrangement of the fibers can be observed in sections of erupting teeth as soon as the teeth are engaged in occlusal contacts. From the pattern and directional orientation of the principal periodontal fibers of teeth in function, it may be assumed that occlusal stress to a great extent is transferred from the cementum of the tooth to the surrounding alveolar bone as pull or tension. The supracrestal periodontal fibers also are arranged in an intricate interwoven functional pattern, extending from tooth to tooth, from tooth to alveolar crest, and in various directions from the tooth into the free and attached gingiva. The arrangement of the periodontal fibers provides both maximum stability for the teeth and promotes the self-cleansing action of the normal gingival crevice during function.

Collagenous Fibers

The direction, structural arrangement, and strength of the periodontal fibers depend on the magnitude, direction and frequency of the occlusal stress on the teeth, on the morphologic features of the periodontium, and also to some extent on the systemic status of the individual. The turnover rate of mature collagen is slow, and the collagenous fibers of the periodontium in an adult person, therefore, are not particularly sensitive to changes of a systemic nature unless trauma or other forms of injury establish a need for reparative processes. If a tooth is exposed mainly to vertical stress the principal periodontal fibers will assume an oblique pattern, in some instances almost parallel to the root surface. In such cases very few horizontal fibers can be observed at the alveolar crest. If the occlusal stress is predominantly horizontal or lateral, one can observe heavy groups of alveolar crest fibers with a horizontal arrangement in the region of the alveolar crest and around the apex of the tooth. There is very little evidence of a functional arrangement of the periodontal fibers at the midportion of the root of the tooth.

Lateral stress on teeth is desirable within physiologic limits because it stimulates the development of a strong fibrous periodontal membrane around the neck of the teeth, thus lessening the potential of traumatic periodontal injury from incidental or accidental occlusal forces. It also seems likely that such heavy collagenous fibers should limit the spread of gingival inflammation more effectively than would be the case with a loose, nonfunctionally arranged connective tissue.

Although collagenous "ligaments" exist in the periodontal membrane, and to an increasing extent with increasing function, it is incorrect to speak of them as ligaments since the periodontal membrane has a rich vascular supply and a multipotential loose connective tissue not found in true ligaments.

The thickness or width of the periodontal membrane will increase with an increase in functional demand.[26,51] If the main functional forces are directed horizontally, an increase in periodontal width will be apparent around the cervical and apical parts of the teeth, and there will be a narrower periodontal space at the middle to the apical one-third of the root. A predominantly axially directed force will produce a widening in the bifurcation or trifurcation areas and around the apical areas of the teeth.

Besides the well established concept of resistance and transfer of occlusal stress to the alveolar bone by tension of functionally oriented periodontal fibers, the tissues making up the periodontal membrane resist compression and transmit some of the occlusal forces to the alveolar bone as direct pressure. The relationship between the teeth and the alveolar bone resembles a cone and socket arrangement, with a soft tissue membrane placed between the cone and the socket. Early German investigators described vascular bundles resembling glomeruli within the periodontal membrane and assumed that these structures acted as shock absorbers. Later, it was suggested that hydraulic principles were applicable in the periodontal membrane[19] and that the blood and tissue fluids within the periodontal membrane absorbed the impact of initial occlusal forces. These theories have been revived by recordings of pulse beat expressed as tooth movements,[42] and it appears from mobility studies that the initial "give" when a very light force is applied to teeth may be on the basis of a hydrodynamic system.[67] However, it would be contrary to biological principles existing elsewhere in the body to assume that the vascular channels of the periodontal membrane would have the function of resisting functional compression associated with mastication and bracing of the jaws in swallowing. It appears more likely that the ability of the periodontal membrane to yield or resist to functional compression is dependent upon the physical properties of the tissues that make up the periodontal membrane. The decisive factors in this regard are the amount and state of the collagenous fibers, the degree of polymerization of the ground substance, the vascularity of the periodontal tissues, and, for really heavy forces, the bony housing of the teeth.[70] Since the collagenous periodontal fibers have a somewhat wavy arrangement and the tooth has to be moved slightly before the fibers become taut, the initial impact of an occlusal force results in a slight compression of some part of the periodontal structures. When the fibers become taut most of the stress is transmitted as pull to the alveolar bone.

In teeth with minimum function there is very little or no indication histologically of a functional arrangement of collagenous periodontal fibers and, under these circumstances, it has to be assumed that the light function is carried on mainly on the basis of the resistance of the periodontal membrane to compression. In teeth with heavy function or bruxism, the periodontal membrane structurally has a pronounced functional arrangement. It must be assumed that in such cases the heavy forces are transmitted chiefly through pull on these heavy fiber bundles.

Axial Stress.   Vertical or axially directed occlusal stress tends to have an even impact on the entire periodontal membrane and therefore results in a minimum of pressure or compression upon any given unit area. Also, axial stress engages the maximum number of oblique principal periodontal fibers. Since axial stress has the lowest compression potential and engages the maximum number of fibers, the physiologic tolerance of the periodontium to axial stress is greater than to stress directed in any other direction.

Lateral Stress.   Horizontal or lateral stress compresses relatively small apical and cervical areas of the periodontal membrane and stretches a small number of periodontal fibers opposite the areas of compression. This concentration of compression and tension indicates that horizontal forces have a great potential for injury of the periodontal structures. As the direction of occlusal forces changes from horizontal to a more vertical direction, an increasingly larger part of the periodontal membrane becomes engaged in the transfer of the stress from tooth to bone, thereby lessening the hazard for periodontal traumatic injury. The concentrated impact of horizontal forces in concentrated areas explains the common clinical observation that trauma from occlusion is much more often the sequela of a horizontal than of an axial force; however, it should be recognized that a certain degree of lateral functional stress is normal for the human dentition.

Factors Affecting Physiologic Tooth Mobility

With precise measuring devices it has been found that tooth mobility is highest immediately on arising in the morning and decreases progressively during waking hours.[66] Holding the teeth apart will also increase mobility. This increase in mobility is probably due to slight extrusion of the teeth when stimuli are not produced by tooth contacts.[64] Chewing and swallowing will decrease tooth mobility.[64] Teeth apparently have a diurnal cycle of mobility changes, which are mainly related to frequency of occlusal contacts in sleeping and waking hours. In longitudinal studies on the effect of tube type diets versus normal diets, no change in mobility was found from alteration in masticatory occlusal contacts.[65] It has been presumed that the swallowing contacts are sufficient to maintain the teeth in their normal position.

Stress-inducing situations will increase tooth mobility in persons with bruxism but do not seem to affect mobility in individuals who do not brux.[65] Forceful chewing on periodontally weakened teeth does not seem to increase mobility to any significant degree, or even decrease mobility.[63] Thus splinting of the teeth with a moderate increase in mobility to stabilize the teeth for function may not be indicated. Pathologic tooth mobility will be discussed under trauma from occlusion (pp. 170, 257).

Changes in Periodontal Tissues

The vascularity of the periodontal tissues decreases with an increase in functional demands. As the functionally oriented collagenous fibers increase in size with very heavy function, the periodontal membrane more and more assumes the morphologic and functional characteristics of a ligament. However, there are always some blood vessels and some interstitial loose connective tissues within the periodontal membrane to distinguish it from a compact ligament.

Sharpey's fibers entering the alveolar bone increase in number and assume a better definition in response to heavy function. Increased function also increases the thickness of the alveolar bone plate. The bony trabeculae of the supporting bone of the alveolar process also increase in number and thickness with increasing function. An increase in thickness of the alveolar process, even to the extent of altering the gingival contour, may be seen in patients with bruxism.

The alveolar bone and adjacent structures physiologically undergo a continuous reorganization and rebuilding in association with changes of occlusal forces on the teeth, mesial drift, and compensatory eruption of the teeth. Histologic evidence of intermittent resorption and repair on the surface of the alveolar bone is found on the side toward which the tooth is moving. If the occlusal forces are within physiologic limits, the areas of active bone resorption in any given section constitute only a small part of the surface of the alveolar bone.[75] When such adaptive resorption is initiated, more bone is resorbed than would be needed to reconstitute the normal width of the periodontal membrane. This adaptive resorption results in a concavity on the surface of the alveolar bone, where the periodontal membrane initially is replaced by granulation tissue. Also, active osteoclasts may occasionally be observed in such areas. Repair and regeneration on this surface of the alveolar bone establish attachment for new periodontal fibers and functional connection with the tooth while the process of resorption may be initiated in an adjacent location. In this way only a small part of the total support for the tooth is at any given time involved in resorption and temporary loss of attachment. At the same time, an adequate number of periodontal fibers not involved in this process maintain the functional connection between the bone and the cementum. Associated with bone resorption on the periodontal membrane side of the alveolar bone, one often finds formation of new bone on the endosteal side of the alveolar bone; thus, a functional alveolar bone of normal thickness is maintained.

Physiologic Drift

The side toward which a tooth is being bodily moved is usually called the pressure side, and the opposite side, with pull on the periodontal fibers, is called the tension side. When teeth are undergoing physiologic mesial drift, the mesial side is the pressure side and the distal side is the tension side. The tension side is characterized by a lamellated surface of the alveolar bone, indicating deposition of bone, while simultaneously there may be evidence of resorption on the bone marrow side of alveolar bone in the same area. This again serves to maintain a normal thickness of alveolar bone plate. In the anterior region of the mouth, the alveolar bone is often fused with the cortical surface of the alveolar process to form one thin plate of cortical bone. If such teeth are moved for a limited distance labially by physiologic forces, the bone is resorbed on the periodontal membrane side and new bone is deposited on the labial aspect of the alveolar process. However, if the new bone formation does not keep up with the rate of the resorption on the periodontal membrane side, the tooth may move through the labial bone plate, causing dehiscence or fenestration.

Changes in Cementum

Deposition of cementum is probably a continuous process throughout the lifetime of the tooth. The lamellated structure of cementum presumably is due to a cyclic deposition. Whether the lamellation is related to a change in direction of the forces acting on the teeth with subsequent new requirements for embedding the reoriented fibers[36] is still an open question. As indicated previously, the turnover rate of collagen in the periodontal membrane in adults is slow, and there is no need for frequent change in fiber attachment on the root surface. Besides that, the functional adjustment to altered tooth position and occlusal force takes place mainly on the surface of the alveolar bone rather than on the surface of the tooth. The Sharpey's fibers entering the cementum are very stable structures, and this stability accounts for the very slow rate of increase in thickness of cementum. The physiologic continuous deposition of cementum may be interrupted by minor traumatic injuries to the periodontal tissues that are evident microscopically as areas of resorption and repair of the cementum. It has been shown by serial sectioning that practically every tooth from adults exhibits such manifestations of previous minor traumatic injuries.[40] Although this is histologic evidence of previous trauma from occlusion, often no clinical and radiographic sign or symptoms of trauma from occlusion may be present.

The cementum decreases in thickness toward the cementum-enamel junction, and it has been assumed that the thicker layer of cementum in the apical area represents, in part, compensation for the continuous eruption which follows occlusal wear of teeth. Functional hyperplasia of cementum may also be seen in the apical areas of teeth that have been exposed to heavy function. Thus, the surface area of the root is increased, allowing for attachment of more functional fibers and thereby increasing the functional capacity of the tooth.

Adaptive Capacity of Periodontal Structures

The adaptive capacity of the periodontal structures (with regard to occlusal stress) varies greatly from individual to individual and even in the same individual from time to time. The occlusal stresses may also vary on the basis of both somatic and psychic changes in the individual. Signs and symptoms of traumatic occlusion may develop in a person's mouth without anything having been done to his occlusal relations.

Protein or vitamin C deprivation in experimental animals, especially during growth and development, leads to impairment of the periodontal tissues and markedly reduces the functional capacity of these structures on the basis of inadequate collagen and bone formation.[91] Other severe experimental nutritional and hormonal deficiencies have also resulted in alterations of the periodontal structures. However, such changes have been minimal or absent in full-grown animals. The alteration of polymerization of the ground substance of connective tissue associated with pregnancy may lead to increased mobility of the teeth.[58] The significance of this increased mobility in the etiology of traumatic occlusion and periodontal disease is not known.

The adaptive capacity or tolerance level of the periodontal tissues to occlusal stress sets the individual border between physiologic and traumatic occlusion.

NORMAL VERSUS IDEAL OCCLUSION

A description of normal occlusion is usually centered around occlusal contacts, alignment of teeth, overbite and overjet, the arrangement and relationship of the teeth within and between the arches, and the relationship of the teeth to osseous structures. Conformity to certain standard values for these criteria is commonly used to determine whether an occlusion is normal, and the descriptions of normal occlusion become very complex and somewhat controversial from one reference to another.

"Normal" implies a situation commonly found in the absence of disease, and normal values in a biological system are given within a physiologic adaptive range. Normal occlusion, therefore, should imply more than a range of acceptable values; it should also indicate physiologic adaptability and the absence of recognizable pathologic manifestations. Such a concept of normal occlusion emphasizes the functional aspect of occlusion and the capability of the masticatory system to adapt to or compensate for some deviations within the range of tolerance of the system.

The functional adaptation of the dentition is well recognized; i.e., the occlusion undergoes certain changes with moderate wear[9] that appear to be beneficial to the health of the entire masticatory system. Such adaptive changes in the temporomandibular joint, at least for adults, appear to be very unlikely.[78]

The neuromuscular mechanism seems to have a great potential for adaptation to imperfections in the relationships among the various factors that align the masticatory system. However, the adaptive capacity of the neuromuscular system depends to a great extent upon the irritability threshold of the central nervous system (fusimotor activity), which is influenced by emotional and psychic tension.[77] Therefore, occlusal interferences may or may not lead to neuromuscular or other functional disturbances within the masticatory system since the presence of such disturbances may depend on how a person adapts or reacts to his occlusal interferences.

The intimate relationship between the peripheral and central nervous system is, in the final analysis, one of the most significant factors in the study of occlusion. One may consider a person's occlusion from two viewpoints: (1) the occlusion itself, evident in an examination of the functional relationship of the masticatory system; and (2) how a person's neuromuscular mechanism reacts to his occlusion.

Functional disturbances of the masticatory system may be present on the basis of very severe occlusal interferences and mild psychic tension or severe psychic tension and very slight occlusal interferences, the average tolerance level being between these extremes. Every analysis of occlusion, therefore, should include an evaluation of the patient's reaction to his occlusion and his occlusal interferences. However, it has been found that functional occlusal therapy, if performed with great accuracy, will eliminate dysfunctional manifestations in the masticatory system in spite of persistent nervous tension and high fusimotor activity. This introduces a concept of "ideal occlusion," a state in which there is no (or is minimal) neuromuscular adaptation needed because there are no occlusal interferences present. Ideal occlusion indicates a completely harmonious relationship of the masticatory system for mastication as well as for swallowing and speech.

To understand the difference in concept between normal and ideal occlusion one may consider, for example, that a forward slide from centric relation to centric occlusion of 1 to 2 mm. is normal since such a slide is found commonly without disturbance to any part of the masticatory system when other aspects of the occlusion also are within the range of normal function. Similarly, an occlusion may be considered clinically normal in the presence of occlusal interferences in lateral excursions, provided the interferences are bypassed by neuromuscular adaptation and there are no clinically apparent disturbances of masticatory function or pathologic periodontal changes. Such an occlusion cannot be considered normal, however, if even minute occlusal interferences cannot be bypassed by neuromuscular adaptation and some form of pathologic sequela results. The concept of ideal occlusion goes beyond a consideration of the lack of pathologic sequelae for the sake of establishing criteria for an occlusion where there is no need for neuromuscular adaptation and where the health of the periodontium and the other structures of the masticatory system is perpetuated through ideal function. Ideal occlusion has less relation to anatomic features than to functional characteristics, although good anatomic relationships provide the best background for functional harmony.

Ideal Occlusion

The concept of an ideal or optimal occlusion refers both to an esthetic and physiologic ideal. The emphasis has more and more moved from esthetic and anatomical standards to a current concern with function, health, and comfort. Extensive electromyographic research has confirmed the common clinical observation that esthetic ideals have very limited relationship to optimal function and health of the dentition.

It is essential for functional comfort that neuromuscular harmony prevail in the masticatory system. Certain requirements regarding the relationship between temporomandibular joint guidance and occlusal guidance will assure such harmony. These requirements are as follows.

1. Stable jaw relationship when the teeth make contact in centric relation is necessary.

2. Centric occlusion should be slightly in front of centric relation and in the same sagittal plane as the path made by the mandible in making a straight protrusive movement between centric relation and centric occlusion (Fig. 4–24). Centric relation and centric occlusion contacts do not have to be in the same horizontal plane, but this arrangement has some practical advantages. The distance between centric relation and centric occlusion is about 0.1 to 0.2 mm. in the temporomandibular joints and about 0.5 mm. at the level of the teeth.

3. An unrestricted glide with maintained occlusal contacts between centric relation and centric occlusion is required.

4. Complete freedom for smooth gliding occlusal contact movements in the various excursions both from centric occlusion and centric relation is needed.

5. The occlusal guidance in various excursions should be on the working (functioning) rather than on the balancing (nonfunctioning) side. Steepness of incisal or cuspal guidance is not important for neuromuscular harmony.

Another equally important aspect of ideal occlusion is functional stability of the masticatory system. Stable occlusal relationship refers to self-perpetuating, stable, and harmonious relationships between teeth and temporomandibular joints throughout life.

The first prerequisite for functional stability is that the impact of full intercuspidation closure be in the long axis of all posterior teeth and against the central part of the meniscus of the temporomandibular joints. The second prerequisite is an even degree of wear resistance. Also, the cutting effectiveness of all functionally alike teeth should be the same.

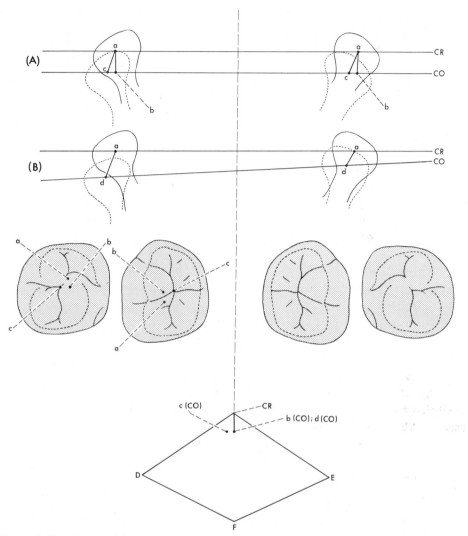

Figure 4–24. Relationship of condyle position to centric occlusion, centric relation, and incisal point in the horizontal plane. In *A* the center of rotation of the condyle *a* is in centric relation closure. At the initial tooth contact at point *a* on the mandibular first molar and maxillary first molar the mandible shifts laterally with the condyle, moving to position *c* with the slide in centric from *a* to *c* on the teeth. This lateral shift and displacement of the condyles is represented at the incisal point as a movement from (CR) centric relation to centric occlusion [point c(CO)]. In order for the condyles to be seated in a more harmonious position at point *b*, which is straight forward of point *a*, point *b* should be established as centric occlusion on the same horizontal plane as point *c*. In an occlusal adjustment or in making restorations this may be accomplished by establishing a long and broad centric. Once established, the incisal point would be allowed to move to b(CO) from (CR). In *B*, asymmetric positioning of the condyles may occur with a lateral shift with the incisal point d(CO) being straight forward of point (CR), especially as a result of improper occlusal grinding or restorative procedures.

A third requirement is that no displacing impact should be present on anterior teeth in centric occlusion closure.

The fourth and fifth requirements are that there should be no soft tissue contact in functional occlusion and that there should be an acceptable interocclusal space.

Orthodontic classifications are more related to anatomical and esthetic standards than to neuromuscular harmony and functional stability. It has not been possible to develop a consensus on a numerical index or system of values that apply both to form and function of the masticatory system.

On the basis of clinical and electromyographic studies it can be summarized that the prerequisites for an ideal occlusion are: (1) a stable and harmonious occlusal relationship in centric relation as well as in the area between centric relation and centric occlusion; (2) equal occlusal facility for bilateral and protrusive excursions; and (3) optimal direction of occlusal forces for stability of the teeth.

Although such a concept of ideal occlusion enables the clinician to help patients who have a low tolerance level to occlusal imperfections or advanced loss of periodontal support for the teeth, it does not mean that such an "ideal" necessarily should be imposed upon all patients with a functionally normal occlusion and healthy periodontium.

TACTILE SENSIBILITY AND OCCLUSAL FORCES

The tactile sensibility of the periodontium is important in the regulation of occlusal forces and reflex opening of the jaw (p. 60). Because of this importance and its relationship to bruxism, traumatic occlusion, and functional disturbances of the masticatory system, the tactile sensibility of the periodontium has been studied recently with renewed interest.[48,50,84] Similarly, recent developments in intraoral telemetry (radio transmitters utilizing transducers) promise to make possible the evaluation of the dynamic occlusal forces involved in mastication, bruxism, and swallowing.[2]

Detection of Changes in Occlusion

In early studies of the "sensory threshold" for foreign bodies between the teeth, Theil[86] and Hollstein[43] reported values of 20μ to 100μ. More recently, Kraft[50] reported that it was impossible to detect bodies of less than 20μ between the occlusal surfaces of the teeth; however, Tryde[88] reported values as small as 10μ. Siirilä and Lane[84] have shown that foreign bodies only as thick as 8μ could be detected by some individuals and that bodies of 60μ were perceived without exception. From these studies it is quite apparent that the periodontal receptors are capable of detecting extremely small changes in the occlusion; they add significance to the clinical observation that minute discrepancies in the occlusion are capable of influencing the masticatory system. Whether basic differences in periodontal sensibility account in part for some individuals' failure to adapt to even minor occlusal interferences is not known. Whether there is a significant difference between the "sensory threshold" for the normal periodontium and the periodontium in periodontal disease or bruxism has not been determined.

In a study by Münch and Schriever[60] it was found that a force on the teeth of as little as 1.5 gm was detectable; however, the results of studies in our own laboratory show that forces of 600 mg. and smaller can be detected by some individuals. Because of the possibility of adaptation of pressoreceptors of the periodontal membrane, a clear picture of the "threshold" for pressoreceptors cannot be given at the present time. It appears likely that the receptors do adapt to light, continuous forces. It does not appear that they adapt to intermittent dynamic forces; this may explain the tolerance of the neuromuscular system to orthodontic forces and the attempt to avoid occlusal interferences associated with traumatic occlusion.

It was shown by Anderson and Picton[8] that when a crown was raised above the occlusal level by 0.5 mm., the load on the tooth was twice as great as normal. This small increase in force was interpreted as indicating the existence of a self-regulating, protective mechanism (presumably the sensibility of the periodontium and neuromuscular regulation). Since it appears unlikely that the receptors in the periodontal membrane adapt to such "high" restorations, a protective avoidance of the restoration or force compensation must take place within the limits and tolerance of the components of the masticatory system.

Stress of Mastication

The stress of mastication varies not only from individual to individual, but from time to time.[5] It has been found, also, that the stress during mastication increases toward the end of the chewing sequence. In a study of stress during mastication, Anderson[6] found that the maxillary whole tooth load was 15 kg. for biscuit, 14 kg. for carrot, and 7 kg. for meat. Also, with the exception of carrots, there was an increased load with swallowing.[5] These studies suggest that the nature of the food controls occlusal forces to some extent and that such forces are greater when closer to centric than out laterally. What regulating effect against nominal stress in mastication occurs in the absence of supporting structures is not clear. The finding that the force (maxillary whole tooth load) was less for meat than for biscuit[5] suggests that the nature of the food may be important in terms of potential excessive forces. An unyielding foreign object, unsuspected in the food, brings about the jaw-opening reflex. However, when hard candy is eaten, there is a tendency to move it around until crushing can be accomplished without excessive force. At least, past experiences dictate in part whether an item can be crushed without excessive force. Such learning may be related to the amount of force necessary to masticate various foods most efficiently when potential excessive forces are considered. A force can be considered to be excessive when it acts as a painful stimulus or produces injury. On the basis of avoidance movements, and less force than might be expected from "high" restorations,[8] it appears logical to assume that occlusal interferences constitute at least the potential for excessive forces, especially if protective mechanisms are bypassed.

Present evidence, based principally on static force measurements, indicates that the average forced biting force is 100 to 150 pounds in adult males, but larger forces have been recorded;[44, 47, 90] for example, the maximum biting force on the first molar in Eskimos has been found to be approximately 350 pounds. It is apparent that biting force is related to the diet and the manner in which the teeth are used. Much larger forces than average could be expected in individuals living on diets requiring the mastication of tough foods. Still, such forces must be within the capacity of the supporting structures to tolerate them. It is rational to assume that the sensibility of the periodontal membrane enters into the management of occlusal forces so that the tolerance level of the supporting structures of the teeth is not exceeded.

REFERENCES

1. Aarstad, T.: The Capsular Ligaments of the Temporomandibular Joint and Retrusion Facets of the Dentition in Relationship to Mandibular Movements (tr. by Halga Christie). Oslo, Akademisk Forlag, 1954.
2. Adams, S. H., and Zander, H. A.: Functional tooth contacts in lateral and in centric occlusion. J. Am. Dent. A., 69:465, 1964.
3. Adler, P.: Sensibility of teeth to loads applied in different directions. J. Dent. Res., 26:279, 1947.
4. Ahlgren, J.: Patterns of chewing and malocclusion of teeth. A clinical study. Acta Odont. Scand., 25:3, 1967.
5. Anderson, D. J.: Measurement of stress in mastication. I. J. Dent. Res., 35:664, 1956.
6. Anderson, D. J.: Measurement of stress in mastication. II. J. Dent. Res., 35:671, 1956.
7. Anderson, D. J., and Picton, D. C. A.: Tooth contact during chewing. J. Dent. Res., 36:21, 1957.
8. Anderson, D. J., and Picton, D. C. A.: Masticatory stresses in normal and modified occlusion. J. Dent. Res., 37:312, 1958.
9. Beyron, H. L.: Characteristics of functionally optimal occlusion and principles of occlusal rehabilitation. J. Am. Dent. A., 48:648, 1954.
10. Beyron, H. L.: Occlusal relations and mastication in Australian aborigines. Acta Odont. Scand., 22:597, 1964.
11. Beyron, H. L.: Optimal occlusion. Dent. Clin. N. Am., 13:537, 1969.
12. Black, G. V.: The force exerted in the closure of the jaws. Dent. Cosmos, 37:469, 1895.
13. Bonwill, W. G. A.: The geometrical and mechanical laws of the articulation of the human teeth — The anatomical articulator. In Litch, W. F.: The American System of Dentistry. Vol. 2. Philadelphia, Lea Brothers, 1887, pp. 486–498.
14. Boos, R. H.: Occlusion from rest position. J. Prosth. Dent., 2:575, 1952.
15. Boos, R. H.: Vertical centric and functional dimensions recorded by gnathodynamics. J. Am. Dent. A., 59:682, 1959.
16. Bosma, J. F.: Deglutition: Pharyngeal stage. Physiol. Rev., 37:275, 1957.
17. Boucher, C. O.: Current Clinical Dental Terminology. St. Louis, The C. V. Mosby Co., 1963.
18. Box, H. K.: Twelve Periodontal Studies. Toronto, University of Toronto Press, 1940.
19. Boyle, P. E.: Kronfeld's Histopathology of the Teeth. 4th ed. Philadelphia, Lea & Febiger, 1955.
20. Brewersdorff, H. J.: Electrognathographie. Deutsch. Zahn. M. Kieferhk., 48:99, 1967.
21. Brietner, C.: Alternation of occlusal relations induced by experimental procedures. Am. J. Orthodont., 29:277, 1943.
22. Brill, N., Lammie, G. A., Osborne, J., and Perry, H. T.: Mandibular positions and mandibular movements. Brit. Dent. J., 106:391, 1959.
23. Brill, N., Schübeler, S., and Tryde, G.: Influence of occlusal patterns on movements of the mandible. J. Prosth. Dent., 12:255, 1962.
24. Burstone, C. J., Baldwin, J. J., and Lawless, D. T.: Application of continuous forces of orthodontics. Angle Orthodont., 31:1, 1961.
25. Butler, J. H., and Zander, H. A.: Evaluation of two occlusal concepts. Parodont. Acad. Rev., 2:5, 1968.
26. Coolidge, E. D.: The thickness of the human periodontal membrane. J. Am. Dent. A., 24:1260, 1937.
27. Davenport, H. W.: Physiology of the Digestive Tract. Chicago, Year Book Medical Publishers, 1961.
28. Dempster, W. T., Adams, W. J., and Duddles, R. A.: Arrangement of the roots of the teeth. J. Am. Dent. A., 67:779, 1963.
29. Dempster, W. T., and Duddles, R. A.: Tooth statics: Equilibrium of a freebody. J. Am. Dent. A., 68:652, 1964.

30. Eggleston, W. B., and Echelberry, J. W.: An Electromyographic and Functional Evaluation of Treated Orthodontic Cases. M.S. thesis, University of Michigan, 1961.

31. Gillings, B. R. D., Kohl, J. T., and Zander, H. A.: Contact patterns using miniature radio transmitters. J. Dent. Res., 42:177, 1963.

32. Gillings, B. R. D., Kohl, J. T., and Graf, H.: Study of tooth contact patterns with the use of miniature radio transmitter. Digest, 4th Internat. Conf. on Med. Elect., 1961.

33. Glickman, I., Pameijer, J., Roeber, F., and Brion, M.: Functional occlusion as revealed by miniaturized radio transmitters. Dent. Clin. N. Am., 13:667, 1969.

34. Graf, H., and Zander, H. A.: Tooth contact patterns in mastication. J. Prosth. Dent., 13:1055, 1963.

35. Guichet, N. F.: Applied gnathology: Why and how. Dent. Clin. N. Am., 13:687, 1969.

36. Gustafson, A-G., and Person, P. A.: The relationship between the direction of Sharpey's fibers and the deposition of cementum. Odont. Tidsk., 65:452, 1956.

37. Gysi, A.: The problem of articulation. Dent. Cosmos, 52:1, 1910.

38. Haack, D. C., and Weinstein, S.: Geometry and mechanics as related to tooth movement, studied by means of two-dimensional model. J. Am. Dent. A., 66:157, 1963.

39. Halderson, H., Johns, E. E., and Moyers, R.: Selection of forces for tooth movement. Am. J. Orthodont., 39:25, 1953.

40. Henry, J. L., and Weinman, J. P.: The pattern of resorption and repair of human cementum. J. Am. Dent. A., 42:270, 1951.

41. Hildebrand, G. Y.: Studies in the masticatory movements of the human lower jaw. Skand. Arch. Physiol., 61:190, 1931.

42. Hofmann, V. M.: Zur Oszillographie des gingival Pulses. Deutsche zahnärztl. Ztschr., 19:765, 1964.

43. Hollstein, W.: Untersuchungen über das "Dickenunterscheidungsvermögen" bei natürlichen Zähnen und insbesondere bei festsitzendem und herausnehmbarem abgeslützten Ersatz. Deutsche. Monatsschr. Zahnheilk, 51:385, 1933.

44. Howell, A. H., and Manly, R. S.: An electronic strain gauge for measuring oral forces. J. Dent. Res., 27:705, 1948.

45. Ingervall, B.: Retruded contact position of the mandible. A comparison between children and adults. Odont. Rev., 15:130, 1964.

46. Jankelson, B., Hoffman, G. M., and Hendron, J. A.: Physiology of the stomatognathic system. J. Am. Dent. A., 46:375, 1953.

47. Jenkins, G. N.: The Physiology of the Mouth. Oxford, Blackwell Scientific Publications, 1953.

48. Kawamura, Y., and Watanube, M.: Studies on oral sensory threshold. Med. J. Osaka Univ., 10:291, 1960.

49. Kerr, A. C., Lea, C. S., and Moody, S.: A method of measuring the frequency of swallowing in man. J. Dent. Res., 39:668, 1960.

50. Kraft, E.: Raum und Ordnungsgefühl and Tastsinn in der Mundhöhle. Deutsche zahnärztl. Ztschr., 17:365, 1962.

51. Kronfeld, R.: Histologic study of the influence of function on the human periodontal membrane. J. Am. Dent. A., 18:1242, 1931.

52. Lucia, V. O.: The gnathological concept of articulation. Dent. Clin. N. Amer., 183, March, 1962.

53. Mann, A. W., and Pankey, L. D.: Oral rehabilitation. J. Prosth. Dent., 10:135, 1960.

54. Manly, R. S.: Factors affecting masticatory performance and efficiency among young adults. J. Dent. Res., 30:874, 1951.

55. Manly, R. S., Pfaffman, C., Lathrop, D. D., and Keyser, J.: Oral sensory thresholds of persons with natural and artificial dentitions. J. Dent. Res., 31:305, 1952.

56. Messerman, T., Reswick, J., and Gibbs, C.: Investigation of functional mandibular movements. Dent. Clin. N. Am., 13:629, 1969.

57. Möller, E.: The chewing apparatus. An electromyographic study of the action of the muscles of mastication and its correlation with facial morphology. Acta. Physiol. Scand., 69: Suppl. 28, 1966.

58. Mühlemann, H. R.: Periodontometry, a method for measuring tooth mobility. Oral Surg., 4: 1220, 1951.

59. Mühlemann, H. R.: Ten years of tooth-mobility measurements. J. Periodont., 31:110, 1960.

60. Münch, J. V., and Schriever, H.: Sensibility of teeth to loads in different direction. J. Dent. Res., 26:279, 1947.

61. Nevakari, K.: An analysis of mandibular movement from rest to occlusal position; a roentgenographic-cephalometric investigation. Acta odont. scandinav., *14*:Suppl. 19, 1956.
62. O'Leary, T. J.: An instrument for measuring horizontal tooth mobility. J. Periodont., *1*:249, 1963.
63. O'Leary, T. J.: Tooth mobility. Dent. Clin. N. Am., *13*:567, 1969.
64. O'Leary, T., Rudd, K., Nabers, C., and Stinupf, A.: The effect of mastication and deglutition on tooth mobility. Periodontics, 5:26, 1967.
65. O'Leary, T., Rudd, K., Nabers, C., and Stinupf, A.: The effect of a "tube type" diet and stress-inducing conditions on tooth mobility. J. Periodont., *38*:222, 1967.
66. O'Leary, T., Rudd, K., and Nabers, C.: Factors affecting horizontal tooth mobility. Periodontics, *4*:308, 1966.
67. Parfitt, G. J.: The dynamics of a tooth in function. J. Periodont., *32*:102, 1961.
68. Parfitt, G. J.: Measurement of the physiological mobility of individual teeth in an axial direction. J. Dent. Res., *39*:608, 1960.
69. Picton, D. C. A.: Tilting movements of teeth during biting. Arch. Oral Biol., *7*:151, 1962.
70. Picton, D. C. A.: Some implications of normal tooth mobility during mastication. Arch. Oral Biol., *9*:565, 1964.
71. Pommerenke, W. T.: A study of the sensory areas eliciting the swallowing reflex. Am. J. Physiol., *84*:36, 1928.
72. Posselt, U.: The physiology of mastication. J. West. Soc. Periodont., *9*:40, 1961.
73. Posselt, U.: Studies in the mobility of the human mandible. Acta odont. scandinav., *10*:Suppl. 10, 1952.
74. Powell, R. N.: Tooth Contact during Sleep. Thesis, University of Rochester, 1963.
75. Ramfjord, S. P., and Kohler, C. A.: Periodontal reaction to functional occlusal stress. J. Periodont. *30*:95, 1959.
76. Ramfjord, S. P.: Bruxism, a clinical and electromyographic study. J. Am. Dent. A., *62*:21, 1961.
77. Ramfjord, S. P.: Dysfunctional temporomandibular joint and muscle pain. J. Prosth. Dent., *11*:353, 1961.
78. Ramfjord, S. P., and Hiniker, J. J.: Distal displacement of the mandible in adult rhesus monkeys. J. Prosth. Dent., *16*:491, 1966.
79. Rix, R. E.: Deglutition and the teeth. Dent. Rec., *66*:103, 1946.
80. Schumacker, G. H.: Morphologische und funktionelle Studien an den Kaumuskeln bei verschiedenen Gebissanomalien. Deutsch. Zahn. Mund. Kieferheilk., *39*:272, 1963.
81. Schweitzer, J. M.: Transograph and transographic articulation. J. Prosth. Dent., *7*:595, 1957.
82. Schweitzer, J. M.: Masticatory function in man. J. Prosth. Dent., *11*:625, 1961.
83. Shanahan, T. E. J., and Leff, A.: Mandibular and articular movements. II. Illusion of mandibular tracings. J. Prosth. Dent., *12*:82, 1962.
84. Siirilä, H. S., and Lane, P.: The tactile sensibility of the periodontium to slight axial loadings of the teeth. Acta odont. scandinav., *21*:415, 1963.
85. Tallgren, A.: An electromyographic study of the response of certain facial and jaw muscles to loss of teeth and subsequent complete denture treatment. Odont. Tidsk., *69*:383, 1961.
86. Theil, E.: Bis zu welchem Grade kann die Tastfähigkeit der menschlichen Zahnreihenglieder festgestellt werden? Deut. Monatsschr. f. Zahnh., *49*:270, 1931.
87. Trapozzano, V. R.: Test of balanced and nonbalanced occlusions. J. Prosth. Dent., *10*:476, 1960.
88. Tryde, G., Frydenberg, O., and Brill, N.: An assessment of the tactile sensibility in human teeth. Acta odont. scandinav., *20*:233, 1962.
89. Tulley, W. J.: Methods of recording patterns of behaviour of the oro-facial muscles using the electromyograph. Trans. Brit. Soc. Study Orthodont., 88, 1953.
90. Uhlig, H.: Über die Kaukraft. Deutsche zahnärztl. Ztschr., *8*:30, 1953.
91. Waerhaug, J.: Effect of C-avitaminosis on the supporting structures of the teeth. J. Periodont., *29*:87, 1958.
92. Weinstein, S., Haack, D. C., Morris, L. Y., Snyder, B. B., and Attaway, H. E.: On an equilibrium therapy of tooth position. Angle Orthodont., *33*:1, 1963.
93. Wictorin, L., Hedegaard, B., and Lundberg, M.: Masticatory function. A cineradiographic study. III.—Position of the bolus in individuals with full complement of natural teeth. Acta Odont. Scand., *26*:213, 1968.

Functional Disturbances of the Masticatory System

Functional disturbances of the masticatory system include any disharmony occurring in the functional relationship of the teeth and their supporting structures, the jaws, the temporomandibular joints, the muscles attached to the mandible, the muscles of the lips and tongue, and the vascular and nervous supply of these tissues. Dysfunction may be evidenced by injury to the periodontium or the temporomandibular joints, the teeth, hypertonicity and myalgias of the masticatory muscles, and by injury to the oral mucosa. An understanding of such disturbances is best achieved by first considering bruxism and its relation to neuromuscular disturbances and then the subjects of traumatic occlusion and temporomandibular joint and muscle disturbances. The diagnosis and treatment of bruxism, traumatic occlusion, and temporomandibular joint disturbances will be discussed in Section III, Diagnosis and Treatment of Functional Disturbances of the Masticatory System. An outline of the factors to be considered in functional disturbances follows.

OUTLINE FOR CONSIDERING FUNCTIONAL DISTURBANCES OF THE MASTICATORY SYSTEM

Etiology of Bruxism

ECCENTRIC BRUXISM
CLENCHING OF TEETH (CENTRIC BRUXISM)
OCCLUSAL HABITS RELATED TO BRUXISM
SIGNIFICANCE OF BRUXISM

113

Etiology of Traumatic Occlusion

INITIATING FACTORS
PREDISPOSING FACTORS

Tissue Response to Traumatic Occlusion (Trauma from Occlusion)

HISTOPATHOLOGY OF TRAUMA FROM OCCLUSION
CLINICAL SIGNIFICANCE OF TRAUMA FROM OCCLUSION

Functional Disturbances of Temporomandibular Joints and Muscles

ETIOLOGY
PATHOGENESIS OF FUNCTIONAL TEMPOROMANDIBULAR
  JOINT DISTURBANCES AND RELATED CONDITIONS
OBSERVATIONS RELATED TO DYSFUNCTIONAL
  TEMPOROMANDIBULAR JOINT AND MUSCLE PAIN
HISTOPATHOLOGY OF TRAUMATIC ARTHRITIS AND
  OSTEOARTHRITIS OF THE TEMPOROMANDIBULAR JOINT

CHAPTER 5

ETIOLOGY OF BRUXISM

The term *bruxism* is derived from the French "la bruxomanie," suggested by Marie and Pietkiewicz in 1907.[16] Frohman[8] was probably the first to actually use the word "bruxism" in 1931. Although Karolyi[11] did not use the term "bruxism," he introduced most of the current concepts of this condition in 1901. Bruxism is commonly defined as "a gnashing and grinding of the teeth for nonfunctional purposes" and has been discussed in the dental literature under many other names. The following are some terms that have been used frequently: "neuralgia traumatica" (Karolyi),[12] "Karolyi effect" (Weski), "occlusal habit neurosis" (Tishler)[28] and, most recently, "parafunction" (Drum).[3,4] Miller[17] suggested differentiating between nocturnal grinding of the teeth, which he called bruxism, and habitual grinding of the teeth in the daytime, which he called bruxomania.

The tendency to gnash and grind the teeth in association with anger or aggression has been recognized and described both for animals and humans.[20] Gnashing of the teeth was linked to tense or unhappy circumstances in early historical records, which indicates that bruxism was recognized hundreds of years ago.

A transient tendency to press or clamp the jaws and teeth together briefly in association with an effort to suppress an emotional outburst such as crying, or to express determination, is very common and probably can be considered normal. Thus, nonspecific acute nervous tension and even physical tension of a high degree (lifting or pushing heavy objects or performance of difficult tasks[30]) is often accompanied by clenching of the jaws and the teeth. Such pressing and bracing of the jaws and teeth with emotional stress or physical exertion should not be considered as bruxism; however, persistent and habitual nonfunctional clenching in centric occlusion without obvious emotional tension or need for bracing should be. Nonfunctional grinding and gnashing and clenching in centric occlusion may be of a different significance both to the teeth and the periodontium than eccentric grinding, and the etiology as well as the treatment may sometimes be different. However, these two conditions are so intimately related that it is preferable to designate both as bruxism, i.e., nonfunctional gnashing and grinding in eccentric excursions as *eccentric bruxism,* and clenching in centric as *centric bruxism.*

Both eccentric and centric bruxism are expressions of an increased muscle tonus. Whether eccentric or centric bruxism dominates depends on the location of the occlusal interferences that act as trigger factors for nonfunctional jaw movements. Eccentric bruxism usually has eccentric interferences for trigger factors, while centric bruxism is more often associated with occlusal instability in the immediate vicinity of centric.

It is often said that bruxism in eccentric excursions involves isotonic muscle contractions, while the more static clenching in centric occlusion represents isometric muscle activity. This differentiation is unscientific because clenching commonly involves minute jaw movements and subsequent changes in the length of the involved muscles. Thus, clenching involves both isotonic and isometric muscle activity.

Another group of conditions, closely related to bruxism, is usually classified as occlusal habits rather than bruxism. These conditions are: biting forcefully into a locked malposition of the jaws; lip, tongue and cheek biting; chewing on objects such as fingernails, pencils, pipe stems and bobby pins; pressing on the teeth with the fingers; and many other habits. Although all these habits or conditions have a definite psychogenic background and serve as outlets for emotional tension, they are not usually classified as bruxism and will be considered here as dysfunctional biting or occlusal habits. Finally, nonfunctional occlusal contact movements may be the sequelae of spastic disorders of a systemic nature.

Eccentric Bruxism

Eccentric bruxism has a dual etiologic background of psychic stress and occlusal interference.[22] The psychic component of repressed aggression, emotional tension, anger and fear has been stressed by many writers as the most important or sole factor in the etiology of bruxism. However, Karolyi,[11] at the beginning of this century, recognized the role of occlusal interferences in addition to the psychic factors in the development of bruxism. He stated that even mild occlusal trauma or minor occlusal defects, such as a sharp cusp, could receive undue attention by neurotic individuals and result in grinding habits. A similar observation was made by Tishler[28] nearly 40 years ago. Recently emphasis has been placed on frustration as the main source of emotional tension, and bruxism appears to be very closely related to frustration. Experimental studies by Hutchinson[10] indicate that frustration, when induced in monkeys, very markedly increased their biting activity.

Although a large number of authors have discussed the etiology and nature of bruxism, there has been almost no research beyond clinical observation until recent electromyographic investigations have provided basic information with regards to the neuromuscular phenomena associated with bruxism.[22] Electromyography has made it possible to observe and record in a documentable way neuromuscular disturbances within the masticating system. Much more detailed and accurate observations can be made by this technique than by clinical investigations alone. Of special importance is the fact that electromyography has provided an opportunity to record alterations in basic muscle tension or tonus associated with nervous tension and with pain.[23]

In order to understand the physiologic nature and mechanism of bruxism it is important to have a clear understanding of the neurophysiology of occlusion; therefore, the chapters in Section I should be reviewed prior to reading this explanation of the neuromuscular mechanism of bruxism.

Muscle Tonus

Bruxism is closely related to increased tonus in the jaw muscles. The muscle tonus can be increased by emotional or nervous tension, by pain or discomfort, and by occlusal interferences. An interplay of these three mechanisms provides the neuromuscular basis for bruxism.

The postural or antigravity tonus contractions within the masticatory muscles are dependent upon the myotatic reflex activity, to which is added the gamma efferent or fusimotor activity.[9] The myotatic reflex center is closely related to the control of the conditioned reflex patterns of jaw movements, which have been developed as a result of nervous impulses from the various proprioceptors and sensory nerve endings in the masticatory system. The influence of the central nervous system on muscle tonus is mainly through the fusimotor system. A state of hypertonicity of the masticatory muscles might therefore be due to either (1) central nervous system influence through the fusimotor system, or (2) local disharmony between the functional parts of the masticatory system acting upon the reflex mechanism which controls subconscious jaw movements. Usually, increased tonus and bruxism are the result of disturbances in both these mechanisms.

Physiologic Adaptation. In every individual there is a limit for physiologic adaptation to imperfection or disharmony in occlusal relationships. When this limit is surpassed, either because of increased occlusal disharmony or increased central nervous system tension, a hypertonic response in the masticatory muscles follows. The hypertonic response may be on the basis of facilitation of nervous impulses of occlusal origin and/or lowered threshold of neuron excitability from nervous tension or pain. An increase in neuromuscular activity may lead to injury to the periodontium or the temporomandibular joint, or may produce pain and discomfort within the tense muscles. Such injury or discomfort will result in increased afferent stimuli to the nerve center of the reflex system, with subsequent tendency for increased efferent activity and increased injurious impact.

Relation to Nervous System. Discomfort from occlusal interference or pain may also affect the central nervous system. A statement sometimes heard from a patient is, "This new filling is driving me crazy." Such central nervous system irritation will lower the irritability threshold of the nerve components associated with the reflex controlled jaw movements, as well as increase the muscle tonus through the fusimotor system directly. Fatigue and subsequent pain from sustained contractions within the jaw muscles also will lower the irritability threshold and enter into the unfavorable "feedback" mechanism. This vicious cycle of self-perpetuating increase in muscle tension related to functional disturbances of the teeth, periodontium, oral tissues, temporomandibular joint, and masticatory muscles is the basis for bruxism in persons under psychic or emotional stress.[22] The brain mechanism of simulated bruxism has been studied in rabbits,[18] and lateral jaw movements have been initiated by electric stimulation of various areas of the brain such as the anteromedial cortical area, internal capsule, subthalamus, and the amygdaloid nucleus. However, it is not possible at the present time to relate the significance of these studies to human bruxism.

Myalgia. The hypertonic and sometimes painful status of the jaw muscles in bruxism is of the same nature as the "occupational" myalgias in the arm and neck muscles of typists under mental stress, or the postural myalgias manifested as "backache" in persons under psychic tension who have postural anomalies. The electromyographic similarity is striking when Lundervold's[15] observations on typists are compared with Ramfjord's[22] observations on jaw muscles in patients with bruxism. Forsberg[7] found that of 157 patients with bruxism, 76 per cent had complaints referable to other muscles. Eggen[5] reported that of 136 patients with bruxism and temporomandibular joint disturbances, 37 per cent had undergone previous treatment for occupational myalgias or pain in the back, shoulder, occipit, arms, or legs. In a control group without a history of bruxism, only 6 per cent had a history of previous muscle pain. Using the Cornell Medical Index, Thaller[26] found a correlation between bruxism and the anxiety state of the patient.

In patients with muscle hypertonicity and bruxism, as well as in patients with myalgias, it appears that the normal regulating influence upon muscle activity from proprioceptive and sensory impulses as well as the reflex activity within the muscles are not functioning normally, or may be lacking.[14]

Occlusal Interferences

It has been shown experimentally and observed innumerable times clinically that occlusal interferences may precipitate bruxism. Clinically, it has been found that bruxism can be alleviated or eliminated by correction of occlusal disharmony—at least to the extent that bruxism cannot be recognized by the patient and its effects on the masticatory system are minimized.[22] Of course, bruxism may be induced again at any time by insertion of a restoration with an occlusal interference. Electromyographically, a marked reduction in muscle tonus and harmonious integration of muscle action follows the elimination of occlusal disharmony.

Any type of occlusal interference may, when combined with psychic stress, initiate and maintain bruxism. A discrepancy between centric relation and centric occlusion is the most common trigger factor for bruxism. Electromyographically, such a discrepancy is manifested as asynchronous contractions or sustained strain in the temporal or masseter muscles at one time or another during swallowing. The second most significant occlusal trigger factor for bruxism is occlusal interferences on the balancing side. Although of much less significance than centric and balancing interferences, interferences in working or protrusive excursions may also trigger bruxism.

Some kind of occlusal interference will be found in every patient with bruxism. However, it is often extremely difficult to locate occlusal interferences, especially in the retrusive range between centric occlusion and centric relation in patients with hypertonic jaw muscles and bruxism. This may explain the claim made by several writers that they have observed numerous patients with bruxism who were free of occlusal interferences. Other investigators refuse to accept occlusal disharmony in the retrusive range between centric occlusion and centric relation as occlusal interferences and, since this is the most common cause of bruxism, such an approach would preclude recognition of the most potent occlusal factor in the etiology of bruxism.

Other Factors

There also may be local factors other than occlusal interferences that contribute to hypertonicity of the jaw muscles and initiate abnormal jaw movements. Such conditions are: gingival flaps of third molars; gingival hyperplasia or any type of periodontal disease, especially if pain is present; surface irregularities of the lip, cheek, and tongue; and pain or discomfort in the temporomandibular joint and jaw muscles.

Bruxism is performed on a subconscious reflex controlled level and is, therefore, in most instances, unrecognized by the patient unless it has been called to his attention by someone else. Because of this, it has been difficult to study the prevalence and incidence of bruxism until recently when recording devices were introduced that can record and store information about the activity of the jaw muscles day and night. The most severe bruxism usually occurs at night, but many individuals also gnash their teeth during the daytime when they are under stress. It appears that gnashing or grinding of the teeth is most common during the night, while pressing or clenching is more common in the daytime. However, both these conditions may occur in the daytime as well as during sleep.

In an extensive electromyographic study of 167 patients, Kraft[13] reported that about half the patients were gnashing their teeth during sleep and the others were only biting or pressing them together. The muscle activity during sleep varied greatly from a few contractions to as many as 259 during 8 hours of sleep. The muscle contractions were usually less than 1 second in duration. Only 11 per cent of the patients had sustained, long contractions lasting from 2.5 seconds to 1 minute. The muscle action was distributed fairly evenly throughout the night in 67 per cent of the patients; in the remaining patients most of the action took place just before sleep and after awakening in the morning.

Our emotional life goes on during sleep, often to an exaggerated extent, and is manifested in dreams. It is also well known that the teeth make contact in deglutition during sleep. The swallowing movements are most numerous in the light sleep associated with going to sleep or waking and with movements during sleep. If a person sleeps on his back and brings his teeth together (with swallowing or otherwise), and the jaw is in a retrusive position, the teeth are apt to close to centric relation and trigger bruxism if interferences are present in the retrusive range. When the person sleeps on his side, interferences in lateral excursions will come into initial contact during closure and interferences in these areas may also trigger bruxism. It has been found[21] that bruxism occurs mainly during the second level of sleep (dream state) and is correlated with rapid eye movements, body movements, and increased heart rate.[24] Verbal reports of mental activity in experimental awakening implied no association between bruxism and any specific mental content.[24]

Since bruxism is an expression of combined psychic and occlusal factors, there naturally will be certain times or conditions in an individual's life during which bruxism is more apt to be present. Bruxism may be present on the basis of a severe occlusal interference and a moderate degree of psychic or emotional tension; it can also be the result of very severe psychic stress and very little occlusal interference. The psychic stress often varies greatly from one period to another in a person's life, and it also varies from one situation to another during daily life. Occlusal interferences that are avoided and of no consequence most of the time can assume important dimensions, trigger bruxism, and become very annoying during periods of psychic stress. It is a common observation in student populations that bruxism is much worse during examination periods than other times. Premenstrual tension is another common precipitating factor for cyclic bruxism. The most common daily stress that brings on bruxism is fast driving, especially in heavy traffic. It can be readily observed that stress situations can evoke bruxism only if local trigger factors are present in the occlusion.

Clenching of Teeth (Centric Bruxism)

It already has been stated that clenching of the jaws may be a normal manifestation of generally increased muscle tonus in emotional and psychic stress, or part of a bracing action associated with physical stress or emergency. To draw a definite separation between normal and pathologic clenching of the teeth is sometimes impossible. Abnormal clenching or centric bruxism refers mainly to habitual clenching of the jaw muscles without the presence of any obvious psychic or physical emergency situation. Such habitual tension clenching of the jaw muscles may go on for long periods of time during the waking hours and is probably more common during the day than at night, but it may go on at night, too. Since this clenching is subconscious and without audible sounds, the patient is almost always unconscious of the habit.

Although there are no apparent jaw movements associated with habitual clenching, it is often accompanied by a very slight movement of some teeth. It may also be accompanied by a slight jaw movement from centric position to centric occlusion or elsewhere around centric occlusion. It is extremely difficult, either by occlusal adjustment or by restorative procedures, to establish an absolutely stable occlusal relationship in which every tooth receives exactly the same pressure at exactly the same time when the teeth are brought together. When it is remembered that touching a tooth with a force of 1.5 gm. or less is perceptible (p. 107),[25] and an occlusal discrepancy of 0.02 mm. or less can be perceived,[2] it is understandable how difficult it is to eliminate all "play" factors of uneven touch from the dentition.

Occlusal wear is mainly the result of occlusal contacts. The firmness of these occlusal contacts when the teeth function together depends on the character of the supporting structures of the teeth, the shape of the roots, the crown-root ratio, tooth position, and the hardness of the contacting occlusal surfaces, including restorative materials. All these factors may be slightly mismatched, which would result in some unevenness of occlusal wear and subsequent uneven occlusal contact relationships. This would explain uneven touch as an occlusal trigger factor when the teeth are brought into contact and would place the etiology of clenching on a similar basis as bruxism. This concept can be supported by clinical evidence of a diminished tendency to clench the jaws following very precise occlusal adjustments or the use of acrylic splints, and by electromyographic evidence of decreased muscle tonus following such procedures. However, the evidence for a direct relationship between an occlusal trigger factor and clenching is not so well established as the evidence of a definite relationship between a trigger factor and eccentric gnashing of the teeth. More basic knowledge about muscle tonus and interocclusal space is needed before the entire mechanism of teeth clenching can be understood.

Occlusal Habits Related to Bruxism

Habitual clenching of the jaws in locked malpositions, biting on objects brought into the mouth and lip, tongue and cheek biting are all outlets for emotional and psychic tension. However, these conditions do not necessarily have any association with occlusal disharmony, as is the case in bruxism. The only indirect effect of occlusal interferences upon these conditions is possibly an increase in muscle tonicity; conversely, muscle tonus may be decreased by occlusal therapy and removal of irritating factors from the mouth. Removal of occlusal interferences may, therefore, make it easier to overcome some of these habits; but lip, tongue, cheek and fingernail biting may also be taken up as a substitute outlet for tension when the previous outlet mechanism through bruxism has been eliminated by removal of the occlusal trigger factors. Several of these habits have a typical cyclic occurrence similar to bruxism. The precipitating factors may be overwork, worry, and premenstrual or other tensions having frustration as the common background.

Other occlusal habits may be associated with a person's occupation, viz., biting thread by seamstresses, holding nails between the teeth by upholsterers or carpenters and holding glass between the teeth by glass blowers. In these instances, there is not necessarily either psychic or occlusal disharmony involved in the occlusal habit.

Gnashing or pressing the teeth together may be precipitated by spastic disorders of local or systemic nature. It has been found that removal of occlusal interferences serves to decrease both the incidence and significance of spastic clenching and gnashing and helps in the control of the spastic jaw movements.

SIGNIFICANCE OF BRUXISM

Bruxism may have a significant influence upon the periodontal tissues, teeth, masticatory and/or adjacent muscles, temporomandibular joints,[23] initiation of headache,[1,19] and the irritability of the central nervous system.

Karolyi[11] was the first to postulate that nocturnal contractions of the masseter muscles might be a main factor in the etiology of "pyorrhea." He also emphasized the damaging role of spastic contractions of the lip and tongue muscles to the periodontium and the disturbing effect of such contractions upon the oral comfort of the patient.[12]

Periodontal Tissue Changes

Any tissue changes associated with traumatic occlusion may, of course, be the result of bruxism. However, since these tissue changes are confined mainly to the periodontal tissues apical to the alveolar crest, it is generally believed at the present time that bruxism does not initiate gingivitis or pocket formation. The role of bruxism and associated traumatic occlusion in the etiology of periodontal disease is controversial and not fully understood.

It is emphasized that bruxism does not necessarily lead to pathologic changes in the periodontal tissues. In most individuals with fairly normal periodontal support, the common sequelae of bruxism are compensatory hypertrophy of the periodontal structures, thickening of the alveolar bone, increased trabeculation of the alveolar process, wider than normal periodontal membrane made up of heavy collagenous fibers, and a well-developed fiber attachment to the cementum. The effect of severe bruxism, at least in most younger individuals, closely resembles the adaptive periodontal reaction to heavy function reported in Eskimos and Australian aborigines.

Periodontal Injury. The potential for periodontal injury from bruxism is generally dependent upon the factors that predispose to traumatic occlusion. Thielemann[27] observed that the greatest amount of periodontal damage from bruxism occurred in patients with steep cusps when lateral stress was applied to the tips of these cusps. Stress on the tip of a cusp has a longer arm of leverage than stress applied to the central fossa, and the stress on the cusp is often directed outside the supporting tissues of the tooth. Buccolingual stress is also of greater significance than mesiodistal stress if the teeth have good inter-proximal support from normal contacts. If the stress is placed on a few teeth, either because of loss of teeth or severe occlusal disharmony, the potential for injury from bruxism increases. The same potential for injury is present when there is lost periodontal support resulting from advanced periodontal disease. It is conceivable, although not proved, that bruxism increases the potential for periodontal injury in such systemic conditions affecting the collagenous support of the teeth as scurvy and protein deficiency, especially in young individuals. The significance of bruxism in the cause of periodontal disease depends on whether bruxism results in trauma from occlusion. It is generally thought, al-though not scientifically proved, that trauma from occlusion is a contributing factor in the progress of destructive periodontal disease, and of increasing significance with the advancement of the periodontal destruction.

It has been claimed by Eschler[6] and others that periodontal disease pre-disposes an individual to bruxism by increasing the tonus of jaw muscles. Oral discomfort and movement of the teeth associated with gingival and perio-dontal inflammation may initiate occlusal interferences and thereby provide a "trigger" for bruxism. The increased muscle tonus from the discomfort asso-ciated with the inflammation increases the likelihood for this triggering factor to precipitate bruxism. Under these circumstances, it may be said that perio-dontal disease initiates bruxism.

Crown Damage

Significant damage from bruxism is often greater to the crown of the teeth than to the periodontium. Wearing away of the teeth from bruxism may result in an unsightly reduction in the length of the crown, disturbances in interproxi-mal contact relationships, and may lead to pulpitis, pulp exposure or pulp death. Sharp, irritating enamel margins, fractured teeth or restorations, and even apical strangulation of the pulp are other possible dental sequelae of bruxism.

Dysfunctional Pain

Bruxism is of utmost significance in the occurrence of dysfunctional muscle and temporomandibular joint pain. This relationship will be discussed separately under functional temporomandibular joint and muscle disturbances in Chapter 13.

Headache

It has been shown by Berlin and Dessner[1] and Monica[19] that bruxism may lead to chronic headache. Although the correlation is not entirely clear, it has been postulated by Wolff[29] and others that the basis for the pain or ache is a disturbed circulation in the muscles.

Discomfort from the teeth, muscles, and temporomandibular joints in association with bruxism will often increase psychic tension and irritability, and further increase muscle tonus and bruxism.

REFERENCES

1. Berlin, R., and Dessner, L.: Bruxism and chronic headache. Odont. Tidsk., *68*:261, 1960.
2. Brill, N., Schübeler, S., and Tryde, G.: Aspects of occlusal sense in natural and artificial teeth. J. Prosth. Dent., *12*:123, 1962.
3. Drum, W.: Neue Wege in der sozialen Prothetik. Zahnärtzl. Mitt., *48*:10, and 44, 1960.
4. Drum, W.: Paradentose als Autodestruktions-vorgang und Hinweise für die Prophylaxe. Berliner Artzbl., *71*:300, 1958.
5. Eggen, S.: Nevromuskular spenning som aarsak til kjeveleddslidelser. Norsk Tand. Tidsk., *64*:123, 1954.
6. Eschler, J.: Bruxism and function of the masticatory muscles. Parodontologie, *15*:109, 1961.
7. Forsberg, A.: Parodontalsjukdom som led i ett psykomotorisk syndrom. Sv. Tand. Tidsk., *49*:681, 1956.
8. Frohman, B.: The application of psychotherapy to dental problems. Dent. Cosmos, *73*:1117, 1931.
9. Garnick, J. J., and Ramfjord, S. P.: Rest position. J. Prosth. Dent., *12*:895, 1962.
10. Hutchinson, R., Azrin, N., and Hunt, G.: Attack produced by intermittent reinforcement of a concurrent operant response. J. Comp. Physiol. Psychol., *11*:489, 1968.
11. Karolyi, M.: Beobachtungen über Pyorrhea Alveolaris. Oesterr.-ungar. Vrtljschr. Zahnh., *17*:279, 1901.
12. Karolyi, M.: Zur Therapie der Erkrankungen der Mundschleimhaut. Oesterr.-ungar. Virtljschr. Zahnh., *22*:226, 1906.
13. Kraft, E.: Über eine Untersuchung der menschlichen Kaumuskeltätigkeit während des Nacht-schlafes. Stomatol., *12*:213, 1959, and *13*:7, 1960.
14. Lipke, D., and Posselt, U.: Parafunctions of the masticatory system (bruxism). West Soc. Periodont. J., *8*:133, 1960.
15. Lundervold, A. J. S.: Electromyographic investigations of position and manner of working in typewriting. Acta physiol. scandinav., *24*:Suppl. 84, Oslo, 1951.
16. Marie, M. M., and Pietkiewicz, M., Fils.: La bruxomanie. Rev. de Stomat., *14*:107, 1907.
17. Miller, S. C.: Oral Diagnosis and Treatment Planning. Philadelphia, Blakiston Co., Inc., 1936.
18. Miyoshi, K.: Studies on brain structures concerning bruxism. J. Osaka Univ. Dent. Soc., *13*: 381, 1968.
19. Monica, W. S.: Headaches caused by bruxism. Ann. Otolaryng., *68*:1159, 1959.
20. Nadler, S. C.: Bruxism, a classification: Critical review. J. Am. Dent. A., *54*:615, 1957.
21. Orland, F., and Robinson, J.: Bruxism and its study during the sleep cycle. Inst. Med., Chicago, *25*:319, 1965.
22. Ramfjord, S. P.: Bruxism, a clinical and electromyographic study. J. Am. Dent. A., *62*:21, 1961.
23. Ramfjord, S. P.: Dysfunctional temporomandibular joint and muscle pain. J. Prosth. Dent., *11*:353, 1961.
24. Reding, G., Zepelin, H., Robinson, J., Zimmerman, S., and Smith, V.: Nocturnal teeth-grinding: All-night psychophysiologic studies. J. Dent. Res., *47*:786, 1968.
25. Siirilä, H. S., and Lane, P.: The tactile sensibility of the periodontium to slight axial loadings of the teeth. Acta odont. scandinav., *21*:415, 1963.
26. Thaller, J. L.: Use of the Cornell Index to determine the correlation between bruxism and the anxiety state: A preliminary report. J. Periodont., *31*:138, 1960.
27. Thielemann, K.: Biomechanik der Paradentose insbesondere Artikulationsausgleich durch Einschleifen. 2nd. ed. Munich, J. A. Bartk, 1956.
28. Tishler, B.: Occlusal habit neuroses. Dent. Cosmos, *70*:690, 1928.
29. Wolff, H. G.: The nature and causation of headache. J. Dent. Med., *14*:3, 1959.
30. Yemm, R.: Irrelevant muscle activity. Dent. Pract., *19*:51, 1968.

CHAPTER 6

ETIOLOGY OF TRAUMATIC OCCLUSION AND TRAUMA FROM OCCLUSION

The term "traumatic occlusion" was introduced by Stillman[16,17] in 1917, and later, in 1922, Stillman and McCall[18] stated, "Traumatic occlusion is an abnormal occlusal stress which is capable of producing or has produced an injury to the periodontium." Both the term "traumatic occlusion" and the broad sweeping definition of Stillman and McCall have been criticized for reasons of ambiguity inasmuch as trauma means a wound or injury, and occlusion means the act of closure or state of being closed. Box[3] maintained that the term traumatic occlusion literally means an act of closure or an occlusion which is the sequela of a traumatic injury, e.g., faulty occlusion following the healing of a fractured jaw. He suggested the term "traumatogenic occlusion" to indicate periodontal injury with genesis or origin in the occlusal relations of the teeth.

Other terms used to describe the relationship of occlusal forces to traumatic injury of the periodontium include "occlusal trauma," "occlusal traumatism," "periodontal traumatism," "traumatism," "trauma from occlusion," "dynamic irritation," and "Karolyi effect." "Traumatogenic occlusion" has been used mainly in the Canadian and British literature. "Karolyi effect" has been used extensively in the dental literature of continental Europe in deference to Karolyi,[10] who in 1901 claimed a cause and effect relationship between bruxism and periodontal disease. However, none of these terms is used to any appreciable extent at present.

Admittedly, terms such as "periodontal traumatism" or "trauma from occlusion"[5] are the most correct etymologically, but the term "traumatic occlusion" is so entrenched in the dental literature that it is used in this book as a matter of convenience to indicate an occlusion that produces trauma. The injury itself is called trauma from occlusion.[5] The implication or meaning of "traumatic occlusion" has in most publications been restricted gradually to indicate an occlusal–periodontal relationship in which evidence of traumatic injury is present. The potential for traumatic injury often cannot be assessed, and it is not logical to make the diagnosis of an injury just because some predisposing factors are present.

Trauma from occlusion is often classified as either primary or secondary. Primary trauma from occlusion refers to the effect of abnormal forces acting upon basically normal periodontal structures, while secondary traumatic occlusion refers to the effect on already reduced or weakened periodontal structures by occlusal forces which may or may not be abnormal but are excessive for reduced or weakened supporting structures. A more recent trend[20] is to include in the term trauma from occlusion, or occlusal trauma, injury to any part of the masticatory system resulting from abnormal occlusal contact relations and/or abnormal function of the masticatory system. Trauma from occlusion thus may be manifest in the periodontium, hard structures of the teeth, pulp, temporomandibular joints, soft tissues of the mouth, and the neuromuscular system.

INITIATING FACTORS

When the masticatory system is functioning under normal conditions, the reflex controlled neuromuscular mechanism will protect its parts from traumatic injury as explained under Physiology of Occlusion, Chapter 4. This normal protective mechanism has to be disturbed in order for trauma from occlusion to develop. Since the source of traumatic force in traumatic occlusion is the muscles of the jaws, it is rational to consider neuromuscular disturbances and traumatic forces as a major factor in the cause of trauma from occlusion.

Neuromuscular Disturbances and Traumatic Forces

Electromyographic studies by Moyers,[11] Perry and Harris,[12] and others[9] all indicate that individuals with malocclusion or occlusal interferences have an asynchronous contraction pattern of the masticatory muscles. Furthermore, occlusal interferences have the potential to increase muscle activity at rest and between functional occlusal contacts, and also to increase the magnitude and frequency of the contractions of the jaw muscles.[14]

Movements of the jaw are initiated when a certain number of motor units come into action; but when occlusal interferences are touched, an inhibition of the normal reflex action occurs from the untimely and disorganized excitation of proprioceptors or sensory endings within the periodontal membrane of the involved teeth. Under such conditions a continuous effort is made by the reflex controlled nerve centers to establish a compromise pattern of occlusal contacts to avoid or minimize irritation and injury to the various tissues of the masticatory system. Inasmuch as the excitability thresholds for the neurons which govern occlusal contact movements on a reflex basis are variable, impulses both of peripheral and central origin may, augmented by facilitation in nerve conduction, elicit what seems to constitute a widely exaggerated contraction of the jaw muscles. This phenomenon of aberrant contraction occurs in association with local discomfort or pain and with general stress and nervous or emotional tension.

Hypertonicity and disorganized contraction patterns of the masticatory muscles provide the basis for bruxism, in which occlusal interferences in the presence of nervous tension act as triggers for abnormal muscle activity.[14] A combination of an abnormally strong and asynchronous contraction pattern may, for instance, initiate heavy contractions of the masseter muscles before proper positioning of the mandible by the temporal muscles has been completed. This type of asynchronous contraction pattern may result in forces that are unfavorably directed and located upon the contacting teeth and their supporting structures.

The threshold for proprioception and sense of touch may be lowered easily by the numbing action of abnormally heavy and long-lasting pressure associated with bruxism or clenching. This means that the protective reflexes based on proprioception and touch within the masticatory system are not operating normally. The reduced periodontal sensitivity to touch and pain, combined with an abnormally increased activity of the jaw muscles, may conceivably lead to injury to the periodontal structures. However, more important probably is that bruxism is not governed by the same neuromuscular principles of protective reflexes that prevent trauma from occlusion from occurring during normal function. With bruxism occlusal interferences are sought out and force applied as an outlet for nervous tension. Pain seems to attract more application of force rather than avoidance of the interferences. Thus the dysfunctional action of bruxism has been called autodestruction,[4] and this mechanism is by far the most common origin of trauma from occlusion to any part of the masticatory system.

Only a small fraction of the potential capacity of the masticatory muscles is used for mastication of food and bracing the jaw during swallowing (usually less than 25 pounds pressure compared to a maximum biting force of 200 to 300 pounds).[1] In bruxism there is an abnormal increase in magnitude, frequency and duration of the occlusal force. The impact of the bruxing force in eccentric bruxism is to a much greater degree directed horizontally than the impact of normal masticatory forces. Furthermore, the attack point of the bruxing force is often close to the incisal edge or cusp tip, where the potential for traumatic injury to the periodontium is much greater than from forces centrally applied and in the direction of the long axis of the teeth.

When all the factors are considered, it is easy to understand the prominent role usually ascribed to bruxism in the pathogenesis of trauma from occlusion, especially the primary type of trauma from occlusion. It is generally conceded that trauma from occlusion is seldom, if ever, the result of masticatory forces in an intact dentition with adequate periodontal support; rather, such injury is an indication of dysfunctional forces that are usually associated with bruxism or other pernicious habits. It must be emphasized that bruxism will strengthen rather than weaken the periodontal structures in most instances, especially if the habit is started in young individuals with adequate periodontal support.

The diagnosis of bruxism does not, by any means, presuppose a diagnosis of trauma from occlusion, although the abnormal forces associated with bruxism provide a hazard for traumatic injury and necessitate a very careful appraisal of the supporting structures of the teeth.

Trauma from occlusion may occur as the result of a number of unfavorable occlusal and periodontal conditions combined with increased muscular tonus and varying degrees of emotional stress. The presence of trauma from occlusion indicates that the adaptive capacity of the masticatory system has been exceeded; in the final analysis, whether this capacity is exceeded depends on how a person has been able to adapt, adjust and live with his occlusion. The adaptive capacity must be significant since primary trauma from occlusion is uncommon and very few individuals have ideal occlusal relations. Trauma from occlusion may be the result of severe occlusal disharmony and a moderate amount of psychic tension, as well as severe psychic disharmony and minor occlusal discrepancies.

PREDISPOSING FACTORS

There are many dysfunctional factors of the masticatory system that predispose to trauma from occlusion. One such factor, bruxism, has already been discussed. (See also Chapter 5.) Trauma from occlusion does not necessarily or usually result from the presence of predisposing factors unless the occlusal forces exceed the adaptive responses or resistance of the supporting tissues. In most instances, even though predisposing factors are present, the protective response of the neuromuscular system and the resistance of the supporting tissues prevent trauma from occlusion from occurring. Even so, the recognition of predisposing factors and their role in the etiology of trauma from occlusion is important in the treatment of trauma from occlusion and periodontal disease.

Malocclusion

Malocclusion has been defined as any deviation from normal occlusion (both from the morphologic and functional standpoint). Malocclusion also refers to an unstable occlusion resulting from unbalanced counteracting forces of mastication and bruxism, and the forces of tongue and lip pressure. In such instances, the teeth may be moved in one direction by occlusal forces and in another direction by lip or tongue pressure ("jiggling of the teeth"). The result of such movement is hypermobility of the teeth and trauma from occlusion (Fig. 6–1).

In other instances, an individual's occlusion may show significant deviations from orthodontic standards of normal occlusion and still enjoy excellent function with no evidence of injury to the periodontal structures. Although combined periodontal and neuromuscular adaptation may have established convenience patterns of occlusal movement with no obvious ill effect to the masticatory system, malocclusion will, in most instances, complicate and restrict the occlusal movement patterns. Even though a patient has a useful convenience pattern, the

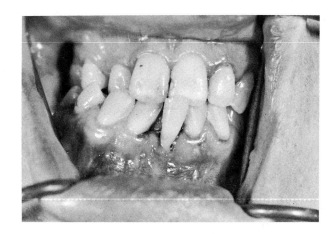

Figure 6–1. Mandibular incisor in labial version being pushed outward by occlusal forces and lingually by lip pressure when the mandible is in rest position. This tooth is loose and had advanced bone loss associated with deep pockets. No other teeth had periodontal pockets in spite of the malocclusion in other areas of the mouth. The patient has adapted to the malocclusion and developed a masticatory pattern that allows for stability of the other teeth. However, "jiggling" of the central incisor cannot be avoided, since this tooth cannot wear or move out of traumatic occlusion.

presence of occlusal interferences in unused ranges represents complicating factors for the neuromuscular system which, when combined with psychic tension, have a tendency to induce hypertonicity and abnormal muscular forces that may subsequently lead to trauma from occlusion.

Occlusion should always be evaluated on the basis of functional potential rather than simply on the basis of the common morphologic classifications often used in orthodontics. For instance, a cross bite may represent optimal functional occlusal relationships in a person with a small maxilla and a large mandible. The absence of pathologic manifestations and the presence of unhindered functional movements are factors which are of much greater importance in the evaluation of occlusion than the standard of cuspal interdigitation used as a basis for the diagnosis of malocclusion. Morphologic and static classifications of malocclusion have a much greater esthetic than functional significance.

Occlusal–Temporomandibular Joint Disharmony

As already discussed, according to Hanau's[6] classic concept of occlusion there are five basic factors which have to be correlated in any analysis of occlusal interrelationships: inclination of condylar guidance, prominence of compensating curve or curve of Spee, inclination of plane of occlusion, cusp height or steepness of functional cuspal inclines, and inclination of incisal guidance. Obviously, the numerical values for any of these factors depend upon reference planes. The relationship between the five basic factors has been expressed in Hanau's and, later, Thielemann's[19] formula. These formulas connot be used for mathematical evaluation of the relationship between the various factors governing occlusion in individual cases since so many of the factors can be given only relative values because of a lack of established methods and standards for their quantitative assessment. The formulas are therefore used as an expression of the relative interrelationship of the five basic factors governing occlusion.

Disharmony of the relationship between the occlusion and the temporomandibular joints may originate from unsatisfactory relationship in two or more of the complex groups of basic factors which govern occlusal relations, or from disharmony between the separate units which make up for the complex factors (for instance, variations of cuspal inclination of teeth within the same dentition, variation in prominence of the curve of Spee from one side of the mouth to the other, etc.). Although minor occlusal discrepancies commonly are present when the teeth reach their initial contact in the plane of occlusion, function and normal attrition combined with adaptive repositioning of the teeth should lead to harmonious occlusal relationships. Unfortunately, the soft diets used in many parts of the world today are not conducive to such adaptive wear, and some occlusal disharmony is almost universally present in dentitions with little or no evidence of occlusal wear. However, occlusal disharmony is not by any means synonymous with trauma from occlusion, since a combination of neuromuscular adaptation and periodontal resistance may compensate for the occlusal irregularities. The significance of occlusal irregularities in the etiology of abnormal muscle contractions has already been presented in Chapter 4.

Restricted or Unilateral Patterns of Mastication

The two main guiding factors in the development of habitual patterns of masticatory movements are convenience of function and avoidance of pain. With the common occurrence of occlusal interferences and the lack of functional demand upon the masticatory system, one will often see a unilateral or restricted convenience pattern of mastication. A unilateral pattern of mastication may originate at the time the teeth erupt and reach occlusal contact, as a result of occlusal interferences and subsequent lack of attrition of the occlusal surfaces; or it may be caused by pulpal or gingival pain later in life. Occlusal irregularities associated with a loss of teeth, movement of teeth by habits or orthodontic therapy, and improper dental procedures may induce unilateral mastication.

The unfavorable sequelae of unilateral mastication have been discussed by Beyron,[2] who pointed out the tendency to develop increasingly severe occlusal disharmony from uneven occlusal wear. Furthermore, calculus and plaques tend to accumulate much more on the nonfunctional than on the functional side, and thus jeopardize the periodontal health of the nonfunctioning teeth. It is also likely, although not proved by controlled experimentation, that tissue metabolism and resistance to local irritation are enhanced by normal function.

Loss of Teeth

A loss of deciduous molars without use of space retaining appliances and the extraction of permanent teeth without replacement are common causes of occlusal disharmony.[7] The classical example of occlusal disharmony following the loss of teeth may be observed in the undesirable sequelae to the masticatory system following the loss of the mandibular first molar (Fig. 6–2, *A*). A few of the most common sequelae include: lingual and mesial tipping of the lower second and third molars; extrusion of the maxillary first molar; and protrusion of the anterior segment of the maxillary arch with opening of the contacts between the mandibular first and second bicuspids, especially in patients with deep overbite. In longstanding cases it is common to see resorption of bone around the maxillary molars and the anterior teeth.

Several of the sequelae of extraction of a mandibular first molar have been attributed to a loss of vertical dimension or so-called "collapse of the bite." It is likely that the open contacts in the maxillary anterior teeth are caused by tipping of the posterior teeth, with an increased slide in centric hitting the front teeth, and by abnormal occlusal relations that have induced a change of masticatory habits and muscle tonicity as well as loss of vertical dimension. Open contacts in the maxillary anterior region will often close following occlusal adjustment and replacement of the missing teeth without attempt to change the vertical dimension (Fig. 6–2, B-D). No long term study under controlled conditions has been reported with regards to changes in vertical dimension following a loss of first molars.

Tipping of the mandibular second and third molars will result in an unfavorable direction of the major occlusal stress upon the maxillary molars in centric occlusion. Tipped molars often engage in balancing interferences between the distobuccal cusps on the mandibular molars and the lingual cusps of the maxillary molars (Fig. 6–3).

Other sequelae resulting from the loss of mandibular first molars such as food impaction,[7] open contacts, uneven marginal ridges, and lack of functional cleansing of the teeth during mastication are not directly related to traumatic occlusion and will not be discussed in detail here.

Another example of far-reaching consequences to the dentition resulting from the loss of a single tooth without replacement may be seen following the extraction of a mandibular incisor in an attempt to relieve crowding of mandibular anterior teeth (Fig. 6–4). The factors that were active in the crowding of the mandibular incisors will be exaggerated by this loss in the continuity of the arch. Such extraction will, therefore, be followed by further lingual tipping of mandibular cuspids and bicuspids, followed by narrowing of the maxillary arch in the bicuspid region, subsequent buckling in the anterior segment of the maxillary arch, and often labial overlapping of central incisors by the lateral incisors. The lingual movement of the mandibular anterior teeth leads to a loss of centric stops, some extrusion of the mandibular and maxillary anterior teeth, and an increase in the amount of overbite. As the maxillary lateral incisors move labially and overlap the maxillary incisors, they will engage the lip more heavily than before. The lip pressure will be transmitted to the maxillary central incisors as a lingual thrust which will persist until contact has been established between the maxillary and mandibular incisors. As a consequence of these changes there develops not only an increase in overbite but also a steeper incisal guidance than before that results in an additional tendency for occlusal interference in lateral and protrusive excursions.

The loss of any functional tooth within the occlusal arrangement will have a tendency to create a disturbance in occlusal relations between the remaining teeth. The effect of the loss is not restricted to the area in the immediate vicinity of the lost tooth or teeth, but changes may be observed in distant areas of the

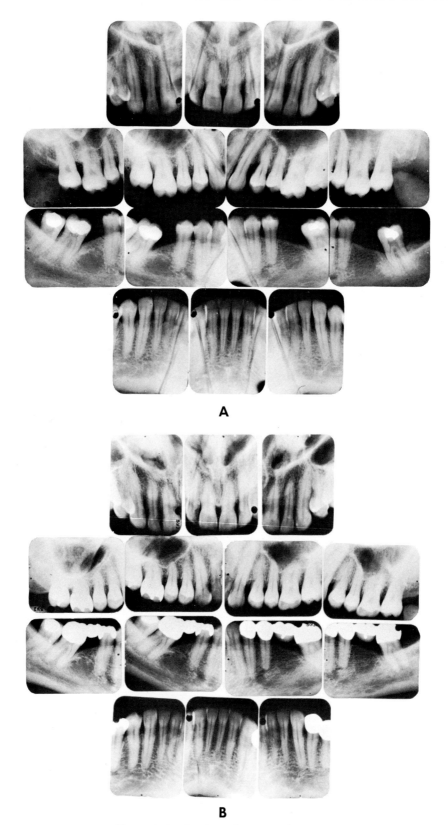

A

B

Figure 6–2. See legend on opposite page.

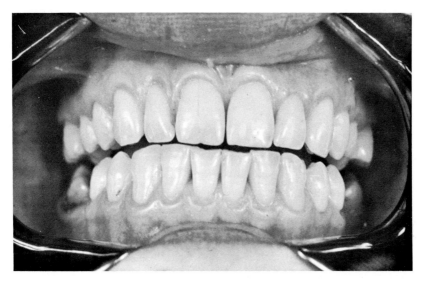

C

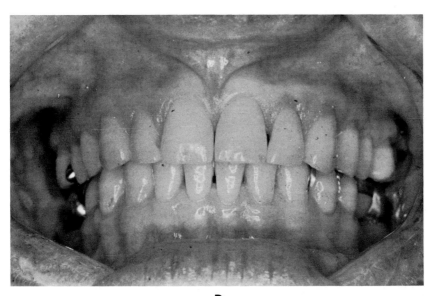

D

Figure 6–2. The effects of the loss of mandibular first molars at the age of 14. *A,* At the age of 33 there is tipping of mandibular molars, hypereruption of maxillary molars, open contact, hypermobility and bone loss in the maxillary anterior segment. *B,* After treatment, including elimination of slide in centric by occlusal adjustment, periodontal surgery, and replacement of the lost molars by fixed bridges, but without alteration of vertical dimension. *C,* Clinical picture prior to treatment. *D,* Clinical picture 14 years after treatment. Note closed contacts of anterior teeth and cured periodontal disease.

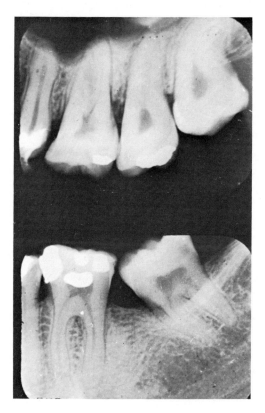

Figure 6-3. The effects of tipped molar and restricted chewing. The maxillary second molar was tender to contact and hypermobile due to loss of lamina dura around the entire tooth. A cavity in the maxillary second bicuspid forced the patient to chew on the opposite side. This restriction of chewing resulted in a severe balancing interference between the maxillary second molar and the tipped mandibular third molar. The interfering forces are more axially directed and less traumatic for the mandibular than for the maxillary tooth.

dentition (Fig. 6–5). This effect has been described by Thielemann[19] and is commonly referred to as Thielemann's diagonal law: "If an interference such as a hypererupted or tipped tooth, third molar gum flaps, etc., restricts the functional gliding movement of the mandible, elongation of the anterior teeth, and often periodontal disease will develop in the anterior region diagonally opposite to the interference." Such extrusion of the anterior maxillary teeth will occur only if these teeth do not have a well-defined cingulum or worn-in centric stop on

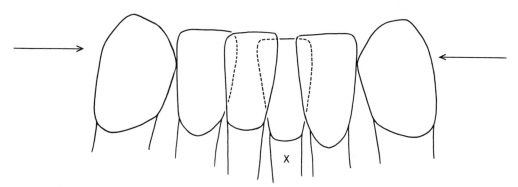

Figure 6-4. Line drawing to illustrate the effects of the extraction of a mandibular central incisor in an attempt to treat anterior crowding of the tooth. The extraction of tooth marked "X" would allow further tipping mesially and lingually of the remaining mandibular anterior teeth and lead to eruption and crowding of the maxillary incisors.

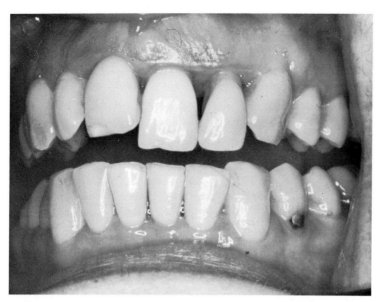

Figure 6-5. Hypereruption of maxillary central and lateral incisors subsequent to loss of third maxillary molar and hypereruption of mandibular third molars on the opposite side with restriction of masticatory pattern.

the lingual aspect of the maxillary anterior teeth. Periodontal disease will often develop in the most distal maxillary molar under these conditions associated with occlusal interferences in the molar regions (Fig. 6–6). The extrusion of the anterior teeth is probably due to the development of a restricted masticatory pattern caused by the molar interference. The extrusion of the anterior teeth resulting from unilateral mastication is, in part, relative since these teeth do not wear as much as the teeth that are maintaining functional contact. As explained previously, the maxillary molars are much more vulnerable to traumatic occlusion following tipping of mandibular molars than the mandibular molars since the main occlusal forces maintain more of an axial direction in the mandible than in the maxilla. A common source of trauma from occlusion is loss of several posterior teeth with a tendency for closure of vertical dimension and an inevitable forward movement of the mandible as it is closing on a hinge path determined by such unyielding structures as the temporomandibular joints. This sequence of events may lead to trauma from occlusion in the maxillary anterior segment as well as for the few remaining posterior teeth. The latter teeth have the burden of maintaining vertical dimension. Such a situation may also lead to impinging trauma to soft tissues.

The dynamics of occlusal forces following extraction of teeth merits a very careful study in each individual case. Occasionally, the occlusion may be so balanced that the changes that have been described will not occur. In other instances, the effects of lost teeth may, after some years, become stabilized and compensated for by rearrangement of the occlusal relations to a point where the occlusion is no longer traumatic.

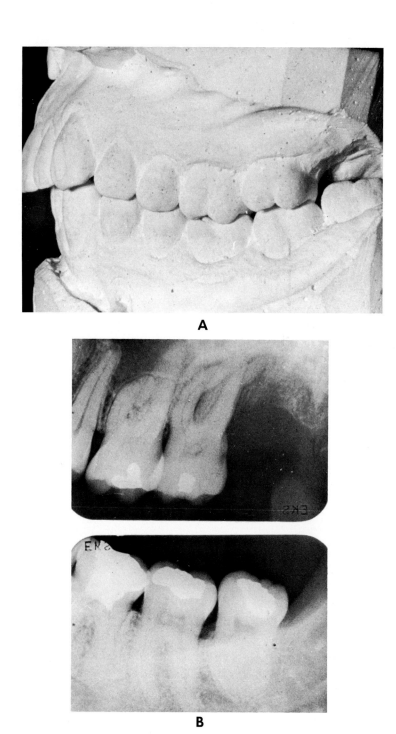

A

B

Figure 6–6.   *A,* Loss of maxillary third molar and hypereruption of mandibular third molar. *B,* Roentgenograms showing the extensive bone loss around the maxillary second molar.

Loss of Periodontal Support

A loss of periodontal support, inadequate periodontal structures following the loss of teeth, or weakened tissue tolerance often leads to secondary traumatic occlusion without any changes in the occlusion or in the nature of the occlusal forces. Secondary trauma from occlusion may be precipitated by heavy normal or even subnormal occlusal forces, depending upon the degree of weakening or inability of the periodontal tissues to withstand such forces.

The periodontium is a functional organ and, like other functional organs of the body, its maximal functional capacity is not needed in normal function. The teeth can carry out normal functions even after a rather large part of the periodontium has been lost; however, when enough advanced loss of periodontal support has occurred, normal functional activity will result in traumatic injury to the periodontium even with the most ideal occlusal relations. Every patient with far advanced periodontal disease will eventually reach a stage where biting through a sandwich or even occlusal contact with swallowing may produce traumatic injury to inadequate residual periodontal structures (Fig. 6-7).

The leverage ratio between the unsupported and the supported part of the tooth will increase with a loss of periodontal support. Besides the obvious increase in length of the active leverage in lateral excursion, the impact of the

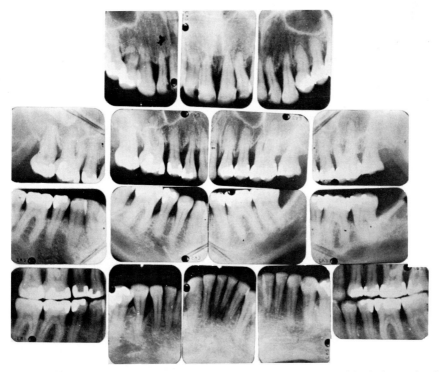

Figure 6-7. Advanced periodontitis and traumatic occlusion aggravated by faulty occlusal adjustment (grinding off incisal edges of mandibular incisors). The patient complained of pain associated with the mastication of tough food.

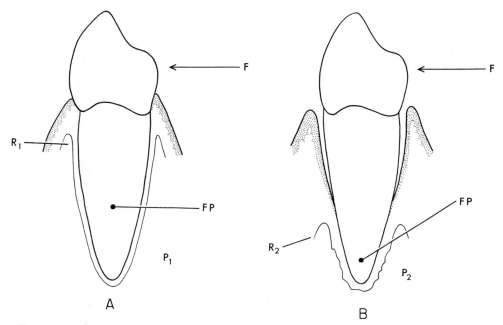

Figure 6-8. Increased tendency for trauma from occlusion with loss of periodontal support. FP, fulcrum point; F, direction of force; R_1R_2 and P_1P_2, areas of resorption and pressure, respectively.

force will also be concentrated over a smaller and smaller area as periodontal support is lost (Fig. 6-8). Destructive periodontal disease may, therefore, eventually reach a stage where trauma from occlusion will accompany functional activity, although the occlusal relationships and the functional forces are unaltered. It is often exceedingly difficult to decide whether teeth have adequate periodontal support for normal functional activity in patients with advanced periodontal disease. This cannot be determined on the basis of a mathematical formula since biologic factors of tissue reaction and psychic alterations of muscle tonus with subsequent change of occlusal force cannot be assessed in terms of reliable figures.

Periodontal support may also be reduced significantly by the loss of several or all posterior teeth. Under such circumstances normal force of occlusal closure in mastication and swallowing will be distributed over only a few teeth and often in an unfavorable direction. Functional relationships often are unfavorable when only a few teeth are present for mastication. This may require distorted neuromuscular manipulations of the jaws in attempts to achieve a semblance of function. Such disturbed functional relationships resulting from loss of teeth increase the potential for trauma from occlusion.

Dental Caries

Occlusal caries may undermine and eliminate areas of occlusal stops in centric occlusion. Such a loss of centric stops may allow for eruption or tipping of the teeth with subsequent occlusal interference in lateral excursions (Fig.

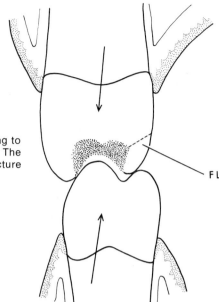

Figure 6-9. Loss of centric stop due to caries leading to eruption of tooth and interference in lateral excursion. The dotted line across lingual cusp indicates tendency for fracture of the cusp.

6-9). Interproximal caries may alter the position of the teeth due to a loss of interproximal contact, altering occlusal relations with the possibility of occlusal interferences. Pain from caries may occur in the preferred path of occlusal movements and force the patient to chew into an area of occlusal interferences since pain takes precedence over convenience in determining the pattern of occlusal movement. Furthermore, pain will tend to increase the tonicity of the masticatory muscles and, therefore, predispose to abnormal muscle contraction, with the potential for injury to the periodontal tissues.

Faulty Dental Restorations and Appliances

A major goal of restorative dentistry is to design and construct dental restorations in harmony with the guiding factors of the masticatory system. This goal should be accomplished by providing for the transfer of functional occlusal forces to the remaining teeth and their surrounding structures with assurance that the forces are within the physiologic tolerance level of these structures. Transient trauma from occlusion is commonly associated with newly placed dental restorations and appliances, but these transient forces are usually alleviated when the tooth has been repositioned or the restorations worn down to the point where occlusal harmony has been re-established. However, if the involved tooth cannot reach a stable, harmonious occlusal relationship, chronic trauma from occlusion will ensue. For example, faulty carving of occlusal amalgam restorations and failure to allow for some eruption may subsequently lead to occlusal interferences on the cuspal inclines in lateral excursions (Fig. 15–5). Also, teeth with thick maxillary anterior three-quarter crowns may be pushed out of position by the occlusion and lingually by the lip when the mandible is assuming rest position. If the entire dentition is present, the potential for adaptive movement of a tooth to a stable position without interference is greater in the buccolingual direction than it is in the mesiodistal direction. In order for mesiodistal movement to occur in the presence of interproximal contacts, very extensive reorganization of the teeth would be required to eliminate interference by tooth movement.

The common result of occlusal interferences, regardless of the source, is increased muscle tonus in the jaw muscles and the introduction of abnormal occlusal forces. For instance, a faulty marginal ridge on a single occlusal inlay (Fig. 6–10) may significantly alter the direction of occlusal forces during swallowing, not only on the involved tooth, but on the rest of the teeth and the other components of the masticatory system such as the temporomandibular joints and the muscles. A slide in centric induced by occlusal interferences may get worse instead of better as time goes by, due to spreading of the maxillary incisors, and may thereby increase the magnitude of the slide. The teeth that receive the impact of a slide from centric relation to centric occlusion often are exposed to a much stronger and more traumatic force than the posterior tooth with the premature contacts; the posterior teeth are often supported in a mesiodistal direction by interproximal contacts. In addition, there will be an increase in muscle discomfort, the development of muscle spasms, and an ever-increasing slide in centric perpetuated by the increasing magnitude of occlusal force. Thus, in a relatively short time, the occlusal relations of all the teeth may change to a great extent and induce muscle spasms and temporomandibular joint pain. If not remedied, these types of occlusal disturbances become extremely difficult to correct.

Uneven wear of occlusal surfaces resulting from uneven hardness of the teeth, restorations, or both, may also induce traumatic occlusion. For instance, an MOD amalgam restoration that is poorly condensed will predispose to greater wear of the amalgam than the adjacent cuspal enamel and thus may induce excessive stress and fracture of these cusps, especially in patients with a tendency for bruxism.

The potential for periodontal and dental adaptation to minor occlusal discrepancies is greater in single-rooted than in multirooted teeth. In cases of large fixed bridges with multiple abutments, there is only minimal potential for occlusal harmony being achieved by adaptive tooth movement. The dental restorations that most often lead to traumatic occlusion are free-end saddle partial dentures (Fig. 6–11) and cantilever bridges (Fig. 6–12); often, perfectly healthy periodontal tissues are gradually destroyed by such appliances.

Another example of a traumatic and unstable occlusion is seen where there is an inadequate overjet related to a deep overbite in a patient with bruxism (Fig. 6–13). The maxillary anterior teeth are moved labially, resulting in a loss of the centric stops of the mandibular incisors. With the loss of centric stops there is subsequent extrusion of the mandibular incisors and the development of interferences in lateral and protrusive excursions of the mandible.

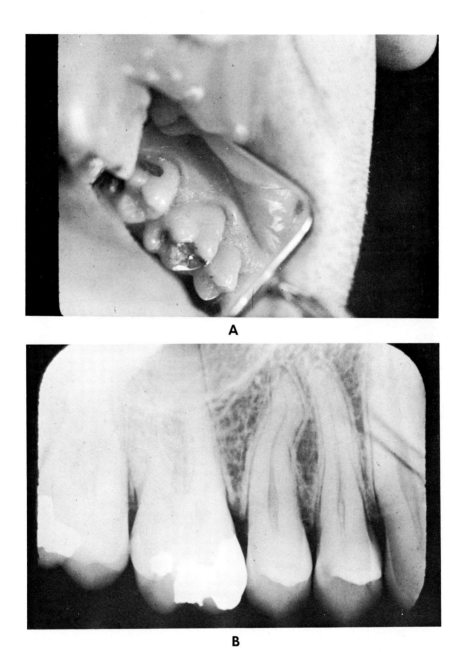

A

B

Figure 6–10. *A,* High marginal ridge on mesial restoration of a maxillary first molar. *B,* The most traumatic effect, clinically and radiographically, is on the mesial aspect of the second bicuspid from the impact of a slide in centric induced by the inlay on the molar.

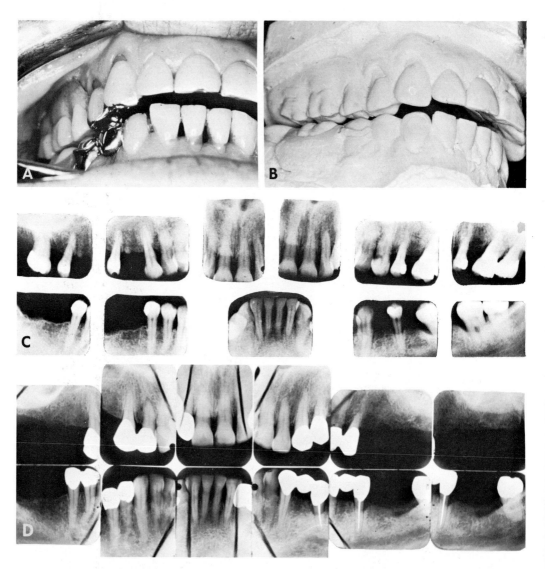

Figure 6–11. *A* and *B,* Faulty occlusion on clasped mandibular and precision attachment maxillary partial dentures. The pictures are taken with the mandible in centric relation. In centric occlusion all of the teeth make even contact. *C,* Before treatment. *D,* Two years after treatment, extensive additional bone loss on right side in spite of splinting of abutment teeth. Intrabony periodontal pockets also have developed around these abutment bicuspids. The left side was not touching in centric relation and shows no additional bone loss. Radiograph viewed from lingual aspect.

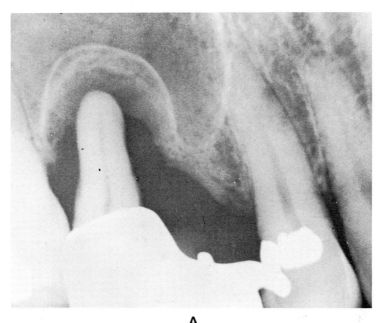

A

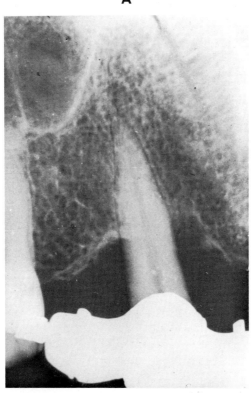

B

Figure 6-12.   *A* and *B*, Cantilever bridges with extensive bone loss.

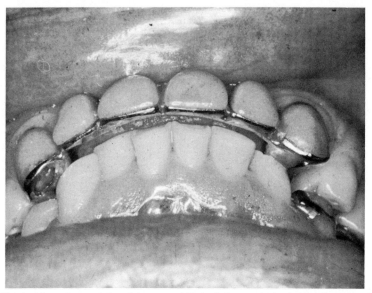

Figure 6-13. Inadequate overjet and deep overbite built into anterior bridge for esthetic reasons. The patient had severe bruxism and drove the bridge labially, resulting in loss of occlusal support for the mandibular incisors and leading to hypereruption of these teeth. Thus, these conditions resulted in a sequence of continuous interferences and hypereruption of the incisors.

Faulty Orthodontic Therapy

The unavoidable transient trauma associated with orthodontic procedures is usually of minor significance if normal periodontal conditions can be established following the orthodontic therapy. To be discussed here is the orthodontic tooth movement that is a source of chronic traumatic occlusion resulting from an unsolved conflict after treatment between functional and morphologic or esthetic requirements. Any tooth that is placed in an unharmonious position (where its occlusal surfaces do not fit into the optimal pattern of occlusal movements for the patient) tends to challenge the neuromuscular system to move the tooth into a harmonious position. Even so, orthodontic retainers are often used to maintain a tooth in a desired orthodontic position in spite of occlusal interference (Fig. 6-14). A functionally inadequate result is sometimes obtained in that occlusal interferences are avoided through the establishment of a restricted pattern of movement. Such a restricted, and often times unilateral, function is an undesirable end result of any dental therapy. When there is a tendency for bruxism, such a result will not prove stable unless the bruxism serves to wear away the occlusal interference while the retainers are still being worn.

An example of posttreatment occlusal problems can be found in malocclusion Class II Division I. In such cases the incisal guidance is commonly made steeper by lingual movement of the maxillary anterior teeth and the cuspal inclination made less steep by the expansion of the maxillary arch in the bicuspid region. Although bodily movement of the teeth is attempted, quite often

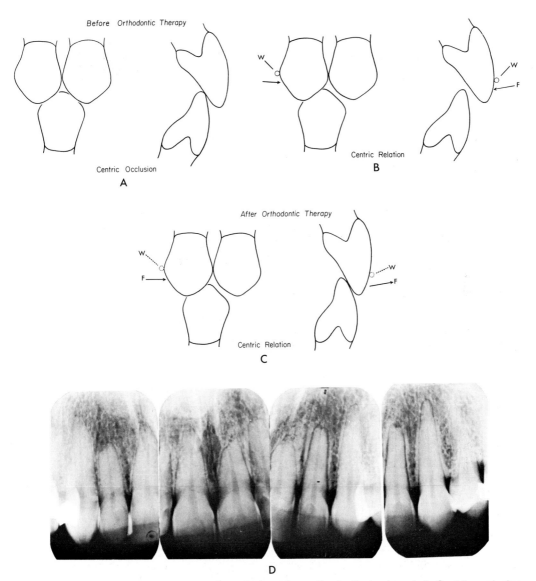

Figure 6–14. Unstable and traumatic occlusion after orthodontic treatment. *A,* Centric occlusion before treatment. *B,* Centric relation before treatment. *C,* After anterior teeth have been moved lingually by Hawley appliance or retainer with reciprocal action within the arch. Biting will force maxillary anterior teeth labially, while the labial arch wire will move them lingually, setting up a "jiggling" action. This is a common source of relapse of diastemas between maxillary anterior teeth following orthodontic treatment. *D,* Roentgenograms of traumatic root resorption following such faulty orthodontic treatment.

some buccal tipping of the teeth occurs. After the maxillary and mandibular front teeth have been brought into contact, the new, relatively steep, incisal guidance may cause interference in the anterior region when the patient attempts to make lateral jaw movements.

Another example of perpetual trauma from occlusion associated with orthodontic therapy occurs in adult patients when attempts are made to extrude molars and bicuspids while anterior teeth are being intruded by a bite plane or

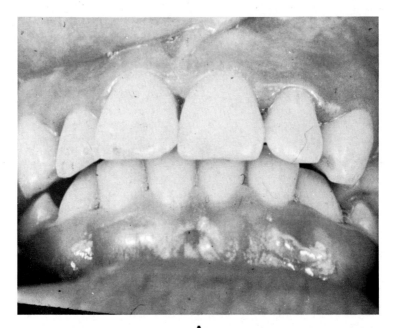

A

B

Figure 6-15. After four years of orthodontic treatment in female, age 23. *A,* The functional and esthetic result in centric occlusion appeared to be good, but the patient had severe temporomandibular joint and muscular discomfort. *B,* In centric relation the mandible moves laterally from centric occlusion. This lateral shift or slide from centric relation to centric occlusion was not tolerated by this patient and had to be eliminated before her symptoms subsided.

similar appliance. Patients are sometimes told to wear the appliances at night for an indefinite period of time. This type of therapy will produce a state of perpetual traumatic occlusion, i.e., intrusion of the anterior teeth and extrusion of molars and bicuspids in the nighttime, and extrusion of anterior teeth and intrusion of molars and bicuspids in the daytime. All dental therapy should have as its goal a stable occlusion at the end of the treatment; any compromise solution short of that goal may result in traumatic occlusion.

A great challenge in orthodontics, as well as in restorative or prosthetic dentistry, is to establish an acceptable relationship between centric occlusion and centric relation (Fig. 6–15). In some instances, the result of the orthodontic therapy may appear to be excellent when the patient bites together in centric occlusion; however, there may be great discomfort associated with bruxism and temporomandibular malfunction because of an unacceptable discrepancy between the centric occlusion and the centric relation.

Faulty Occlusal Adjustment

Faulty occlusal grinding may induce severe trauma from occlusion, oral discomfort, hypertonicity and pain in the masticatory muscles, bruxism, and headache. The common complaints after faulty occlusal grinding are soreness of the teeth, food impaction, decreased masticatory effectiveness, temporomandibular pain and, sometimes, drifting of the teeth. Hypermobility of the teeth and even root resorption have been observed following faulty occlusal adjustment (Fig. 6–16). Excessive reduction of the cusp height on the working side is

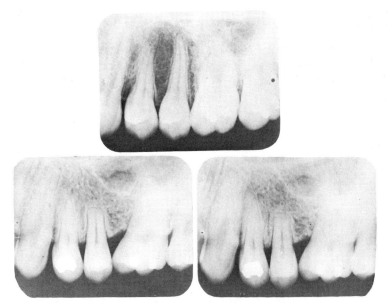

Figure 6–16. *Upper radiograph,* Prior to occlusal adjustment. *Lower left,* Two months after adjustment. The bicuspids had been left with occlusal interferences and the patient, with bruxism, had managed to grind the teeth so that they were loose and sore. Note root resorption. *Lower right,* Follow-up after readjustment of occlusion; there is no further resorption.

a common mistake and may create balancing side interferences that are almost impossible to eliminate by additional grinding. Grinding so as to remove the tips of buccal cusps of lower molars and bicuspids, thereby inducing lingual tipping of these teeth, is another mistake that may subsequently lead to occlusal interferences.

There is a common tendency to grind on anterior teeth to alleviate trauma to these teeth from a slide in centric (from centric relation to centric occlusion). This type of occlusal grinding increases the magnitude of, rather than correcting, the slide. Trauma to the anterior teeth is corrected by grinding on the posterior teeth in order to eliminate the slide and to assure correct posterior positioning of the jaw. A few extreme cases have been observed in which it was necessary to perform a complete mouth rehabilitation with inlays and crowns on practically every tooth in the maxilla or the mandible in order to re-establish oral comfort following faulty occlusal adjustment.

Occlusal and Other Habits

Since biting habits are usually performed on a subconscious level, it is very difficult to obtain a reliable history with reference to such practices. Occlusal habits are often related to a patient's occupation, and may include biting on common foreign objects such as pencils (Fig. 6–17), bobby pins, rims of eye glasses, pipes (Fig. 6–18), thread (Fig. 6–19), toothpicks and fingernails.[15] Some of these habits, such as biting of fingernails, are frowned upon socially, and a patient may be hesitant to admit the practice because of embarrassment. The traumatic effect of an occlusal biting habit is usually localized to one or two areas with only a few teeth involved. In some instances, the patients place their jaws into occlusal interlocking positions far out of the functional range of occlusion and press the teeth together into traumatic occlusion (Fig. 6–20). There are often notches and cracks in the enamel of the teeth that are used to bite into hard objects. It should also be emphasized that such habits do not necessarily induce trauma to the periodontium. Instead, in some instances, the habit induces functional hypertrophy, which results in increased strength of the periodontal structures. The teeth that are used in habitual biting of foreign objects may be out of normal occlusion contact, and foreign objects may be used for interproximal wedging or pressing on the teeth instead of biting. The traumatic force in such instances cannot be characterized as trauma from occlusion. When a habit pattern is suspected, the patient as well as his family should be alerted for its presence. When the patient has been made aware of the habit, it may be overcome by autosuggestion.

Lip, Tongue and Cheek Biting.   Lip, tongue and cheek biting may cause malpositioning of the teeth and muscular discomfort and thereby predispose to traumatic occlusion (Fig. 6–21). In such instances, any resulting traumatic injury to the periodontal structures can hardly be considered to be produced as a direct effect of lip, tongue and cheek biting; however, resulting trauma can be considered to be the effect of altered or too few occlusal contacts (Fig. 6–22).

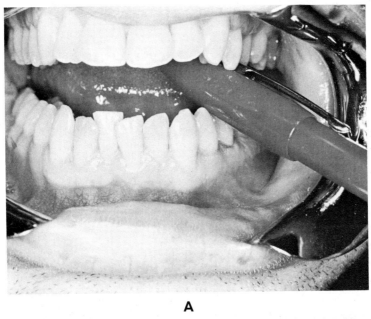

A

B

Figure 6-17. *A,* Habitual biting on pencil. *B,* Resultant periodontal damage. There were pockets as well as bone loss.

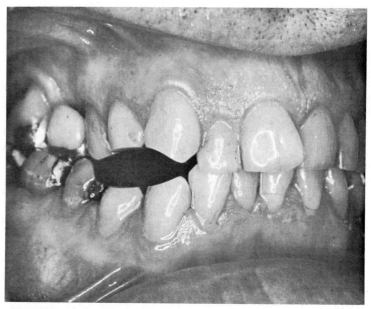

Figure 6-18. Excessive wear and some intrusion of the involved teeth, caused by pipe biting.

Habitual injury to soft oral tissues from biting also has to be characterized as trauma from occlusion. Such soft tissue injury is seen not infrequently in association with bruxism.

Inflammatory and Neoplastic Displacement of Teeth

Swelling associated with inflammation or tissue proliferation of progressive or neoplastic nature may move the teeth into a position of occlusal interference or premature contact. Simple gingivitis, especially of the hyperplastic type, will often lead to slight movements of the teeth, especially in the anterior region of the mouth. In dilantin hyperplasia of the gingiva, or hereditary gingival fibromatosis, the anterior teeth are commonly moved from their normal relationships. In advanced periodontal disease, a so-called pathologic migration of teeth is commonly found, and teeth with bi- and trifurcation involvement often register premature contacts in occlusion. Gingival inflammation and soreness of the gingival tissue may initiate tongue pressing habits which also may move teeth into a traumatic position.

It is often stated in the periodontal literature that gingival inflammation will not extend into the periodontal membrane proper. Although this might be true for cases of mild chronic gingivitis or periodontitis, it has been found in reviewing extensive autopsy material that severe gingivitis or actively progressing periodontitis often exhibits inflammatory changes extending into the periodontal membrane proper. Clinically associated are soreness and hypermobility of the involved teeth resulting from the swelling and edema that accompany

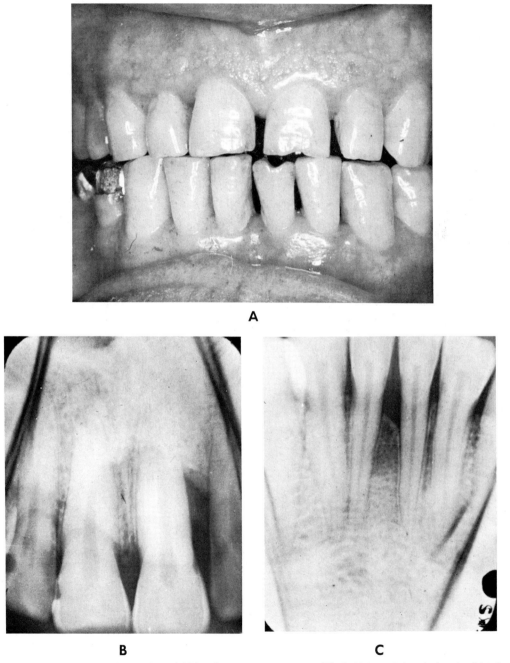

Figure 6–19. Results of thread biting in a seamstress, age 55. *A*, Note notches in involved teeth. *B* and *C*, Radiographs of the involved teeth showing vertical bone loss.

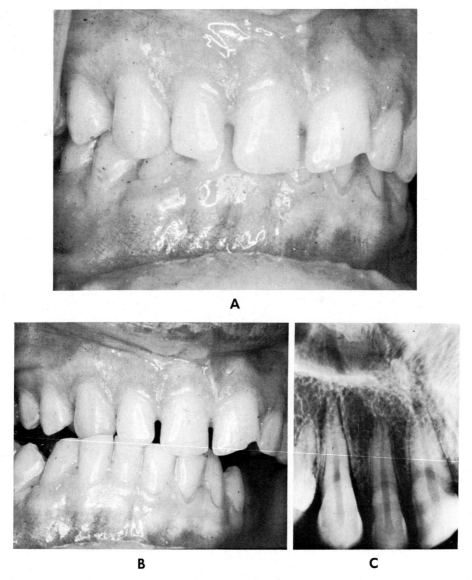

Figure 6-20. A, Female, age 20, with complaint of loose and sore maxillary cuspid. No occlusal interference could be found. B, Patient revealed that during tension she interlocked her teeth and pressed them together forcibly. C, Radiograph showing widened periodontal space around the involved tooth.

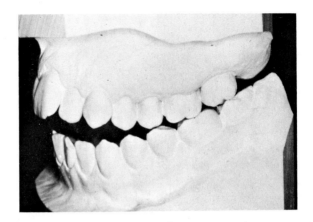

A

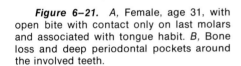

Figure 6–21. *A,* Female, age 31, with open bite with contact only on last molars and associated with tongue habit. *B,* Bone loss and deep periodontal pockets around the involved teeth.

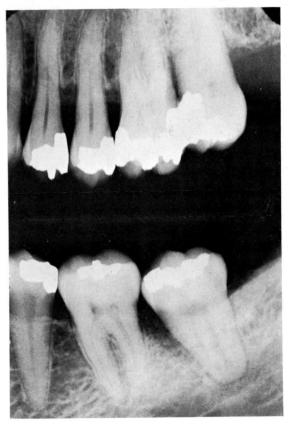

B

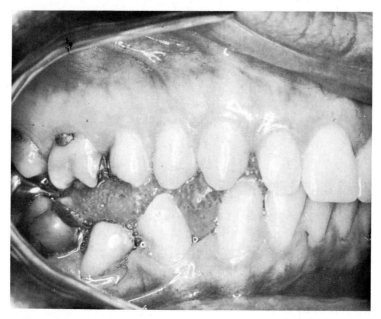

Figure 6-22. Occlusal relationship disturbed by tongue pressing in woman, age 29.

the inflammation. In such instances, the occlusal relationship will be altered and the teeth forced into a traumatic position. Conversely, it may often be found that teeth move back into a normal nontraumatic position following successful treatment of the gingival inflammation. For the same reason, one should not try to complete an occlusal adjustment in the presence of severe gingival inflammation, since the teeth at that time may not be in their optimal position.

Accidental Fractures and Surgical Mandibular Resections

Occlusal disharmony can often be observed following fractures of the jaws (Fig. 6–23). Occlusal adjustment or occlusal adjustment combined with orthodontic or restorative procedures should always follow healing of jaw fractures or partial mandibular resections in patients with Class III malocclusion.

Inadequate Form and Position of Teeth

Small tapered roots, especially on teeth with large crowns, predispose to trauma from occlusion (Fig. 6–24). Fractured or inadequately developed roots and the results of apicoectomy provide a reduced support for the teeth and therefore predispose to trauma from occlusion. During the shedding of deciduous teeth there is always evidence of trauma from occlusion that increases in degree as the root–crown ratio becomes more and more unfavorable.[13] Malposi-

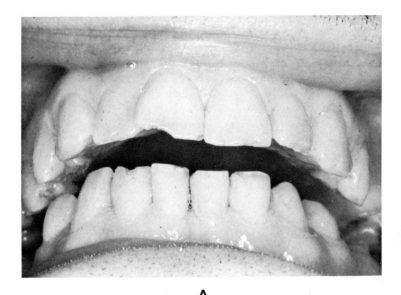

A

B

Figure 6–23. *A,* Male, age 34, with contact in centric only on the last molars after healing of jaw fracture. *B,* After occlusal adjustment an acceptable occlusion was re-established.

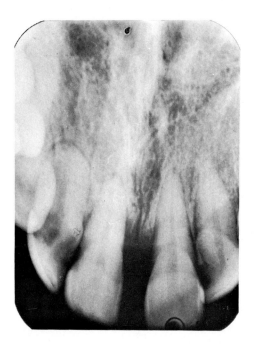

Figure 6-24. Large crowns and small tapered roots predisposing to traumatic occlusion.

tion of teeth and poor arch relations may also predispose to trauma from occlusion from unfavorable stress distribution during occlusal function. Malposed teeth may be the result of developmental and systemic disturbances; e.g., cleft palate, Cooley's anemia, various craniofacial dysostoses, and acromegaly.

REFERENCES

1. Anderson, D. J.: Measurements of stress in mastication. J. Dent. Res., *35*:664, 1956.
2. Beyron, H. L.: Occlusal changes in the adult dentition. J. Am. Dent. A., *48*:674, 1954.
3. Box, H. K.: Traumatic occlusion and traumatogenic occlusion. Oral Health, *20*:642, 1930.
4. Drum, W.: Autodestruction of the masticatory system. Paradontologie, *16*:155, 1962.
5. Glickman, I. et al.: The combined effects of inflammation and trauma from occlusion in Periodontics. Int. Dent. J., *19*:393, 1969.
6. Hanau, R. L.: Full Denture Prosthesis. Intraoral Technique for Hanau Articulator Model H. (n.p.) Buffalo, 1930.
7. Hirschfeld, I.: Food impaction. J. Am. Dent. A., *17*:1504, 1930.
8. Hirschfeld, I.: The individual missing tooth: A factor in dental and periodontal disease. J. Am. Dent. A., *24*:67, 1937.
9. Jarabak, J. R.: An electromyographic analysis of muscular and temporomandibular joint disturbances due to imbalances in occlusion. Angle Orthodont., *26*:170, 1956.
10. Karolyi, M.: Beobachtugen über Pyorrhea Alveolaris. Oesterr.-ungar. Vrtljschr. Zahnh, *17*:279, 1901.
11. Moyers, R. E.: Temporomandibular muscle contraction patterns in angle Class II, Division I malocclusions: An electro-myographic analysis. Am. J. Orthodont., *35*:837, 1949.
12. Perry, H. T., and Harris, S. C.: Role of the neuromuscular system in functional activity of the mandible. J. Am. Dent. A., *48*:665, 1954.
13. Ramfjord, S.: Effects of acute febrile diseases on the periodontium of rhesus monkeys with reference to poliomyelitis. J. Dent. Res., *30*:615, 1951.

14. Ramfjord, S.: Bruxism, a clinical and electromyographic study. J. Am. Dent. A., *62*:21, 1961.
15. Sorrin, S.: Habit, an etiologic factor of periodontal disease. Dent. Digest, *41*:290, 1935.
16. Stillman, P. R.: The management of pyorrhea. Dent. Cosmos, *59*:405, 1917.
17. Stillman, P. R.: Traumatic occlusion. Nat. Dent. A. J., *6*:691, 1919.
18. Stillman, P. R., and McCall, O. J.: A Textbook of Clinical Periodontia. New York, The Macmillan Co., 1922.
19. Thielemann, K.: Biomechanik der Paradentose. Leipzig, Herman Meusser, 1938.
20. World Workshop in Periodontics, Ramfjord, S., Kerr, D., and Ash, M. (Eds.). Ann Arbor, University of Michigan, 1966.

CHAPTER 7

PERIODONTAL RESPONSE IN TRAUMA FROM OCCLUSION

Whether injury occurs to normal periodontal structures from abnormal occlusal forces or occurs to already weakened periodontal structures from normal or excessive occlusal forces depends (1) on the resistance and response of the tissue to the forces and (2) on those morphologic features of the teeth, arches and supporting structures which resist or modify the forces. Impairment of tissue resistance or response may occur from alteration of the metabolic activity and structural integrity of the tissues as a result of local or systemic disturbances. Such morphologic features as root form, crown form, crown-root rotation, arch form, and tooth position can affect or modify the magnitude of forces capable of producing injury to the tissues. The response of the periodontal structures to physiologic occlusal forces was presented in Chapter 4. An excellent comprehensive review of periodontal response to occlusal forces by Reitan[29] is recommended.

Many attempts have been made to study tissue changes associated with trauma from occlusion in animals.[2, 3, 5, 11, 14, 19, 33, 35, 36] Although these experiments have not entirely duplicated the conditions in humans, they have supplied basic knowledge with regards to tissue reaction associated with trauma and repair within the periodontal structures. Histopathology of traumatic occlusion has also been studied in autopsy material.[1, 4, 6, 13, 16, 20, 22] However, lack of clinical history for the autopsy specimens with regard to previous occlusal relations and function makes interpretation of such tissue sections somewhat speculative. A few experimental investigations of limited scope in humans have been reported.[17, 25, 27, 28, 31] However, the long term histopathological changes and the clinical significance of trauma from occlusion have not been studied under controlled conditions.

Both metabolic activity and structural integrity of the periodontal tissues can be altered by a number of systemic deficiency states and diseases. It has been reported that scorbutic monkeys with normal teeth and no periodontal pockets, but weak periodontal structures, could not chew food of normal consistency.[34] Such extreme conditions have been observed only in growing animals, and chances of trauma from occlusion occurring in humans because of systemic weakening of the supporting structures of the teeth appear to be very small.

HISTOPATHOLOGY OF TISSUE CHANGES

Minor Trauma

Capillary and phase microscopy have been utilized in recent years to study the effect of minor injuries to living tissue. Such methods have provided an opportunity to study mild traumatic tissue changes that are not recognizable by conventional microscopy. Following minor injury, the cells of living tissue release cytoplasmic substances that may cause dilatation and increased permeability of the adjacent capillaries.[15, 37] Subsequent transudation of plasma into the tissue spaces will lead to edema. An accumulation of waste products from the overburdened connective tissue cells in an area of repeated mild trauma may also have an irritating effect upon the capillary walls and may disturb the normal fluid exchange. Furthermore, slight injury to the endothelial lining of the vessel walls may provoke subtle cellular changes manifested as roughness of the vessel walls. Such roughness will promote adherence of platelets, agglutination, clotting and possibly thrombosis of capillaries. Neurogenic vasoconstriction from injury can also produce stasis in capillaries. All these minor and usually transient changes associated with slight traumatic injury may contribute to metabolic changes[32] and lowered periodontal resistance to concomitant local irritation around the teeth that are in traumatic occlusion.

Severe Trauma

The histologic changes in the periodontal tissues following occlusal trauma have been described by several investigators.[3, 6, 11, 12, 14, 16, 23, 24, 29, 35] The common findings in an area of recent severe trauma are extravasation of blood cells, hematoma, thrombosis, ischemic necrosis, and sometimes, rupture of the walls of small vessels (Fig. 7–1). Areas of compression or necrosis resulting from crushing can be observed, especially in the bifurcation or cervical areas where the teeth have been pressed hard against the alveolar crest. The crushed necrotic tissue is gradually replaced by granulation tissues, and the boundary between necrotic and living tissue is well defined. However, if the occlusal trauma is minor, there is no well defined border between necrotic and living cells. The removal of dead cells and their replacement takes place simultaneously (Fig. 7–2). Severe trauma may result in complete necrosis of parts of the periodontal membrane, including the cementoblasts and the osteoblasts in these areas (Fig. 7–3). In such instances, elimination of the dead tissues and

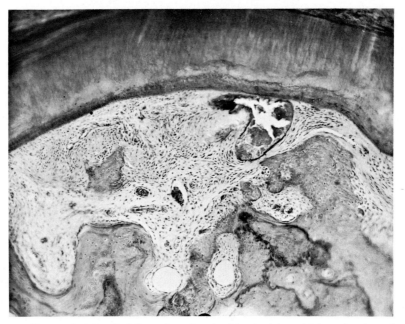

Figure 7-1. Traumatic injury in bifurcation of molar (monkey) from high occlusal amalgam restoration. Present are necrosis, thrombosis, and rupture of vessel wall.

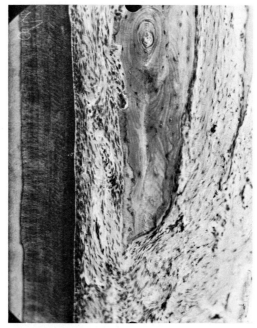

Figure 7-2. Mild trauma with simultaneous resorption and repair in alternating areas. Human maxillary incisor following loss of posterior teeth.

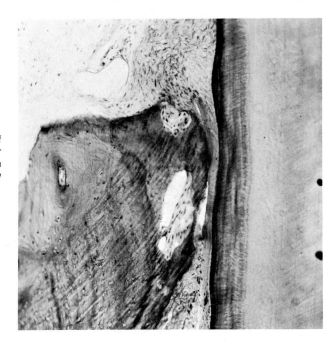

Figure 7–3. Crushing necrosis of periodontal membrane at alveolar crest with beginning resorption from adjacent periosteum and marrow spaces (human autopsy material).

repair will be initiated in adjacent areas of living periodontal membrane, endosteal cells, bone marrow, and in the haversian canals leading into the periodontal membrane. In cases of extreme trauma the crushed tissues may undergo liquefaction necrosis (Fig. 7–4) and subsequent replacement by vascular granulation tissue (Fig. 7–5). Practically none of the cells commonly seen associated with inflammatory exudate are present in an area of periodontal trauma (Fig. 7–6). The necrotic and necrobiotic tissues are dissolved and removed by enzymatic or humoral processes with very little evidence of phagocytosis, and without any manifestation of exudative inflammation. Less severe trauma may lead to degenerative changes in the periodontal membrane. Such changes are hyaline (Fig. 7–7) or mucoid degeneration (Fig. 7–8), dystrophic calcific deposits (Fig. 7–9) and lack of normal osteoblastic and cementoblastic activity.

Alternating areas of resorption and repair of the alveolar bone are common with mild traumatic pressure (Fig. 7–2), while in severe trauma the resorption is initiated from the marrow spaces. (See Fig. 7–3 for rear resorption.) Fibrosis of the adjacent marrow spaces is often present. Severe trauma may also lead to resorption of the cementum and extension of this resorption into the dentin. The cementoblasts have the highest tolerance to pressure of all of the cells in the periodontal membrane, but if the trauma has been severe enough to disrupt the life of these cells, subsequent resorption of the cementum will ensue. When the source of the trauma is eliminated, repair goes on with apposition of alveolar bone, formation of new periodontal fibers, and the formation of cementum on the root surface. However, if the length of the root has been shortened by resorption, regeneration of the root will not occur. Severe root resorption start-

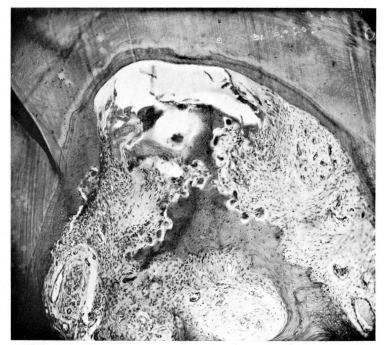

Figure 7-4. Severe trauma in bifurcation of molar (monkey) following insertion of very high occlusal amalgam restoration. Note liquefaction necrosis, resorption of bone and cementum, formation of granulation tissue, and fibrosis of marrow spaces.

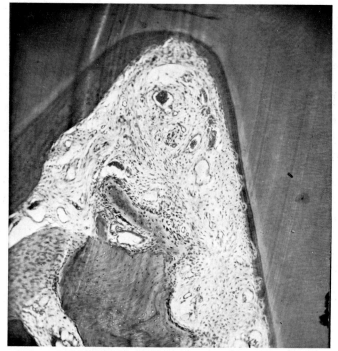

Figure 7-5. Healing stage of trauma from occlusion in bifurcation of molar (monkey) after high amalgam filling had been worn down by bruxism. Present is vascular granulation tissue, osteo- and cementogenesis, and beginning formation of collagen fibers.

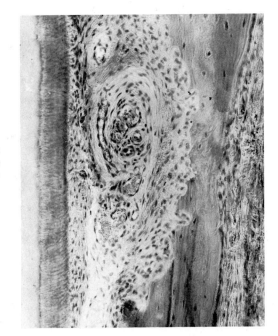

Figure 7-6. Trauma from occlusion, human lateral incisor after loss of posterior teeth. There is resorption of alveolar bone and vascular granulation tissue, but there are no inflammatory cells.

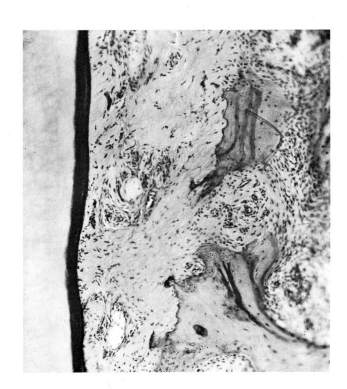

Figure 7-7. Hyaline degeneration associated with trauma from occlusion and widened periodontal space (human autopsy material).

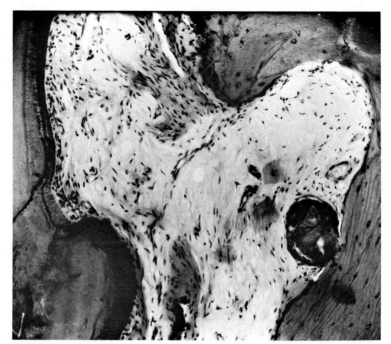

Figure 7–8. Mucoid degeneration associated with trauma from occlusion (human maxillary incisor).

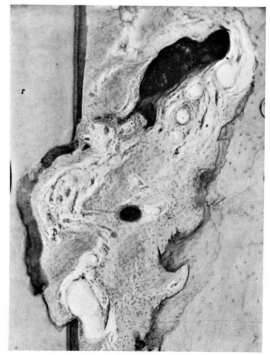

Figure 7–9. Dystrophic calcification and cementicle in area of previous traumatic cemental tear (human autopsy material).

ing from the periodontal membrane side may sometimes be followed by new bone formation and ankylosis of the tooth (Fig. 7–10). Such a case may roentgenographically be indistinguishable from so-called "internal resorption," and the pulp may be undamaged and have normal vitality.

Rocking or jiggling of a tooth by traumatic occlusion over a long period of time may produce a thicker than normal periodontal membrane without any direct evidence of traumatic injury (Fig. 7–11).

Only very inadequate and inconclusive studies have been reported of histopathological changes in the pulp associated with traumatic occlusion.[21, 33] It has been observed clinically that severe occlusal trauma may lead to necrosis[15] of the pulp[7] and sometimes to calcification of a large part of the pulp.

Disuse Atrophy

Tissue resistance to occlusal stress can be impaired by degeneration associated with disuse atrophy or hypofunction of the periodontal structures. Disuse atrophy of functionally oriented periodontal fibers develops slowly in adults. It was reported[27] that gingival and alveolar crest fibers of anterior teeth maintain a distinct functional orientation for approximately 6 months following the loss of opposing teeth. The presence of several bundles of well defined oblique fibers was also observed within the periodontal membrane in the same specimen. However, there was a tendency for young fibroblasts to appear parallel to the root surface, while the old fibers with thin, spindle-shaped nuclei maintained their previous functional arrangement (Fig. 7–12). In some instances, the collagen fibers were replaced by a meshwork of reticulum-like fibers in a seemingly edematous or mucoid environment. These areas of so-called "mucoid degeneration" contained a few plasma cells and lymphocytes (Fig. 7–13).

In autopsy material from long term nonfunctioning teeth, part of the periodontal membrane has sometimes been replaced by fatty bone marrow (Fig. 7–14). In such cases, the periodontal membrane is thin (0.10 to 0.12 mm.) and fairly even. In short term disuse atrophy there is marked osteoblastic activity on the periodontal membrane side of the alveolar bone and some cementoblastic activity (Fig. 7–15). In long term disuse there is practically no osteoblastic or cementoblastic activity, but one can see numerous incremental lines from previous depositions of calcified structures both on the surface of the alveolar bone and the cementum. However, the alveolar bone appears to be thin, probably as a result of a loss of bone from the marrow side of the alveolar plate. In some areas the alveolar bone is completely missing and the bone marrow extends into an area normally expected to be periodontal membrane (Fig. 7–14). Even in such instances of replacement of the periodontal membrane by bone marrow, the surface of the root is always covered by fibrous connective tissue. The supporting bone of teeth in hypofunction has fewer and thinner trabeculae than the supporting bone of teeth in normal function.

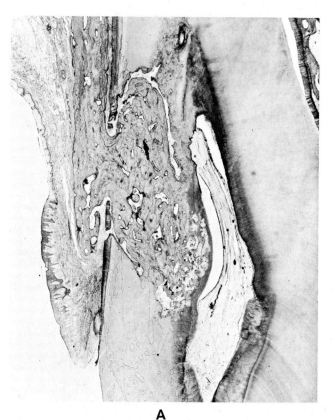

A

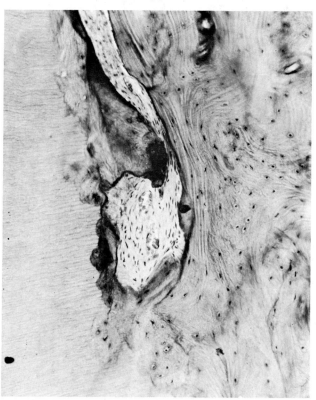

B

Figure 7–10. *A*, External root resorption and replacement by bone with ankylosis of the tooth. This tooth was the single terminal abutment of a 6-unit fixed bridge. Normal pulp (human autopsy material). *B*, High magnification of area of ankylosis.

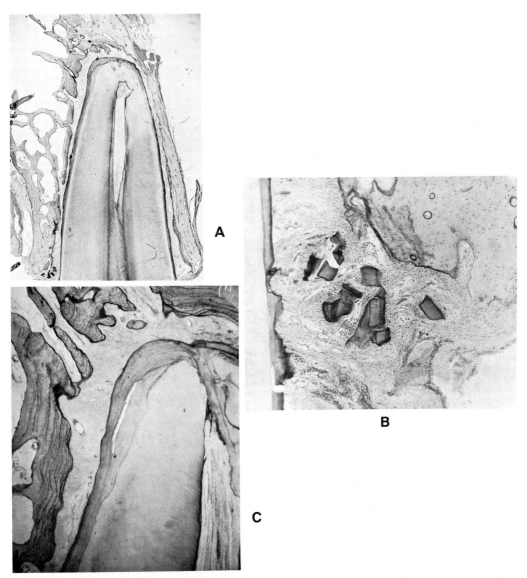

Figure 7–11. *A,* Central incisor with very severe attrition and pulpal calcification. Thick alveolar bone and widening of periodontal space in cervical and apical areas (human autopsy material). *B,* High magnification shows cemental tears and repair at alveolar crest, but no indication of active trauma. *C,* High magnification of apical area. Numerous layers of bone and cementum formed in the process of compensatory eruption of this "worn-down" tooth. No evidence of trauma; only compensatory hypertrophy of periodontal structures in response to unusually heavy occlusal forces.

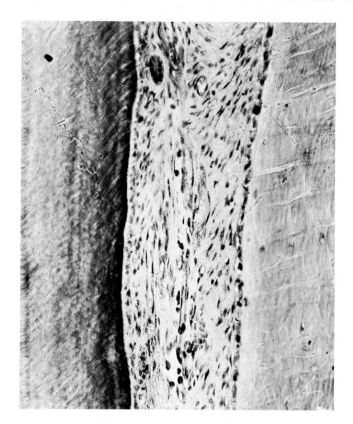

Figure 7–12. Loss of functional arrangement of periodontal fibers after six months without opposing tooth (human biopsy material).

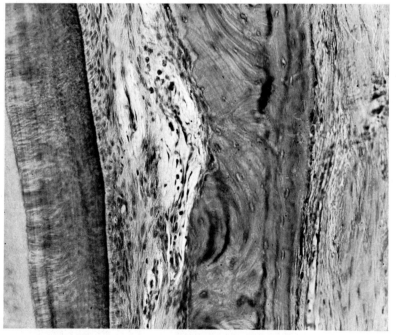

Figure 7–13. Mucoid degeneration and some plasma cells in nonfunctioning periodontal membrane (human biopsy material).

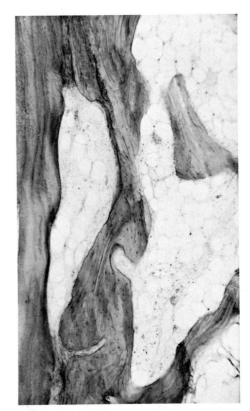

Figure 7-14. Replacement of periodontal membrane by fatty bone marrow in long-term nonfunction of tooth to the left in the picture (human autopsy material).

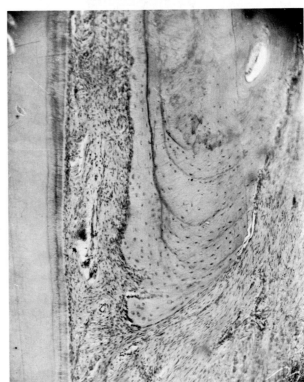

Figure 7-15. New bone formation at alveolar crest and active cementogenesis. This tooth was without an antagonist for two months (human biopsy material).

CLINICAL SIGNIFICANCE OF TISSUE CHANGES

Tooth Mobility

The replacement of dense functional periodontal tissues by granulation tissues in an area of periodontal trauma will lead to increased tooth mobility. This is caused by the softness of the granulation tissue and the widening of the periodontal space following resorption of the alveolar bone (Fig. 7–6). In chronic trauma from occlusion the hypermobility is due entirely to the increased width of the periodontal space, although the tissues may be normal (Fig. 7–11, *A*). Increased mobility may also be caused by root resorption resulting from trauma from occlusion. Traumatic occlusion may reduce the margin of a thin alveolar crest (Fig. 7–16) and thereby decrease the periodontal support for the tooth, resulting in an unfavorable ratio between the supra- and the subcrestal parts of the tooth and an increase in the leverage of occlusal forces. However, new bone will usually form on the outer aspect of the alveolar crest, preventing actual lowering of the level of the bone.

Gingival Inflammation

The significance of traumatic occlusion in the spread of gingival inflammation and downgrowth of the epithelial attachment is not fully known. It has been suggested that extension of gingival inflammation may assume an altered path in the presence of traumatic occlusion, allowing the inflammation to penetrate

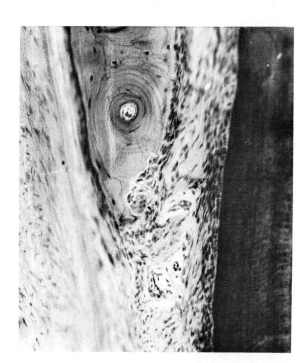

Figure 7–16. Resorption of alveolar crest from traumatic occlusion (human biopsy material).

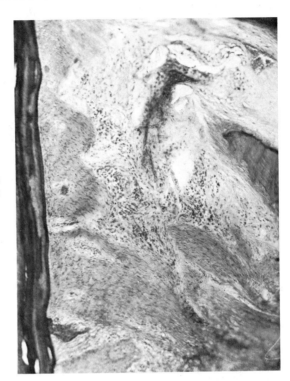

Figure 7-17. Spread of inflammation into periodontal membrane in a case of trauma from occlusion (human autopsy material).

into the periodontal membrane (Fig. 7–17) instead of following the common path on the outside of the alveolar bone or alveolar process.[9,23] However, more experimental work and observation under controlled conditions is needed before definite conclusions can be reached on the significance of traumatic occlusion in the formation of periodontal pockets. At the present time, it is generally conceded that, in the absence of local irritation, traumatic occlusion does not produce gingival inflammation or initiate periodontal pockets, since traumatic occlusion cannot destroy the supracrestal fibers[35] (Fig. 7–18). Such destruction would be necessary before apical migration of the epithelial attachment and pocket formation could occur. However, most investigators imply or believe that traumatic occlusion is an important factor in accelerating and contributing toward pocket formation when local irritants are present.[8,26] In other words, pockets grow deeper faster when traumatic occlusion is added to local irritants (Fig. 7–19).

Intrabony Pockets

Traumatic occlusion seems to be especially significant for the deepening of intrabony pockets since the normal protection of the supracrestal fibers is absent here. It is conceivable, though not likely, that traumatic occlusion against the wall of an intrabony pocket may destroy the attachment of the periodontal fibers at the apical level of the epithelial attachment and allow for a downgrowth of the epithelial attachment and subsequent deepening of the

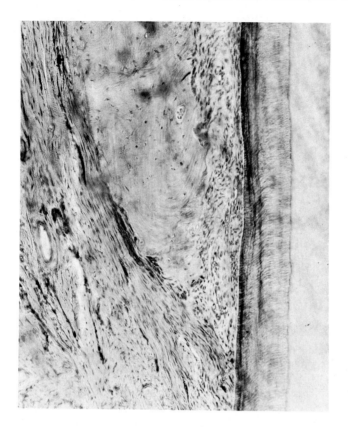

Figure 7–18. Supracrestal fibers unaffected by trauma from occlusion (human biopsy material).

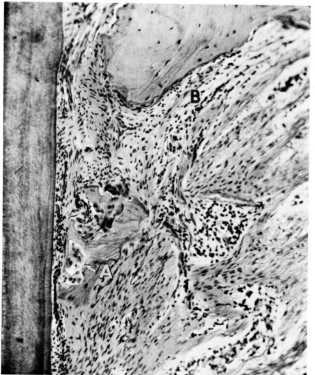

Figure 7–19. Resorption of alveolar crest from traumatic occlusion at A. Spread of inflammation from gingival irritation extending to outside of alveolar crest inducing resorption at B.

pockets. Glickman and Smulow[10] have suggested "that when gingival inflammation and trauma from occlusion occur together, they produce specific types of periodontal pathology, such as angular bone destruction and infrequently pockets." However, this postulate was not confirmed by Stahl[31] in human surgical specimens. Neither did Comar et al.[5] find such a pattern of bone loss in monkeys with experimental trauma from occlusion and marginal irritation. Trauma from occlusion involving teeth with intrabony pockets or pockets extending into the bi- or trifurcation definitely predisposes to the formation of periodontal abscesses. Trauma from occlusion will disturb the metabolism of the tissues in the area of trauma and lower the resistance to bacterial infection. It is inadvisable to increase the occlusal load on teeth with bi- or trifurcation involvement by using such teeth as abutments for bridges or partial dentures. In teeth with bi- or trifurcation involvement a considerable amount of bony support has been lost, and secondary trauma from occlusion may readily ensue if such teeth are exposed to heavy occlusal loads.

It has been stated but not proved that healing of periodontal pockets following subgingival curettage may be disturbed by trauma from occlusion. Whether gingival atrophy or recession and alteration of gingival contour can be the sequelae of trauma from occlusion is still a controversial subject among clinicians. No one has been able to produce either of these manifestations in experimental traumatic occlusion. From current evidence it appears unlikely that trauma from occlusion plays any significant role in either gingival recession or altered gingival contour.

Root Resorption

Root resorption with permanent shortening of the root and decreased functional capacity can be the result of trauma from occlusion. Traumatic occlusion and resorption may result in ankylosis of the teeth (Fig. 7–10). Interference with the pulpal circulation from traumatic occlusion and compression of the periapical tissues may lead to hyperemia of the pulp and associated pulpal sensitivity, especially to cold. In extreme cases, it may lead to strangulation and necrosis of the pulp.[18] The role of trauma from occlusion in the formation of denticles and linear calcification of the pulp is not known. However, calcification of the entire pulpal space has been observed following single incidents of occlusal trauma and in severe bruxism.

Disuse Atrophy

The main clinical significance of disuse atrophy and the associated degenerative changes is related to the functional capacity of the tissues. These tissues have practically no functional capacity, although clinically the teeth appear to be firm because of the narrow periodontal spaces which limit the possibility for noticeable mobility. Trauma from occlusion will readily develop when such teeth are engaged in function either as abutments for restorative dental appliances or by replacement of lost antagonists. Fortunately, the potential for adaptive and reorganizing activity of the periodontal membrane persists to a varying degree throughout the lifetime. Functional adaptive changes in the periodontal membrane have been observed in autopsy material from a 92 year old patient. Although teeth that have been out of function for a long time may feel sore to bite on and initially become loose following inclusion in occlusal function, the periodontal tissues will, if the occlusal relations are good, regain their functional character and strength in a few months.

REFERENCES

1. Bauer, W.: Über traumatische Schädigungen des Zementmantels der Zähne mit einem Beitrag zur Biologie des Zementes. Deutsche Monatsschr. Zahnh. *45*:769, 1927.
2. Bhaskar, S. N., and Orban, B. J.: Experimental occlusal trauma. J. Periodont., *26*:270, 1955.
3. Box, H. K.: Experimental traumatogenic occlusion in sheep. Oral Health, *25*:9, 1935.
4. Box, H. K.: Studies in Periodontal Pathology. Canadian Dent. Res. Foundation, Bulletin No. 7, 1924.
5. Comar, M. D., Kollar, J. A., and Gargiulo, A. W.: Local irritation and occlusal trauma as co-factors in the periodontal disease process. J. Periodont., *40*:193, 1969.
6. Coolidge, E. D.: Traumatic and functional injuries occurring in the supporting tissues of human teeth. J. Am. Dent. A., *25*:343, 1938.
7. Edlin, C.: Pulpal necrosis as a sequel to occlusal trauma. Dent. Pract., *20*:282, 1970.
8. Glickman, I.: Inflammation and trauma from occlusion, co-destructive factors in chronic periodontal disease. J. Periodont., *34*:5, 1963.
9. Glickman, I., and Smulow, J. B.: Alterations in the pathway of gingival inflammation into the underlying tissues induced by excessive occlusal forces. J. Periodont., *33*:7, 1962.
10. Glickman, I., and Smulow, J. B.: Effect of excessive occlusal forces upon the pathway of gingival inflammation in humans. J. Periodont., *36*:51, 1965.
11. Glickman, I., Stein, R. S., and Smulow, J. B.: The effect of increased functional forces upon the periodontium of splinted and non-splinted teeth. J. Periodont., *32*:290, 1961.
12. Gottlieb, B.: Traumatic occlusion. J. Am. Dent. A., *14*:1276, 1927.
13. Gottlieb, B.: Traumatic occlusion and the rest position of the mandible. J. Periodont., *18*:7, 1947.
14. Gottlieb, B., and Orban, B.: Die Veränderungen der Gewebe bei übermässiger Beanspruchung der Zähne, Leipzig. George Thieme, 1931.
15. Häupl, K.: Über die feingeweblichen Veränderungen bei funktionell Bedingtem Knochenumbau. Odont. Tidsk., *60*:209, 1952.
16. Häupl, K., and Lang, F. J.: Die marginale Paradentitis. Berlin, Herman Meusser, 1927.
17. Häupl, K., and Psansky, R.: Histologische Untersuchungen über die Wirkingsweise der in der Functions-Kiefer-Orthopädie verwendeten Apparate. Dtsch. Zahn-, Mund-, Kieferhk., *5*:214, 485, and 641, 1938.
18. Ingle, J. L.: Alveolar osteoporosis and pulpal death associated with compulsive bruxism. Oral Surg., *13*:1371, 1960.
19. Itoiz, M. E., Carranza, F. A., Jr., and Cabrini, R. L.: Histologic and histometric study of experimental occlusal trauma in rats. J. Periodont., *34*:305, 1963.
20. Kronfeld, R.: Histologic analysis of the jaws of a child with malocclusion. Angle Orthodont., *8*:21, 1938.
21. Landay, M. A., Wazimow, H., and Seltzer, S.: The effects of excessive occlusal forces on the pulp. J. Periodont., *41*:3, 1970.
22. Lundquist, G. R.: Connective tissue changes associated with variable occlusal stresses. J. Am. Dent. A., *24*:1577, 1937.
23. Macapanpan, L. C., and Weinmann, J. P.: The influence of injury to the periodontal membrane on the spread of gingival inflammation. J. Dent. Res., *33*:263, 1954.
24. Orban, B.: Tissue changes in traumatic occlusion. J. Am. Dent. A., *15*:2090, 1928.

25. Oppenheim, A.: Human tissue response to orthodontic intervention of short and long duration. Am. J. Orthodont. & Oral Surg., 28:263, 1942.
26. Posselt, U., and Emslie, R. D.: Occlusal disharmonies and their effect on periodontal diseases. Internat. Dent. J., 9:367, 1959.
27. Ramfjord, S. P., and Kohler, C. A.: Periodontal reaction to functional occlusal stress. J. Periodont., 30:95, 1959.
28. Reitan, K.: The initial tissue reaction incident to orthodontic tooth movement as related to the influence of function. Acta odont. scandinav., 9:Suppl. 6, 1951.
29. Reitan, K.: Biomechanical principles and reactions. *In* Graber, T. M. (Ed.): Current Orthodontic Concepts and Techniques, pp. 56–159. Vol. I, Philadelphia, W. B. Saunders Co., 1969.
30. Schärer, P., Butler, J. H., and Zander, H. A.: Die Heilung parodontaler Knochentazchen bei occlusaler Dysfunktion. Schw. M. Zahn., 79:244, 1969.
31. Stahl, S. S.: The response of the periodontium to combined gingival inflammation and occlusofunctional stresses in human surgical specimens. Periodontics, 6:14, 1968.
32. Stallard, R. E.: Tissue changes in the supporting structures in occlusal traumatism using radioisotopes. Periodontics, 2:143, 1964.
33. Stones, H. H.: An experimental investigation into the association of traumatic occlusion with paradontal disease. Roy. Soc. Med. Sect. Odont. Proc., 31:479, 1938.
34. Waerhaug, J.: Effect of C-avitaminosis on the supporting structures of the teeth. J. Periodont., 29:87, 1958.
35. Waerhaug, J.: Pathogenesis of pocket formation in traumatic occlusion. J. Periodont., 26:107, 1955.
36. Wentz, F. M., Jarabak, J., and Orban, B.: Experimental occlusal trauma imitating cuspal interferences. J. Periodont., 29:117, 1958.
37. Westin, G.: Erythrocytic aggregation in vivo with special regard to the local effect of trauma in the pathogenesis of the paradentitis. Paradentologie, 7:165, 1953.

CHAPTER 8

FUNCTIONAL DISTURBANCES OF TEMPOROMANDIBULAR JOINTS AND MUSCLES

Injury from outside sources (extrinsic) or from functional disturbances within the masticatory system (intrinsic) may result in discomfort or pain in the temporomandibular joint and its contiguous structures and in the muscles related to the function of the joint. Functional disturbances of joints and muscles can be understood best by a review of the physiology of the masticatory system, which has been presented in Section I. Closely related are functional disturbances of the jaw muscles, which have been discussed under Bruxism in Chapter 5. The diagnosis and treatment of functional disturbances of the temporomandibular joints and muscles are discussed in Chapter 17.

The functional disturbances related to temporomandibular joint and muscle pain include acute traumatic arthritis, muscle spasms, chronic traumatic arthritis, and osteoarthritis. One or more of these conditions may be present at a given time, and their manifestations may be limited only to the joints and adjacent structures; however, manifestations may involve the entire masticatory system and extend even to other parts of the head and neck.

ETIOLOGY

Various theories have been proposed regarding the causes of dysfunctional pain in the masticatory system, but it is becoming more and more evident that the most common underlying factor is an abnormally increased muscle tonus plus some form of bruxism.[50]

Psychic Tension, Emotional and Physical Stress

The tissues within the temporomandibular joints, as well as other parts of the masticatory system, are normally protected by basic neuromuscular reflexes and, through coordination of muscle function and forces, by the neuromuscular system. Injury to the temporomandibular joints, except that due to external trauma, is therefore the result of an abnormal muscle action and a related imbalance in the alignment of the various parts of the masticatory system. Anything that might increase the basic muscle activity or tonus, such as frustration, psychic stress, emotional tension, occlusal interferences or pain, may lead to functional disturbances and pain in the temporomandibular joints and adjacent muscles.

There is minimal stress upon the components of the temporomandibular joints in "empty movements," provided a harmonious relationship exists between the occlusion and joints and the person has physiologic muscle tonus.[26] "Empty movements" refer to tooth contact during swallowing or tooth contact without anything between the teeth. Although heavy stress may occur on the balancing side in the temporomandibular joint when biting on hard food or other objects,[18] the joint is normally protected from damaging forces by neuromuscular coordination of the biting forces and protective reflexes. However, when there is an abnormal increase in muscle tonus and response to stimulus, there exists the potential for traumatic injury to the joint, as well as to muscles and ligaments. As previously explained (Chapter 5, Bruxism), such an increase in basic muscle activity is associated with psychic tension. Intense reticular stimulation will not only tend to initiate heavy contraction in the masticatory and facial muscles, but at the same time render the nociceptive inflow less effective than with low reticular stimulation.[43] This reduction in efficiency of protective reflexes by way of central nervous system overstimulation may in part explain the interplay between the masticatory system and the central nervous system in the etiology of temporomandibular joint dysfunction[43] (pp. 54, 62 and 178). The increased activity is found to a greater extent in the masticatory and facial muscles than in most other muscles of the body, since the facial and jaw muscles are involved normally in expression of emotions such as anger, fear and aggression. For a more detailed explanation of the relation between muscles and the nervous system, see Chapter 3.

After an injury has been established, the pain from the injured tissues has a tendency to increase muscle activity, which in turn may increase the injurious forces and produce additional trauma. This vicious cycle of "feedback" between muscle tension and injury usually is expressed in one or another form of bruxism and plays an exceedingly important role in the development of traumatic temporomandibular joint arthritis and associated functional disturbances.[50]

Occlusal Interferences, Premature Contacts and Occlusal Instability

The role of occlusion and occlusal interferences in the cause of functional temporomandibular joint and muscle disturbances is controversial.[44] According to recent investigations, patients (as a group) with functional disturbances of joints and muscles do not have any more occlusal interferences than individuals without the disturbances.[27, 62] On the other hand, such disturbances can unquestionably be eliminated in the overwhelming majority of cases by removal of occlusal interferences. Furthermore, the disturbances can very easily be precipitated again by placement of a single occlusal interference in the same patient. A number of patients can also relate their symptoms to insertion of dental restorations or appliances, and muscle pain has been experimentally produced in denture patients by changes in occlusion.[9, 34]

It is evident that the most important factor in the development of these disturbances is the individual patient's lack of adaptation to a less than ideal occlusion.[51] This adaptive capacity is very closely related to a patient's psychic status of stress and emotional tension or tranquility and emotional stability. Onset, remissions and exacerbations of traumatic temporomandibular joint arthritis and muscle pain commonly follow or coincide with episodes of nervous tension (premenstrual tension, emotional conflicts, college exams, etc.). This threshold of psychic irritability, as it relates to occlusal interferences that trigger abnormal action of the jaw muscles, varies from individual to individual and from time to time in the same individual.

As in bruxism,[48] any type of occlusal interference may, when combined with psychic tension, result in traumatic temporomandibular joint arthritis and related muscle pain. However, certain types of interferences are more prone to precipitate this unfavorable situation. The most common occlusal interference to trigger such abnormal muscle action is a "slide in centric" or an unstable area in the retrusive range between centric relation and centric occlusion, and a laterally directed slide seems to be more significant than a straight posterior-anterior slide. The resultant disturbance from occlusal interferences can be observed best electromyographically during unconscious swallowing. Jaw and occlusal instability, both in centric relation, centric occlusion and the area between these two positions, may also lead to traumatic temporomandibular joint arthritis and muscle spasms.[50]

Balancing side occlusal interferences have a very disturbing influence on the function of the masticatory system and often trigger bruxism and associated pain in muscles and temporomandibular joints.

Occlusal interferences on the working side or in protrusive excursion seldom trigger abnormal muscle activity. However, if bruxism is carried out against a ledge or a facet of wear on the tip of a maxillary cuspid or incisal edge of maxillary incisors, trauma and pain occasionally occur in the temporomandibular joint of the balancing side (diagonally opposite to the interfering cuspid.)

There can be no doubt that a definite relationship exists between occlusal disharmony and traumatic temporomandibular joint arthritis,[25, 35, 38, 46] with or without muscle and tendon pain. This relationship can be demonstrated both clinically and electromyographically.[50] However, occlusal disharmony alone will not lead to pain in these structures unless the overwhelmingly important factor of psychic tension also is present. It would, therefore, be misleading to designate occlusion as the primary factor in the etiology of these functional disturbances. Even so, neither will psychic tension in the presence of ideal occlusion lead to the dysfunctional pain. It is the various combinations of psychic tension and occlusal interferences that are responsible for the painful symptoms.[19, 31, 33, 37, 40, 45] In some extreme instances psychic tension may be so severe that very little occlusal interference is necessary to start muscle spasms; or occlusal interferences may be so severe that it takes very little psychic tension to initiate excessive forces and produce injury. The majority of cases are found between these two extremes.

Pain and Discomfort in the Masticatory System or Adjacent Structures

Pain or discomfort from dental,[24] periodontal,[17] sinus, and other diseases[65] increases basic muscle activity and may, therefore, when combined with occlusal interferences, increase the chances for traumatic temporomandibular joint arthritis and muscle pain. It has also been pointed out that muscle spasm, sustained muscle contractions associated with "splinting," and pain may distort the usual patterns of jaw movement and bring out new occlusal interferences which were not interferences when the movement pattern was normal.[1, 55]

Abnormal Biting Habits

Habitual biting and bending on objects brought into the mouth, or "locking" the mandible into extreme nonfunctional position, may precipitate dysfunctional pain unrelated to functional occlusal relationships. These habits serve as outlets for emotional tension and are closely related to bruxism, although they may have no occlusal triggers; and occlusal therapy, consequently, would be of no help for this kind of pain. It has been shown that isometric pressing together of the teeth for three minutes caused pain in all six subjects who participated in the experiment.[64] On the average the onset of pain occurred after 64 seconds of pressing the teeth together, and the pain was most often in the temporomandibular joints, zygomatic arch, and in the temporal region.

Loss of Posterior Teeth

It has been claimed that loss of posterior teeth predisposes to traumatic temporomandibular joint arthritis[47, 61] because (1) more pressure results on the joint from biting on front teeth than on posterior teeth; and (2) loss of posterior teeth may lead to loss of occlusal vertical dimension with subsequent distal displacement and overclosure of the mandible.[29, 41] Although loss of posterior teeth may be one factor predisposing to traumatic temporomandibular joint arthritis and muscle spasms with pain, this is not because of distal displacement and overclosure of the mandible but rather because of the disturbed neuromuscular relationship that follows the change in the occlusion. The mechanism involved in the disturbed relationship will be discussed under pathogenesis of functional temporomandibular joint and muscle disturbances.

External Force or Injury

External injury or extrinsic trauma originating from outside the masticatory system, such as accidents, blows to the jaws, or prolonged opening of the jaw with stretching of the muscles during dental procedures, may also lead to traumatic temporomandibular joint arthritis and muscle pain. According to Hankey,[28] about 20 per cent of his patients with such disturbances gave a history of extrinsic trauma which might have been the cause of the traumatic temporomandibular joint arthritis. Extrinsic trauma is of importance in the etiology of the acute traumatic temporomandibular joint arthritis if one includes the results of poorly aligned, healed jaw fractures, and possibly permanent damage to the meniscus from severe traumatic injury.[21]

Luxation, Subluxation, and Sprain

The anterior range of condylar movement is determined by muscles rather than by a well defined anterior ligament of the temporomandibular joint. It is possible, as a result of serious uncoordination of muscle activity with associated muscle spasms, to dislocate the mandible into a position anterior to the articular tuberculum, and to hold it there by sustained muscle spasm. The dislocation usually involves both condyles and occurs most often in young women.[53] Recurrent dislocation, or habitual luxation, is rare and appears to be related to psychic tension rather than to specific types of dysfunctional occlusion. However, effective treatment of occlusal disharmony will reduce high muscle tonus and may thus minimize the chances for muscle spasms and dislocation of the joints.

Subluxation does not refer to an anatomically well defined partial luxation of the mandible. Rather, the term is used to indicate that the mandible is temporarily "stuck" or locked into a certain position that does not correspond necessarily to full mandibular opening. Subluxation often is related to severe "clicks" in the temporomandibular joint(s). Subluxation is the manifestation of abnormal activity of the jaw muscles (splinting or spastic activity). The abnormality is definitely related to disharmony within the masticatory system as well as to psychic tension. While a dislocation or luxation has to be treated by repositioning the mandible, in subluxation the condyle(s) return to a normal position when the muscle spasms subside. Often the patient with subluxation has learned to treat the problem by massage of jaw muscles and/or specific manipulation or movement of the mandible.

Sprain in the temporomandibular ligaments often occurs both with luxation and subluxation. A sprain is the result of abnormal stress placed on the ligaments by spastic jaw muscles, but may also occur in association with extreme mandibular opening (yawning, biting an apple, etc.). Both luxation and subluxation sprain are apt to occur when jaw muscles are relaxed, as during sleep, and triggering of the jaw-jerk reflex. After a sprain the path of mandibular closure is changed by the splinting action of the muscles in an effort to protect the injured parts of the joint. Thus the patient's occlusion will feel different to him when he bites together. It is difficult for an examiner to determine what the normal joint relations should be until such time as the sprain has healed.

Luxation, subluxation, and sprain may occur occasionally as the result of extrinsic trauma. The exact nature of origin becomes known from the patient's history.

PATHOGENESIS OF FUNCTIONAL TEMPOROMANDIBULAR JOINT DISTURBANCES AND RELATED CONDITIONS

In the classical concept, the pathogenesis of functional temporomandibular joint disturbances has been related to "distal displacement" and "mandibular overclosure." Since Monson's articles in 1920[41] and 1921[42] stated that a back thrust of the mandible could not only encroach on the auditory apparatus but could also elicit pain in the joint area by pressure on nerve endings, the distal displacement theory has provided the generally accepted explanation for the various painful symptoms associated with dysfunction of the masticatory system. Later, Costen[14,15] and Goodfriend[22,23] elaborated on this concept, added their own interpretations, and grouped a number of symptoms and theoretical speculations together that became known collectively as "Costen's syndrome." Although an impingement of the auriculotemporal nerve by distal displacement of the condyle as postulated by Costen has been repudiated by Sicher[58] and others,[66] the distal displacement and mandibular overclosure theory is still used by most authors in attempts to explain the various pathologic and clinical manifestations associated with functional disorders of the temporomandibular joints and adjacent structures. It was Sicher's opinion that the degenerative changes associated with traumatic temporomandibular joint arthritis were the result of a distal impingement of the condyle upon the soft tissues and synovial villi posterior to the normal position of the condyle. Allegedly, distal displacement and overclosure interferes with the production of synovial fluid, which normally provides the joint with nutrition and lubrication. Thus, degenerative changes of the joint, commonly described by histopathologic investigators,[6] have been attributed to an interference with the metabolism and function of the synovial membrane.[58] Adherents to the displacement theory have attributed the pain in areas surrounding the joint to degeneration and irritation of nerve endings entering the joint capsules and periphery. Pain more distant from the joint has been explained on the basis of "referred pain." It has also been suggested that pain in the temporomandibular joint region could be referred pain from sinuses[57] and from muscles[63] of the head and neck.

Another concept of the pathogenesis of the manifestations of traumatic temporomandibular joint arthritis is to consider it a variant of other types of arthritis of unknown etiology (or "arthrosis,"[8] as it usually is called in the European literature). This concept has provided the basis for various types of symptomatic treatment such as heat, diathermy, x-ray, injections of corticoids, hyaluronidase, extirpation of the disc, etc.

A third concept, in which muscle dysfunction and fatigue are considered the source of pain in both the temporomandibular joint and adjacent structures, has gained considerable support during the last decade.[20, 54, 56] From this concept the term "temporomandibular joint pain dysfunction syndrome" has been suggested to describe all such pain of a dysfunctional origin. Occlusion has been assumed to play a minor or secondary role in this syndrome inasmuch as the main emphasis has been on psychic tension and muscle spasms as sources of the pain.

None of the previously mentioned concepts provides a logical and generally applicable explanation for all the following clinical, histopathologic and electromyographic observations regarding dysfunctional temporomandibular joint and muscle pain.

Observations Related to Dysfunctional
Temporomandibular Joint and Muscle Pain

From clinical experience with several hundred patients over the last 20 years it appears that almost every patient has experienced partial or complete relief of symptoms by occlusal therapy without changing vertical dimension. There is actually no scientific evidence to indicate that an increase in interocclusal or freeway space predisposes or contributes to traumatic temporomandibular joint arthritis or muscle pain. To the contrary, it appears that any encroachment upon an existing interocclusal space with procedures designed to raise the bite increases the disturbing input to the neuromuscular mechanism from occlusal interferences. Also, increasing the interocclusal space increases tolerance to occlusal interferences by lowering the disturbing input from these interferences. If there are no interferences present, the difference between the rest vertical dimension and the occlusal vertical dimension may be less critical than previously assumed, especially with regards to an increase in interocclusal space.

As reported by Cobin[12] several years ago, it has been observed that occlusal adjustment or other forms of occlusal therapy which reposition the mandible to a stable centric relation distally or laterally to the previous centric occlusion will often provide relief from the disturbing symptoms. A therapy that allows the mandible to move farther distally could not conceivably give this relief if the symptoms were due to a distal displacement in the first place.

A lateral slide in centric (from centric relation to centric occlusion) will often elicit pain on the side where the condyle moves inward and forward. The condyle is then placed against the anterior and lateral rather than the distal aspect of the joint, representing the opposite to "distal displacement." It has been found in comparative anatomic and radiologic studies[10] that the joint damage is often severe towards the lateral or medial aspects of temporomandibular joints which were previously painful. This finding indicates a lateral pressure component on the joint rather than posterior pressure. In the same study[10] it was also found that most pathologic changes on the lateral aspects of the joints were not seen in roentgenograms.

Most patients with unilateral pain in the temporomandibular joint try to chew on the involved side, since this hurts less than chewing on the opposite side. There is normally less pressure on the condyle on the working than on the balancing side, and the balancing condyle moves forward in lateral function. The fact that a patient avoids the use of an involved side for balancing function because of pain indicates that the pain is elicited from contacts in the anterior rather than the posterior parts of the joint.

In patients with bruxism and wear facets on the tip of the maxillary cuspid, the painful joint is often diagonally opposite to this cuspid. This indicates that bruxing on the cuspid has produced pain from undue stress on the anterior aspect of the joint on the opposite or balancing side, rather than from distal pressure on the joint.[50]

Experimental "anterior displacement" of the mandible in denture construction has brought on muscle and temporomandibular joint pain.[9, 34]

From experimental work on monkeys with occlusal splints which place the mandible in an anterior displacement position,[30] striking bone resorption at the site of insertion of the external pterygoid muscle on the neck of the condyle has indicated that this muscle has been hyperactive as a result of the occlusal displacement. The pain in the joint area may be, in part, from such hyperactivity and abnormal pull on tendons at the site of muscle insertion.

Individuals with only anterior teeth remaining in occlusal contact have a tendency to develop deep overbite and sometimes dysfunctional temporomandibular joint and muscle symptoms. While this development has been considered a proof for the distal displacement and overclosure theory, the fact remains that when such patients are placed on a flat biteplane, their mandible moves farther distally as their symptoms subside. The more plausible explanation of this phenomenon is that the patient has to hold his mandible more and more forward to bite against the maxillary anterior teeth, which under these circumstances move more and more forward. This biting forward by necessity also induces pressure on the anterior aspect of the temporomandibular joint. When the patient can again seat the condyle in the normal position without having to bite forward to contact the front teeth, the symptoms are alleviated. Again the problem seems to be an anterior, rather than a distal, displacement of the condyle.

Condylar position is unquestionably influenced by pain and muscle tension. Electromyographically, an abnormally increased activity in the posterior temporal muscle fibers is usually seen associated with a traumatic temporomandibular joint arthritis.[50] This can be explained as an attempt at splinting or holding the condyle away from painful contact with the injured anterior aspect of the joint. After proper occlusal adjustment or use of biteplanes, this hypertonicity localized to the posterior temporal fibers disappears. There is often a marked change in the location of the recordable stationary hinge axis, and the relationship between the jaws and the teeth in centric relation may thus be drastically changed. The stationary hinge axis moves upward and forward into the glenoid fossa and the last molars make premature contacts while there is anterior open bite.

The adjustment to a normal condylar position after the pain has subsided does not in any way prove that the down and posterior position of the condyle was the cause of the joint pain. Sprained ligaments in the knee joint, for example, will alter the functional movements of the knee, but that does not mean that this altered protective movement pattern caused the painful injury in the first place. That it is possible to record a stationary hinge axis in a patient with temporomandibular joint or muscle pain does not prove that this is the normal centric relation for the patient;[13] this will be discussed in Chapter 17.

An apparent distal position of the condyle in temporomandibular joint roentgenograms also is meaningless because of the normal anatomic variations of these joints.[16, 36, 52] Attempts to place the condyle roentgenographically in the middle of the glenoid fossa by opening the bite, as was advocated several years ago,[39] does not have a rational scientific basis. As discussed under relationship of muscle activity and condylar positions, the condyle may be held back by splinting muscle action and this may also be evident on a roentgenogram; but that again does not prove that this distal position of the condyle caused the pain.

Summary of Observations

The dull ache associated with functional temporomandibular joint and muscle disturbances is either the result of traumatic injury to the joint structures, particularly the peripheral anterior and lateral parts of the joints, or of abnormal muscle activity with muscle spasms.

The stabbing neuralgic type of pain sometimes experienced by patients with functional disturbances is probably the result of irritation of nerve endings associated with the joint structures, but may be referred pain from other parts of the masticatory system.

The "drawing pain" or dull ache at the site of insertion and attachment of the jaw muscles is also the result of overactivity of the muscles, producing pain reaction from the nervous elements of the tendons and their insertions.

The cause of the functional disturbances and the pain is a combination of psychic tension and occlusal disharmony resulting in muscular hyperactivity and producing traumatic injury to the joint structures, tendons and muscles related to the masticatory system.

Distal displacement, overclosure and loss of occlusal vertical dimensions are not specific causes for dysfunctional pain, and the pathologic changes in the joints are the result of direct trauma rather than indirect degeneration associated with any of these often implicated factors.

Most patients have pain both in the joints and in the muscles. An almost equal number of patients have pain only in the joint structures, while a relatively small number of patients (10 to 15 per cent) have muscle pain, discomfort and other peripheral symptoms without any pain in the temporomandibular joint.[50]

HISTOPATHOLOGY OF TRAUMATIC ARTHRITIS AND OSTEOARTHRITIS OF THE TEMPOROMANDIBULAR JOINT

There are only a few reports in the literature on the histopathology of traumatic arthritis and osteoarthritis of the temporomandibular joints in humans, and they are all concerned with chronic cases.[2, 5, 32, 59, 60] Some of the autopsy findings have been supplemented with clinical records taken prior to death.[6, 7] The early pathologic changes are fibrinoid and hyaline degeneration of the meniscus (Fig. 8–1) and the fibrous connective tissues covering the articular area of the condyle and the glenoid fossa. There is an interrupted arrangement of the cells covering the bone, and the cells resemble hyaline cartilage, even in joints in which the growth has long ago ceased (Fig. 8–2). The early degenerative changes also include cracks in the surface of the meniscus and the articular fibrocartilage (Fig. 8–3), followed by foci of necrosis (Fig. 8–4) and bone resorption, while proliferative changes with new bone formation may take place at the periphery. There may also be focal areas of vascularization[11] (Fig. 8–5), proliferation of fibrous tissue and hyaline cartilage (Fig. 8–6), and chronic inflammation in the meniscus (Fig. 8–7). In some instances there is perforation of the central part of the meniscus, fragmentation of the meniscus, and/or erosions on the medial or lateral parts of the meniscus.

Traumatic temporomandibular joint arthritis will eventually develop into osteoarthritis in those individuals with a predisposition for osteoarthritic changes. Osteoarthritis is a local degenerative disease which may develop as a result of heavy exposure to wear and tear or trauma over a long period of time. The pathology of osteoarthritis of the temporomandibular joint is the same as for osteoarthritis in other joints, with severe deformative changes of "lipping" at the periphery of the articular surfaces of the condyle (Fig. 8–8), fragmentation and partial calcification of the meniscus (Fig. 8–9), and exposure of necrotic or eburnated bone on the functional articular surfaces (Fig. 8–10).

The capsules show evidence of degeneration and chronic inflammation. In one case where "sclerosing" solution had been used, these changes were severe (Fig. 8–11). No correlation between the severity of the pathologic changes and the symptoms revealed in the premortem history has been found since the history of pain has been highly inconsistent in these cases.[6, 7]

Experimentally induced trauma to the temporomandibular joint from occlusal disharmony in monkeys has revealed only mild degenerative changes in the articular surfaces of the joints. Also present was transient resorption and new bone formation at the periphery of the articular surfaces, at the insertion of the external pterygoid muscles, and on the anterior surface of the postglenoid spine.[30, 49] Typical osteoarthritic changes have been observed in old monkeys without any apparent occlusal disharmony.

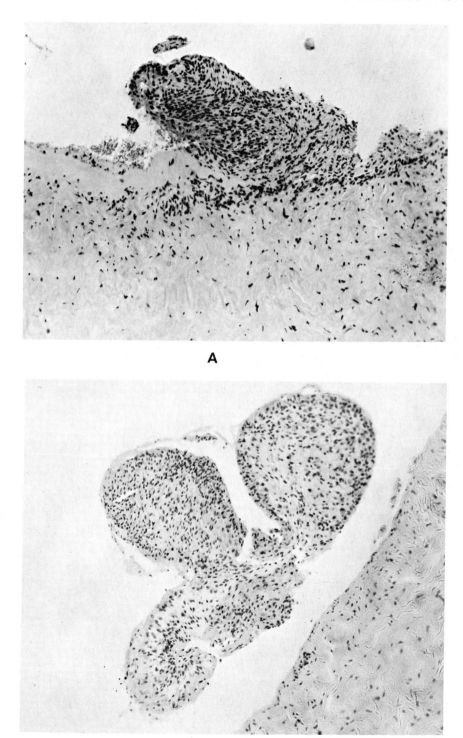

Figure 8–1. *A*, Fibrinoid and hyaline degeneration of meniscus and a nodule of proliferating connective tissue on surface. *B*, Villosynovitis and hyaline degeneration at the periphery of the same meniscus (specimen from surgical meniscectomy in patient with traumatic temporomandibular joint arthritis).

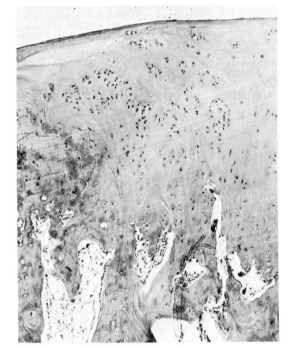

Figure 8-2. Part of articular surface of condyle of male, age 27. Note irregular hyaline cartilage and hyaline degeneration, lack of well-defined cortical bone, and absence of the normal fibrous connective tissue toward the condylar surface (specimen from surgical condylectomy in patient with traumatic temporomandibular joint arthritis).

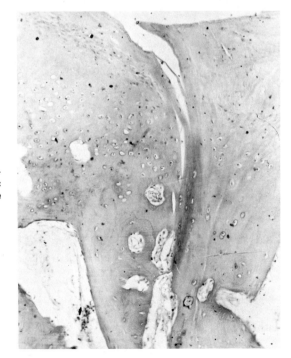

Figure 8-3. Crack in hyaline cartilage surface of articular part of condyle. Traumatic temporomandibular joint arthritis (from same specimen as Figure 8-2).

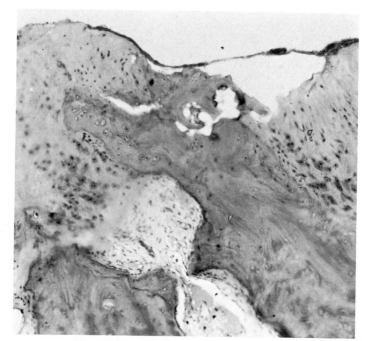

Figure 8-4. Traumatic necrosis on articular surface of condyle. Observe the irregular hyaline cartilage and rough joint surface, also fibrosis of the bone marrow and lack of well defined cortical bone
(specimen from surgically removed condyle in patient with traumatic temporomandibular joint arthritis,
histologically undergoing osteoarthritic changes).

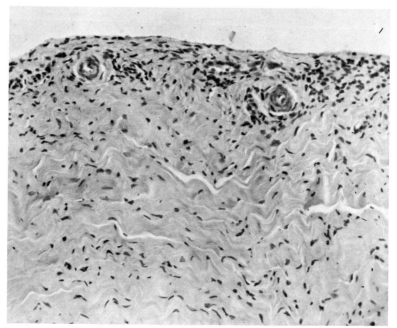

Figure 8-5. Vascularization of traumatized peripheral zone of meniscus and associated mild chronic
inflammation (specimen from surgically removed meniscus in patient with traumatic temporomandibular
joint arthritis).

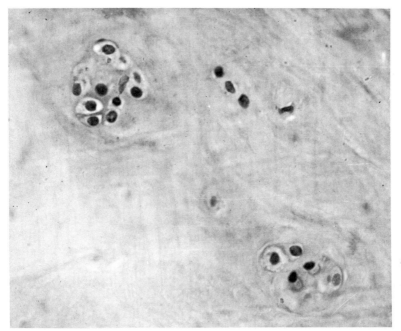

Figure 8-6. Hyalinization and formation of cartilage cells of central part of meniscus (specimen from surgically removed meniscus in patient with traumatic temporomandibular joint arthritis).

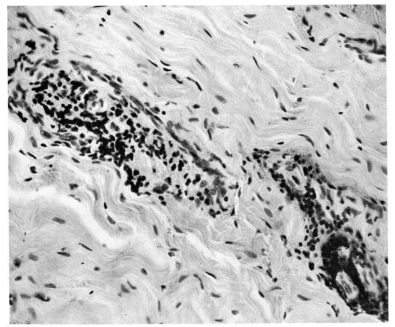

Figure 8-7. Foci of chronic inflammation toward periphery of meniscus (specimen from surgically removed meniscus in patient with traumatic temporomandibular joint arthritis).

A

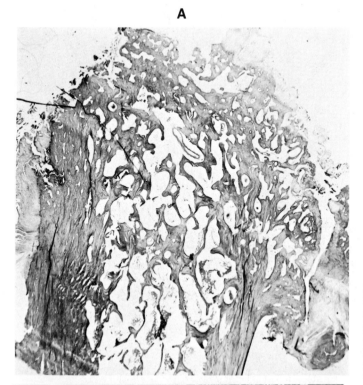

Figure 8–8. A, Irregular bony surface and anterior bony "lipping" of condyle (specimen from condylectomy in patient with osteoarthritis). *B,* Aging changes and early osteoarthritis in temporomandibular joint from old rhesus monkey. Note spur or "lipping" on anterior aspect of condyle.

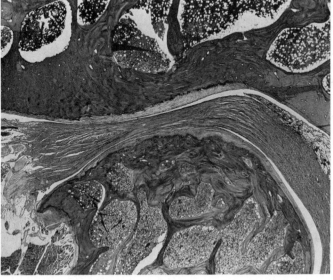

B

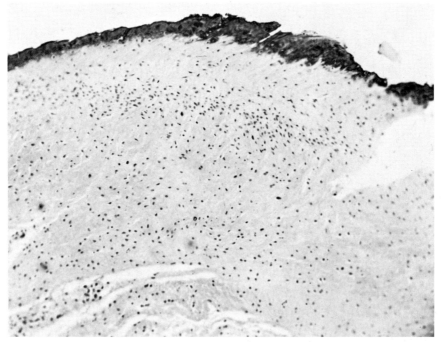

Figure 8–9. Fragmentation of hyalinized and partially calcified meniscus (surgical specimen from meniscectomy in patient with traumatic osteoarthritis).

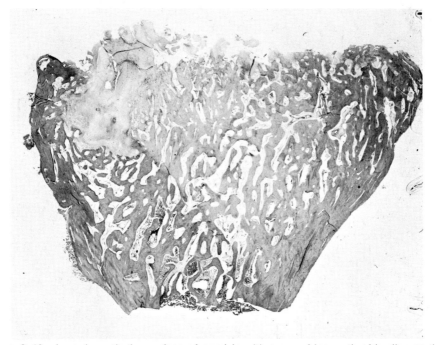

Figure 8–10. Irregular articular surface of condyle with areas of ingrowth of hyaline cartilage (to left) and other areas of eburnated bone (to right). Note heavy bony trabeculation and fibrosis of bone marrow (specimen from surgical condylectomy in patient with traumatic osteoarthritis).

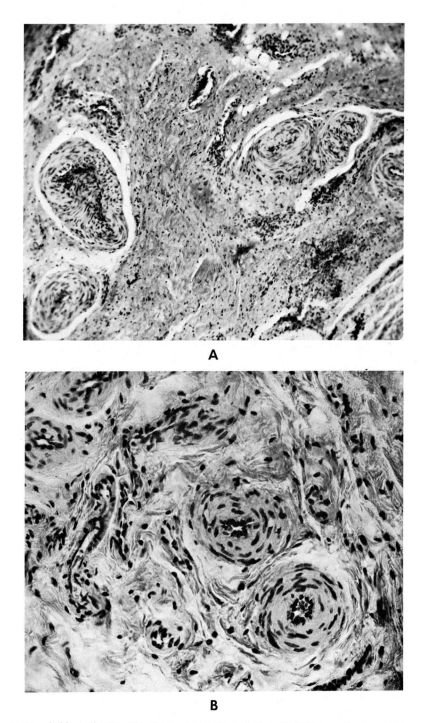

Figure 8–11. *A*, Marked sclerosis of blood vessels and chronic inflammation in anterior aspect of joint capsule. *B*, High magnification from same specimen showing marked sclerosis of vessels (surgical specimen from meniscectomy in patient who previously had sclerosing solution injected into joint).

REFERENCES

1. Arnaudow, M.: Zur funktionellen Theorie der Arthropathia deformans des Kiefergelenkes. Deutche Zahnärztl. Ztschr., *17*:1317, 1962.
2. Axhausen, G.: Des Kiefergelenkknacken und seine Behandlung. Deutsche Ztschr. Chir., *232*:238, 1931.
3. Axhausen, G.: Ein Beitrag zur deformirenden Arthropathie des Kiefergelenkes. Deutsche Zahnärztl. Ztschr. *9*:852, 1954.
4. Axhausen, G.: Pathologie und Therapie des Kiefergelenkes. Fortschr. Zanhlk., *6*:177, 1930; *7*:199, 1931; *8*:201, 1932.
5. Bauer, W. H.: Anatomische und mikroskopische Untersuchungen über das Kiefergelenk mit besonderer Berücksichtigung der Veränderung bei Osteoarthritis deformans. Ztschr. Stomatol., *30*:1136; 1279; 1334; 1932.
6. Bauer, W. H.: Osteoarthritis deformans of the temporomandibular joint. Am. J. Path., *17*: 129, 1941.
7. Blackwood, H. J. J.: Arthritis of the mandibular joint. Brit. Dent. J., *115*:317, 1963.
8. Boman, K. A.: Temporomandibular joint arthrosis and its treatment by extirpation of the disc, a clinical study. Acta chirurgica scandinav., Suppl. 118, 1947.
9. Brill, N., Schübeler, S., and Tryde, G.: Influence of occlusal patterns on movements of the mandible. J. Prosth. Dent., *12*:255, 1962.
10. Carlsson, G. E., Lundberg, M., Öberg, T., and Welander, U.: The temporomandibular joint. A comparative anatomic and radiologic study. Odont. Rev., *19*:171, 1968.
11. Carlsson, G. E., Öberg, T., Bergman, F., and Fajers, C. M.: Morphological changes in the mandibular joint disk in temporomandibular joint pain dysfunction syndrome. Acta Odont. Scand., *25*:163, 1967.
12. Cobin, H. P.: The temporomandibular syndrome and centric relation. New York Dent. J., *18*: 393, 1952.
13. Cohn, L. A.: Factors of dental occlusion pertinent to the restorative and prosthetic problem. J. Prosth. Dent., *9*:256, 1959.
14. Costen, J. B.: A syndrome of ear and sinus symptoms dependent upon disturbed function of the temporomandibular joint. Ann. Otol. Rhin. & Laryng., *43*:1, 1934.
15. Costen, J. B.: Neuralgias and ear symptoms associated with disturbed function of the temporomandibular joint. J.A.M.A., *107*:252, 1936.
16. Donovan, R. W.: A method of temporomandibular joint roentgenography for serial or multiple records. J. Am. Dent. A., *49*:401, 1954.
17. Eschler, J.: Elektrophysiologische und pathologische Untersuchungen des Kausystems. Deutsche Zahnärztl. Ztschr., 7:1333, 1952.
18. Findlay, I. A.: Mandibular joint pressures. J. Dent. Res., *43*:140, 1964.
19. Franks, A. S. T.: The social character of temporomandibular joint dysfunction. Dent. Pract., *15*:94, 1964.
20. Freese, A. S.: The myofascial trigger mechanisms in temporomandibular joint and allied disturbances. Oral Surg., *14*:933, 1961.
21. Gerry, R. G.: Effects of trauma and hypermotility on the temporomandibular joint. Oral Surg., 7:876, 1954.
22. Goodfriend, D.: Dysarthrosis and subarthrosis of the mandibular articulation. Dent. Cosmos, *74*:523, 1932.
23. Goodfriend, D.: Symptomatology and treatment of abnormalities of the mandibular articulation (normal). Dent. Cosmos, *75*:844; 947; 1106; 1933.
24. Gopfert, C.: Über die Einwirkung von Zahnschmerz und von Schmerzriezen der Gesichtshaut auf den reflektorischen Tonus der Kaumuskulatur. Deutche Zahnärztl. Ztschr., *11*:76, 1956.
25. Granger, E. R.: Occlusion in temporomandibular joint pain. J. Am. Dent. A., *56*:659, 1958.
26. Gysi, A.: Modifikation des Artikulators und der Aufstellregelen für Vollprothesen. Bern, Hans Huber, 1958.
27. Hallmann, K.: Kiefergelenk und Okklusion. Oesterr. Ztschr. Stomatol., *59*:185, 1962.
28. Hankey, G. T.: Temporomandibular arthrosis. An analysis of 150 cases. Brit. Dent. J., *97*: 249, 1954.

29. Harris, H. L.: Effect of loss of vertical dimension on the anatomic structures of the head and neck. J. Am. Dent. A., *25*:175, 1938.

30. Hiniker, J. J., and Ramfjord, S. P.: Anterior displacement of the mandible in adult rhesus monkeys. J. Prosth. Dent., *16*:503, 1966.

31. Jarabak, J. R.: An electromyographic analysis of muscular and temporomandibular joint disturbances due to imbalances in occlusion. Angle Orthodont., *26*:170, 1956.

32. Kerr, D. A.: The pathology of traumatic temporomandibular arthritis produced by traumatic occlusion. J. Dent. Med., *4*:190, 1957.

33. Kydd, W. L.: Psychosomatic aspects of temporomandibular joint dysfunction. J. Am. Dent. A., *59*:31, 1959.

34. Lammie, G. A., Perry, H. T., Jr., and Crumm, B. D.: Certain observations on a complete denture patient. Part I: Method and results. J. Prosth. Dent., *8*:786, 1958.

35. Lindblom, G.: Disorders of the temporomandibular joint. Acta odont. scandinav., *11*:61, 1953.

36. Lindblom, G.: On the anatomy and function of the temporomandibular joint; studies on clinical bite-rehabilitation material including arthrosis cases with special references to radiographic findings. Acta odont. scandinav., *17*:Suppl. 28, 1960.

37. McCall, C. M., Jr., Szmyd, L., and Ritter, R. M.: Personality characteristics in patients with temporomandibular joint symptoms. J. Am. Dent. A., *62*:694, 1961.

38. Markowitz, H. A., and Gerry, R. G.: Temporomandibular joint disease. Oral Surg., *2*:1309, 1949.

39. Maves, T. W.: Radiology of the temporomandibular articulation with correct registration of vertical dimension for reconstruction. J. Am. Dent. A., *25*:585, 1938.

40. Moulton, R.: Psychiatric considerations in maxillofacial pain. J. Am. Dent. A., *51*:408, 1955.

41. Monson, G.: Occlusion supplied to crown and bridgework. Nat. Dent. A. J., *7*:399, 1920.

42. Monson, G.: Impaired function as a result of closed bite. Nat. Dent. A. J., *8*:833, 1921.

43. Newton, A. V.: Predisposing causes for temporomandibular joint dysfunction. J. Pros. Dent., *22*:647, 1969.

44. Osing, W.: Untersuchungen über Zusammenhänge von Bissart und Entstellung der Arthropathia deformans im Kiefergelenk. Oesterr. Ztschr. Stomatol., *55*:374, 1958.

45. Perry, H. T., Lammie, G. A., Main, J., and Tuescher, G. W.: Occlusion in a stress situation. J. Am. Dent. A., *60*:626, 1960.

46. Posselt, U., and Addiego, B. J.: A gnatho-thesiometric study of various mandibular positions in individuals with normal and abnormal function of the temporomandibular joints. Odont. Rev., *9* No. 1:1, 1958.

47. Prentiss, H. J.: Preliminary report upon the temporo-mandibular articulation in the human type. Dent. Cosmos, *60*:505, 1918.

48. Ramfjord, S. P.: Bruxism, a clinical and electromyographic study. J. Am. Dent. A., *62*:21, 1961.

49. Ramfjord, S. P., and Hiniker, J. J.: Distal displacement of the mandible in adult rhesus monkeys. J. Prosth. Dent., *16*:491, 1966.

50. Ramfjord, S. P.: Dysfunctional temporomandibular joint and muscle pain. J. Prosth. Dent., *11*:353, 1961.

51. Ramfjord, S. P.: The significance of recent research on occlusion for the teaching and practice of dentistry. J. Prosth. Dent., *16*:96, 1966.

52. Ricketts, R. M.: Variations of the temporomandibular joint as revealed by cephalometric laminography. Am. J. Orthodont., *36*:877–898, 1950.

53. Schwartz, L., and Chayes, C.: Facial Pain and Mandibular Dysfunction. Philadelphia, W. B. Saunders Co., 1969.

54. Schwartz, L.: Conclusions of the Temporomandibular Joint Clinic at Columbia. J. Periodont., *29*:210, 1958.

55. Schwartz, L.: Disorders of the Temporomandibular Joint. Philadelphia, W. B. Saunders Co., 1959, (p. 55).

56. Schwartz, L.: Temporomandibular joint syndromes. J. Prosth. Dent., *7*:489, 1957.

57. Shapiro, H. H.: Differential diagnosis of dental pain. Oral Surg., *4*:1353, 1951.

58. Sicher, H.: Temporomandibular articulation in mandibular overclosure. J. Am. Dent. A., *36*:131, 1948.

59. Steinhardt, G.: Zur Arthropathia deformans der Kiefergelenkes. Ztschr. Laryng. Rhinol. Otol., *30*:475, 1951.
60. Steinhardt, G.: Zur pathologischen Anatomie und Pathogenese einiger akuten und chronischen Kiefergelenkerkrankungen. Deutsche Zahnhlk. Heft, *86*:66, 1933.
61. Summa, R.: The importance of the inter-articular fibro-cartilage of the temporo-mandibular articulation. Dent. Cosmos., *60*:512, 1918.
62. Thomson, H.: Mandibular joint pain. Brit. Dent. J., *107*:243, 1959.
63. Travell, J.: Temporomandibular joint pain referred from muscles of the head and neck. J. Prosth. Dent., *10*:745, 1960.
64. Vestergaard, C. L.: Facial pain from experimental tooth clenching. Tandlagebladet, *74*:175, 1970.
65. Weisengreen, H., and Elliott, H. W.: Electromyography in patients with oro-facial pain. J. Am. Dent. A., *67*:798, 1963.
66. Zimmermann, A. A.: An evaluation of Costen's syndrome from an anatomic point of view. *In* Sarnat, B. G. (ed.): The Temporomandibular Joint. Springfield, Ill., Charles C Thomas, 1951, pp. 82–110.

Diagnosis and Treatment of Functional Disturbances of the Masticatory System

Prior to the diagnosis of any disturbance of the masticatory system, a history and examination of the patient should be completed. No examiner should be content to seek out only the signs and symptoms of bruxism and/or trauma from occlusion; to do so invites an inaccurate diagnosis and incorrect treatment. Although bruxism and trauma from occlusion may be distinct disturbances of the masticatory system, their relationship to the whole masticatory system and to all phases of dental treatment must not be overlooked. For example, to attempt to treat bruxism without recognizing psychoneurosis, pulpal disease, periodontal disease, or other disturbances that may be discovered in a complete examination and that may be significant factors in the cause of bruxism, is an invitation to failure. Similarly, the futile treatment of hopeless, periodontally involved teeth for the correction of bruxism can be avoided by a complete examination.

The treatment of bruxism or trauma from occlusion should be considered in light of the entire treatment plan for the patient. For example, an occlusal adjustment, except for acute conditions, should be rendered after all active inflammation of the periodontal tissues has been eradicated and after completion of orthodontic procedures, but prior to periodontal surgery.

The usual format of including treatment along with diagnosis has not been followed in the chapter on trauma from occlusion. The treatment of trauma from occlusion has been covered in several chapters because it may be eliminated in several ways: (1) a decrease of the total muscular forces applied to the teeth by elimination of bruxism and abnormal muscle tension (this approach is discussed in the chapter on diagnosis and treatment of bruxism); (2) the distribution of the occlusal forces over more teeth by occlusal adjustment or splinting of teeth; (3) changing the direction of the forces from lateral to tolerable axial forces by occlusal adjustment, orthodontic therapy, or restorative dentistry; and (4) an increase of tissue tolerance to occlusal forces by periodontal therapy. (This indirect approach usually is considered to be outside the realm of occlusal therapy and will not be discussed.) The relationship of trauma from occlusion to occlusal adjustment, minor orthodontic therapy, restorative dental procedures, and splinting of teeth will be considered in separate chapters.

OUTLINE FOR CONSIDERING DIAGNOSIS AND TREATMENT OF FUNCTIONAL DISTURBANCES OF THE MASTICATORY SYSTEM

Methods for Diagnosing Dysfunctional Relationships of the Masticatory System

DIAGNOSTIC PROCEDURES

CLINICAL EXAMINATION

LOCATING CENTRIC RELATION

EXAMINATION FOR "SLIDE IN CENTRIC"

EXAMINATION FOR OCCLUSAL INTERFERENCES IN LATERAL AND PROTRUSIVE EXCURSIONS

HABITUAL PATTERN OF MASTICATION

OTHER DIAGNOSTIC METHODS

DIAGNOSIS

Mounting and Analysis of Casts in an Adjustable Articular

PROCEDURES FOR MOUNTING OF CASTS

DISCUSSION OF MOUNTING PROCEDURES

ANALYSIS OF MOUNTED CASTS

Diagnosis and Treatment of Bruxism

DIAGNOSIS

SIGNS AND SYMPTOMS

SIGNIFICANCE OF DIAGNOSIS

SUMMARY

TREATMENT

ADJUNCTIVE THERAPY

OCCLUSAL THERAPY

BITING HABITS RELATED TO BRUXISM

SPASTIC DISORDERS ACCOMPANIED BY BRUXISM

Signs and Symptoms of Trauma from Occlusion

DIAGNOSIS

SIGNS OF TRAUMA FROM OCCLUSION

SYMPTOMS OF TRAUMA FROM OCCLUSION

CHAPTER 9

METHODS FOR DIAGNOSING DYSFUNCTIONAL RELATIONSHIPS OF THE MASTICATORY SYSTEM

The diagnosis of dysfunctional relationships should rest upon observed deviations from accepted principles of what constitutes physiologic or normal occlusal and functional relationships of the masticatory system. Since there is great confusion about what is normal, there are no well defined and generally accepted standards for what constitutes abnormal or dysfunctional relationships. For example, students are still taught to classify occlusion according to Angle's classification, introduced in 1899.[1] However, this classification is based entirely upon morphologic relationships of the teeth, without any regard for the temporomandibular joint and functional relations.

The other common standard for evaluation of occlusal relationships is the classical balanced denture occlusion based mainly on Gysi's ideas.[7] The application of this denture concept to the natural dentition has often had disastrous results and led to mutilation by grinding or "oral rehabilitation" of numerous well functioning and healthy dentitions.

Functional analysis of occlusion or bite analysis was introduced more than 30 years ago (pioneered by Schuyler[18] and Lindblom[11]) and was a worthy attempt to apply physiologic principles to the analysis of the function of the human dentition. Unfortunately, the words "functional" or "physiologic" were not very meaningful until the research of the last two decades established a scientific concept of the physiology of the masticatory system. The methods for diagnosis outlined in this chapter are, therefore, based on the concept of occlusion presented in Chapter 4, Physiology of Occlusion.

DIAGNOSTIC PROCEDURES

History

An adequate history is of basic importance for any clinical diagnosis, and a history should be obtained prior to the examination procedures.

The patient's chief complaint, if any, should first be recorded, and followed by a brief, but meaningful, chronological history of the condition that caused the complaint. Many patients with dysfunctional relationships of the masticatory system have no annoying symptoms relative to these disturbances. Teeth may, for example, have hypermobility and advanced periodontal disease without the patient's knowledge; therefore, a negative history of complaints relative to masticatory dysfunction should not be taken to indicate that no disturbances are present and that further examination would be unnecessary.

A past dental history should always be obtained regardless of the presence or absence of complaints. The history should include an account of loss of teeth, replacements, restorations, orthodontics or any type of previous dental therapy, as well as injuries to the teeth and jaws.

Oral Habits

Masticatory and extramasticatory habits are, in most instances, unrecognized by the patient, but sometimes a positive history can be obtained. Specific problems regarding diagnosis of bruxism, oral habits, muscle and temporomandibular joint disturbances are discussed under diagnosis of these conditions.

Psychic Status

Since the patient's psychic status is extremely important in determining the significance of any disharmony within the masticatory system, one should by careful questioning determine whether the patient has serious tension problems. Some patients who consult dentists regarding occlusal complaints may be much more in need of psychotherapy than dental therapy. It is extremely important that serious psychic disturbances be recognized as early as possible in dealing with patients, otherwise both the patient and the dentist may be wasting time or, even worse, the patient's psychosis may reach a critical stage during the dental treatment. Several cases of suicide have been reported among patients under treatment for occlusal disturbances.[12]

Clinical Examination

The masticatory system is a functional unit rather than an anatomically well defined organ. A clinical examination, therefore, has to include structures directly participating in the function of the masticatory system and also structures indirectly influenced by such function.[15]

The first inspection should include a consideration of the head and neck, posture, facial asymmetries or gross abnormalities.[10] Spastic muscle contractions and hypertrophies should be observed and the temporomandibular joints and adjacent areas palpated at rest and during various jaw movements. Palpate also sites of muscle attachment for the jaw and the neck muscles. Inspect lip position during speech and at rest.

The intraoral examination should include routine inspection and palpation of all intraoral structures, including the internal pterygoid muscles. The periodontal examination should include gingival color, form, density, level of epithelial attachment, pocket depth, and bleeding tendency. The teeth should be examined for mobility, sensitivity to temperature changes and soreness to percussion. Wear facets on the teeth should be noted and related to movement patterns of the mandible.

The clinical examination should be supplemented by roentgenographic evaluation. The roentgenographic and clinical findings associated with occlusal disturbances are discussed in Chapter 12, Signs and Symptoms of Trauma From Occlusion.

The static and functional relationships between the temporomandibular joints and the teeth should be examined thoroughly. Such an examination is usually started with the mandible in rest position. Whether rest position is determined by command relaxation, after swallowing, or after saying words such as Mississippi makes little difference so long as the patient is relaxed, sitting or standing upright, and looking forward at eye level.[5] Under these conditions, this position represents the rest vertical dimension.

Closing from rest position to maximal occlusal contact should be on a straight path. Observe if there are any deviations from the straight path of closure. The vertical dimension with the teeth in maximal occlusal contact is called occlusal vertical. The difference between the rest vertical and the occlusal vertical is called freeway or interocclusal space. It can be assessed clinically by measuring the distance from the nasion (or a mark on the skin immediately under the nose) to the chin point with the jaw in rest position and subtracting the distance between the same two points with the jaws closed. Cephalometric roentgenograms can also be used for this purpose. Because of the great individual variations in interocclusal space, the actual measurements are of limited or no value for analysis of occlusal relations, and the diagnosis of "loss of vertical dimension" should never be made solely on the basis of a wide interocclusal space.

An important consideration in analysis of occlusion is the functional contact relationships between the maxillary and mandibular teeth. The sound effect of a patient tapping his teeth together in centric occlusion should be noted, possibly with the aid of a stethoscope. Stable tooth contact with balanced muscle activity will elicit a sharp, well defined sound; an unstable occlusion will give various and uneven sound effects.[21] Occlusal contact movements in various directions should be smoothly gliding and unhampered or unrestricted by occlusal interferences.[3] However, such examination of occlusal contact relations has to be related to the temporomandibular joints in order to provide a true expression for the functional relationships of the masticatory system. The relationships between the temporomandibular joints and the occlusion are most significantly expressed in centric relation. Although this border position of jaw movements is reached only under certain conditions[6] it is of utmost importance for muscle harmony and functional comfort of the masticatory system. In centric relation it should be possible to obtain harmonious centering of both temporomandibular joints simultaneously.

Locating Centric Relation

By far the most difficult part of an analysis of the masticatory system is to locate centric relation, and in patients with tense jaw muscles and/or temporo-mandibular joint pain it is often impossible to locate the true centric relation with any method available.

Centric relation is normally a "ligamentous position" determined by the ligaments and structures of the temporomandibular joints.[4] However, splinting action by jaw muscles associated with pain, or severe hypertonus of jaw muscle associated with occlusal interferences and psychic tension, may interfere with the placement of the condyle into the glenoid fossa in the most retruded and upper-most stationary hinge position or centric relation. The main prerequisite for accurate determination of centric relation is complete relaxation of the patient's jaw muscles; unfortunately, the patients for whom centric relation is most important are the patients with muscle tension.[16]

In order to succeed in the determination of centric relation the three factors that may induce abnormal muscle tension have to be controlled. These factors are psychic or emotional tension, pain in temporomandibular joints or other parts of the masticatory system, and "muscle memory" or protective reflex action caused by faulty occlusal contacts. A step-by-step procedure has been developed for recording of centric relation which takes all these factors into consideration.

Procedures for Obtaining Centric Relation

Seat the patient comfortably in the dental chair with the backrest reclined to about 60 to 70° and place the headrest under the occipital ridge so there is no tension in the neck muscles when the patient rests his head (Fig. 9–1).

Ask the patient to relax his arms and feet.

Have patient focus his eyes on an object in the line of straight forward vision between 12 and 15 inches away, and have him breathe slowly through his nose.

Ask the patient to open his mouth as far as possible and to hold it open for about one-half to one minute.

Place the right thumb on the patient s mandibular central incisors and the forefinger under the patient's chin (Fig. 9–2). Hold the thumb high enough on the teeth to prevent contact of the opposing teeth in case the patient should try to bite together to swallow.

Speak to the patient in a soft and monotonous voice during the entire procedure. Repeat over and over that he should relax his arms and feet and breathe slowly through his nose.

Tell the patient also that you will guide and move his jaw, and reassure him that he is doing very well (regardless of how tense his jaw muscles may be at that time).

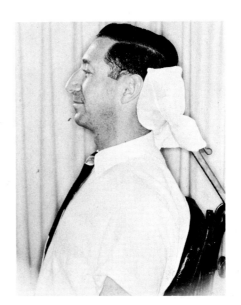

Figure 9–1. Proper position of the patient's head for determination of centric relation.

It is very important that the operator should not cause pain when he starts to move the patient's jaw toward closure. The room should be as quiet as possible, and the operator should concentrate all his efforts toward establishing rapport with the patient. This approach obviously includes features of hypnotic induction or relaxation technique.

Guide the patient's jaw first from maximum opening until the jaw seats back into the most open stationary hinge position. Opening and closing the jaw slightly often helps in obtaining the posterior hinge position. It is important to approach recording of centric relation from wide opening because muscle orientation and protective reflexes associated with faulty contacts are much less active when the teeth are far apart than when they come close together.

As soon as the jaw has been placed in the open hinge position, the operator should move the jaw up and down on the arc of stationary hinge closure, gradually bringing the teeth closer together until the operator's thumbnail strikes the maxillary anterior teeth.

If during these exercises the patient starts to use his tongue to orient his jaw position by touching both the maxillary and mandibular teeth, he should be told either to place the tongue in the floor of the mouth or against the anterior or middle aspect of the hard palate. Do not have the patient roll the tongue back in the pharynx, since this will strain some of the jaw muscles and will have a tendency to bring the condyle down and back from the normal seat in the glenoid fossa.

The operator should gradually move the thumb down on the mandibular incisors while moving the mandible up and down on the path of the stationary hinge axis or centric relation until initial contact is established between the mandibular and maxillary teeth (Fig. 9–3). This can easily be felt and heard and establishes the patient's initial occlusal contact in centric relation. Once this initial contact has been established correctly, it is much easier to guide the patient back to it in subsequent manipulations. There are no pain fibers in the central part of the meniscus and the corresponding parts of the condyle and glenoid fossa, and therefore no painful symptoms can be attributed to these parts of the joint if the condyle is properly seated in centric relation.

Use of Drugs. Barbiturates, "tranquilizers" and muscle relaxants have been tried as supportive adjuncts to location of centric relation, seemingly with some success. However, from limited clinical and electromyographic experiments, it appears that placebo starch pills are equally effective in bringing about relaxation of the jaw muscles if given the proper build-up by the operator. In order to obtain any appreciable effect from relaxants such as meprobamate the patient has to take at least 800 to 1200 mg. a day for several days. Since

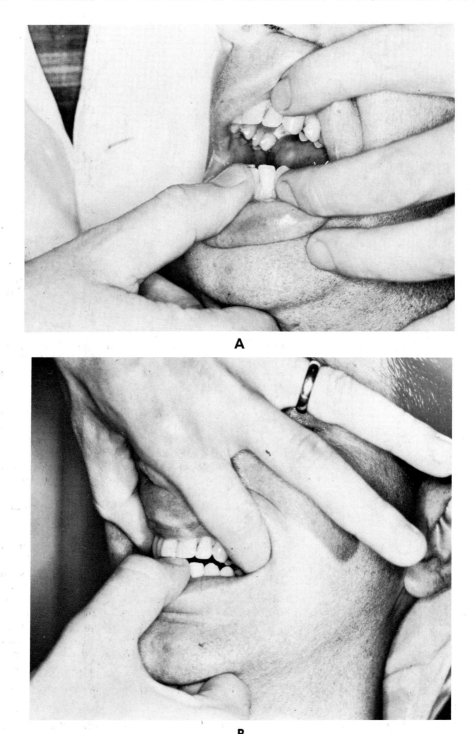

Figure 9-2. *A,* Proper position of the operator's thumb for determining centric relation. *B,* The thumb is placed on the patient's mandibular incisors with light pressure and without any painful pinching or pressing.

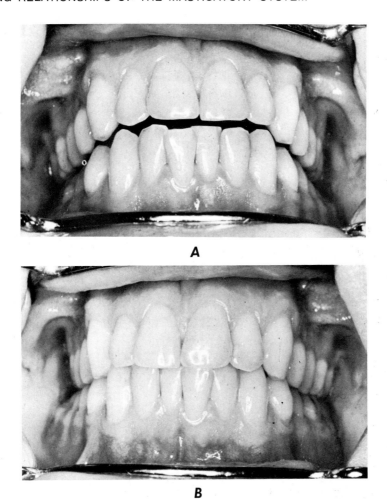

Figure 9–3. *A,* Initial occlusal contact with the mandible in centric relation. *B,* Centric occlusion of the same patient.

patients with such tense jaw muscles often have psychic problems, the use of drugs may result in exaggerated dental problems and requests for more drugs. This result is undesirable from the standpoint of both the dentist and the patient since the dentist by default is then treating an essentially psychiatric problem rather than a dental condition. A much more desirable and effective adjunct to jaw relaxation than drugs is the use of occlusal biteplanes or splints as discussed under treatment of bruxism.

Other Methods for Location of Centric Relation

A number of other techniques have been recommended for location of the terminal hinge position or centric relation; a few will be discussed briefly. The best known method is probably the gothic arch or Gysi's tracing.[7] This method has been adapted for the natural dentition by use of an "occlusolator,"[22] which can be attached to the teeth, and by the use of a combined "central bearing screw" and extraoral tracer, which raises the bite enough to allow for an extra-oral gothic arch tracing. This instrument is somewhat cumbersome, and there is always the real possibility of a false tracing producing a typical gothic arch. Furthermore, it appears from clinical observation that the arrow point jaw position assumed during gothic arch tracing is not necessarily identical to the centric relation obtained by placing the condyle into the glenoid fossa as previously described.

Another method used widely to determine centric relation is to locate the stationary hinge position of the mandible by the use of a kinematic face bow.[13] This is also a rather cumbersome method, and a registered stationary hinge axis may move several millimeters following occlusal therapy in patients with bruxism and temporomandibular joint disturbances.[8] Thus, the location of a stationary hinge axis provides no assurance of an ideal centric relation for the patient, and the use of a kinematic face bow is hardly practical for diagnostic purposes.

Forceful retrusion of the mandible either manually by the dentist or by the use of a retruder is an unreliable way of recording centric relation, since the patient will fight against such forces. Although the force may be symmetrically applied for both sides, muscle pull by the patient can easily be asymmetrical, especially if there is pain or discomfort. There is absolutely no documented evidence,[14] however, that the retruder may bring the mandible into a position distal to centric relation as claimed by numerous authors.[9] The main reason that a retruding device is not recommended is that it interferes with the relaxation of the jaw muscles, which is so essential for recording of the ligamentous centric relation. With forceful retrusion one may or may not be recording centric relation.

Another unacceptable method is to have the patient hold the mandible into a retrusive position either by placing the tongue back toward the pharynx or otherwise pulling the jaw back. This does not tend to seat the condyles into the glenoid fossa and will often place the mandible in a position considerably different from centric relation recorded by other methods.

Since centric relation is reached during swallowing of a mouthful of food, it would be logical to do a functional recording during swallowing, but this is technically impractical in the natural dentition. The best evidence that the true reproducible centric relation has been located is the operator's feeling of a completely relaxed mandible that he easily can move up and down on the retrusive hinge path to tooth contact.

Locating and Marking the Initial Tooth
Contact in Centric Relation

The most common method for marking of premature occlusal contact is the use of various types of carbon paper or ribbon. There are, however, a number of shortcomings to this practice: (1) Carbon paper or ribbon does not mark well

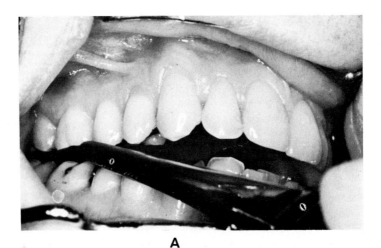

A

Figure 9–4. *A*, Removal of indicator wax using the mesiobuccal cusp of the maxillary first molar as a landmark. *B*, Holding the wax against a source of light makes it easy to locate the penetration marks. The penetration marks can be oriented by noting the relationship of the end-point of the flat-backed forceps to the mesiobuccal cusp of the first maxillary molar.

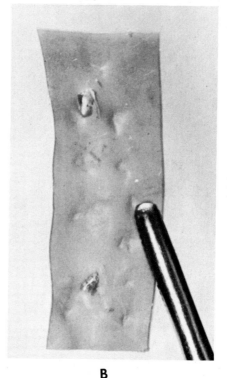

B

on a glossy polished surface and the premature contacts in centric relation are usually on such surfaces. (2) Paper or ribbon is too thick to discriminate between teeth almost or actually making contact. (3) If the carbon paper or ribbon is highly inked, there is a tendency to obtain "false" markings wherever it touches the teeth, regardless of occlusal contacts. (4) If the paper or ribbon is dry or has a low degree of inking, the markings are not visible.

The effectiveness of carbon paper or ribbon is enhanced by drying the occlusal surfaces of the teeth and by heating the paper or ribbon lightly over a flame. When the paper or ribbon has been placed between the teeth, tap the patient's mandibular teeth against the maxillary teeth in the manner described for locating centric relation.

A much more reliable method than paper or ribbon for locating initial tooth contact in centric relation is the use of thin sheets of soft colored wax. Strips of green inlay wax* (28 to 32 gauge) and 1/2 to 3/4 inch wide are heated lightly and placed on the maxillary or mandibular posterior teeth on both sides, and again the patient's mandibular teeth are tapped against the maxillary teeth by the operator. The premature contact will then penetrate the wax The wax can either be inspected while sticking to the teeth or taken out of the mouth and held against a light source. If it is removed from the teeth one should use flat backed pliers or forceps and point the end of the instrument to a landmark such as the mesiobuccal cusp of the first maxillary molar in order to determine the location of the premature contact (Fig. 9–4, *A*). Inlay wax with a sticky coating on one side (occlusal indicator wax*) is also available. This is used in the same manner as the regular inlay wax, but the penetration is marked on the tooth with a soft lead pencil before the wax is removed. However, this is not quite so discriminating in marking as the regular inlay wax held against a light source (Fig. 9–4,*B*).

Another very accurate method for locating premature contact is to dry the tooth off and paint a lacquer on either the maxillary or mandibular occlusal surfaces, let it dry a little, and then tap the patient's teeth together.[19] However, this method is time consuming and somewhat messy.

Examination for "Slide in Centric"

Tap the patient's teeth together in centric relation and ask him to squeeze his teeth together. This will provide a glide or slide from centric relation to centric occlusion. Observe the direction of this slide carefully since a straight, forward slide is of much less significance than a lateral shift. The teeth that make contact during this slide can usually be marked with carbon paper or ribbon. Note also with palpation of the teeth and from carbon markings what teeth are receiving the impact of the slide when it ends in centric occlusion. The traumatic impact of a slide in centric is often much greater upon the teeth engaged at the end of the slide than the teeth that provide the path for the slide. Traumatic occlusion in the maxillary anterior region, for example, is often the result of a slide in centric on posterior teeth that do not exhibit any ill effect from the slide.

Premature Contacts in Centric Occlusion

Premature contacts in centric occlusion can be located best by having the patient bite or tap very lightly on strips of inlay wax or carbon paper. Light

---

*Kerr Dental Manufacturing Company.

palpation with the fingertips on the buccal aspect of the teeth that are in contact when the patient taps or bites together also helps to locate premature contacts in centric occlusion. Do not rely too much on the patient's ability to point out the teeth that make initial or too heavy contact since by changing his muscle pull (in heavy biting especially) he can shift the heavy contacts from one area of the mouth to another without moving the jaws to any observable extent. Observe for occlusal stability related to cusp-fossa relationships. Determine if there is an "open bite" in centric occlusion closure. If the "bite" is open, always try to determine the cause.

Examination for Occlusal Interferences in Lateral and Protrusive Excursions

Occlusal interferences hampering or hindering smooth gliding occlusal contact movements in lateral and protrusive excursion can be located by visual inspection, palpation, carbon paper or ribbon markings, wax, and placement of lacquer. If the patient is simply asked to do lateral excursions with the teeth in contact, there is a tendency for him to follow the convenience paths of minimal hindrance, and the major occlusal interferences may be avoided and not marked. It is therefore advisable to guide lateral movements with the operator's hand on the patient's jaw, starting from centric occlusion and doing bilateral sweeping movements. Since it has been shown now by Adams and Zander[2] that lateral movements in mastication do not go back to lateral tracings from centric relation but stay on the lateral path from centric occlusion, this method would cover the area of possible interferences during mastication. However, it is not known how far back the mandible goes during lateral bruxism, so in order to be sure that all possibilities for occlusal interferences in lateral excursions have been covered, the lateral excursions from centric relation should also be investigated by moving the jaw on the retrusive lateral paths of a Gysi's tracing. If the teeth are loose, inspection and palpation will locate the interfering teeth better than occlusal markings.

The steepness of cuspal and incisor guidance and the amount of overbite are not very important for the function of the natural dentition so long as the various occlusal and incisor contact movements can be performed in an unrestricted, smooth, gliding fashion. Measurement of overbite and overjet, therefore, are not very meaningful for an analysis of occlusal function or dysfunction except for extreme cases with soft-tissue impingement.

Quite often there is splinting action of the muscles from protective reflexes associated with occlusal interferences that makes it difficult to examine lateral and protrusive excursions. A technique similar to the one recommended for location of centric relation can also be used to induce guided lateral movements. Sometimes it also helps to start lateral movement with the teeth apart and gradually bring in occlusal contacts.

Habitual Pattern of Mastication

The patient should be given a piece of soft wax and asked, first, to chew in the most convenient way, then instructed to chew in various excursions. This is done in order to determine if a restricted convenience pattern of mastication is present and what this pattern is. There should also be a careful examination for possible signs of occlusal habits such as notching and chipping of teeth not related to occlusal contact.

Other Diagnostic Methods

Roentgenograms

Roentgenograms and other laboratory aids are of value in the diagnosis of dysfunction of the masticatory system. The value of roentgenograms in diagnosis of temporomandibular joint disturbances is discussed in Chapter 17, and the roentgenologic signs of trauma from occlusion have been outlined under Signs of Trauma From Occlusion (p. 257). It can be stated in summary that roentgenograms of the temporomandibular joints, because of anatomic variations, are of limited value for the diagnosis of dysfunctional relations of the temporomandibular joints and the teeth. Jaw movements can be recorded on roentgenograms, but this yields very little information that cannot be observed better by clinical examination. Roentgenograms of the joints have their greatest value in the differential diagnosis[20] of pathologic disturbances other than those involving the occlusion. Thus, one cannot diagnose faulty centric relation or occlusion from roentgenograms of the joints. Neither can "distal displacement" or "anterior displacement" be diagnosed from roentgenograms. The old concept of hypermobility or subluxation as diagnosed by roentgenologic evidence of the condyle positioned anterior to the articulate tuberculum in maximal opening is not tenable since more than one-third of the people with normally functioning joints have this characteristic.[17]

Electromyography

Electromyography is a laboratory method for evaluating muscle function that has received considerable attention in the literature on occlusion during the last 10 to 20 years. It offers an opportunity to observe and record in a documentable way functional disturbances within the masticatory system, but at the present time electromyography has to be considered a research tool rather than an aid in routine clinical diagnosis of occlusal disturbances. There are too many potential sources of uncontrollable variations and artifacts in electromyography to make it a clinical method for dental use. Electromyography supplies supportive evidence for clinical observations and has to be combined with other devices to record actual occlusal contact relations.

DIAGNOSIS

The findings made when the described examination techniques are utilized should be related to the many subsequently described signs and symptoms of dysfunction of the masticatory system to provide the basis for the diagnosis. The diagnosis should be derived from interviewing, examining, and synthesizing the descriptive features of diseases and the facts obtained from the examination and interview. The data obtained from the history and examination of the patient will usually provide the information necessary to make a positive diagnosis. Some experience in the diagnosis of functional disturbances is necessary if the proper significance is to be placed on the signs and symptoms noted in the history and examination. It is to be emphasized that the temporomandibular joints and masticatory muscles are only a part of the functional unit described as the masticatory system. An analysis of functional disturbances of the system may show that one or more interrelated disturbances are present and, thus, one or more diagnoses should be made. Finally, the diagnosis or diagnoses should be evaluated for significance to the prognosis and plan of treatment. It is sometimes assumed that a diagnosis automatically provides the information for evaluating the prognosis and for planning treatment. Although a diagnosis provides identification of the disturbances encountered, only a basic knowledge of the principles underlying the disease and clinical judgment can assure that proper treatment is given.

REFERENCES

1. Angle, E. H.: Classification of malocclusion. Dent. Cosmos, *41*:248, 305, 1899.
2. Adams, S. H., and Zander, H. A.: Functional tooth contacts in lateral and in centric occlusion. J. Am. Dent. A., *69*:465, 1964.
3. Beyron, H. L.: Characteristics of functionally optimal occlusion and principles of occlusal rehabilitation. J. Am. Dent. A., *48*:648, 1954.
4. Brill, N., Lammie, G. A., Osborne, J., and Perry, H. T.: Mandibular positions and mandibular movements. A review. Brit. Dent. J., *106*:391, 1959.
5. Garnick, J., and Ramfjord, S. P.: Rest position. J. Prosth. Dent., *12*:895, 1962.
6. Graf, H., and Zander, H. A.: Tooth contact patterns in mastication. J. Prosth. Dent., *13*:1055, 1963.
7. Gysi, A.: The problem of articulation. Dent. Cosmos, *52*:1, 1910.
8. Hughes, H. J.: The Terminal Hinge-axis of the Mandible. Thesis, University of Michigan, May, 1963.
9. Ingle, J. D.: Determination of occlusal discrepancies. J. Am. Dent. A., *54*:6, 1957.
10. Kerr, D. A., Ash, M. M., and Millard, H. D.: Oral Diagnosis. 2nd ed. St. Louis, The C. V. Mosby Co., 1965.
11. Lindblom, G.: I St. Appolonias vald. Stockholm, Nordiska Bokhandels Förlag, 1946.
12. Lipke, D., and Posselt, U.: Parafunctions of the masticatory system (bruxism). Panel discussion. J. West. Soc. P., *8*:133, 1960.
13. McCollum, B. B.: Fundamentals involved in prescribing restorative dental remedies. Dent. Items Interest, *61*:522; 641; 724; 852; 942; 1939.
14. Posselt, U.: Studies in the mobility of the human mandible. Acta odont. scandinav. *10*:19, Suppl. 10, 1952.
15. Ramfjord, S. P.: Diagnosis of traumatic temporomandibular joint arthritis. J. Calif. State D. A., *32*:300, 1956.

16. Ramfjord, S. P.: Dysfunctional temporomandibular joint and muscle pain. J. Prosth. Dent., *11*:353, 1961.
17. Ricketts, R. M.: Variations of the temporomandibular joint as revealed by cephalometric laminography. Am. J. Orth., *36*:877, 1950.
18. Schuyler, C.: Fundamental principles in the correction of occlusal disharmony: Natural and artificial. J. Am. Dent. A., *22*:1193, 1935.
19. Troest, T.: Diagnosing minute deflective occlusal contacts. J. Prosth. Dent., *14*:71, 1964.
20. Updegrave, W. J.: Radiography of the temporomandibular joint. *In* Schwartz, L., and Chayes, C. M.: Facial Pain and Mandibular Dysfunction. Philadelphia, W. B. Saunders Co., 1969.
21. Watt, D. M.: Classification of occlusion. Dent. Pract., *20*:305, 1970.
22. Zander, H. A., and Hurzeler, B.: Diagnosis of occlusal disharmonies. J. So. Calif. State D. A., *26*:382, 1958.

Film

"Examination of Occlusion"
 May be loaned through:
  V. A. Central Office Film Library
  810 Vermont Avenue, N.W.
  Washington, D.C. 20420

  Film Library
  American Dental Association
  211 East Chicago Avenue
  Chicago, Ill. 60611

CHAPTER 10

MOUNTING AND ANALYSIS OF
CASTS IN AN ARTICULATOR

Accurate stone casts are helpful for the study of the morphology of the teeth and their intra-arch relationship.[2] Number, form, attrition facets, contact relations, position of the teeth and arch form can all be studied to some advantage from good casts. Even centric occlusion relationships between the maxillary and mandibular teeth can be viewed. However, centric relation and functional relationships cannot be studied with any semblance of accuracy unless the casts are mounted correctly on an individually adjustable articulator.

Properly mounted casts constitute an important aid in the analysis of functional occlusal relationships as well as in diagnosis and treatment planning. However, technical limitations regarding reproduction of the complicated jaw movements in articulators tend to restrict the significance of functional analysis in an articulator.[13]

Mounted casts provide an opportunity to study occlusal relations from the lingual side and give a detailed view of occlusal facets and their functional relations. Such studies of mounted casts are of great help for treatment planning and patient education as well as for teaching and self-learning for the dentist. In cases of extensive oral rehabilitation, mounting, adjustment of the casts and trial waxing of the restorations is a must for the novice and of great help for the experienced operator.

Some very complicated articulators have been constructed in attempts to reproduce mandibular movements accurately.[1, 4, 10] However, the time and effort that are required in the use of such instruments is hardly justified for diagnostic purposes since the added information from such mountings compared with conventional methods and instruments can be obtained directly in the mouth with even greater reliability than in any instrument. Therefore, when the advantages and disadvantages inherent in the use of various articulators for diagnostic purposes are considered, it appears that mounting casts in a Hanau

215

or Dentatus articulator with a conventional face bow provides all the essential information that can be gained from a study of mounted casts. Furthermore, the unavoidable errors associated with the use of such articulators have been found to be within the adaptive range of the temporomandibular joint, jaw muscles and the periodontium of practically every patient if the articulators are used to their best advantage.

The more complicated and unquestionably more accurate instruments should be reserved for research and possibly for patients with a poor adaptive capacity for minute discrepancies within the masticatory system.

PROCEDURES FOR MOUNTING OF CASTS

Before the casts are made, a preliminary examination of the occlusion should be done and gross occlusal interferences in centric relation removed.

The impressions for the casts should be made with alginate, hydrocholoid or rubber base materials. The casts should be made with a thick mix of very hard colored stone and carefully checked for air bubbles or any other signs of distortion. It is especially important that the occlusal anatomy, including the base of the sulci, be reproduced distinctly and accurately. The materials and equipment needed for mounting of casts are given in the outline that follows. The adjustable articulator (Hanau H2-0 or H2-X, or Dentatus ARH or ARL) with an infraorbital plane recording is preferred for the occlusal analysis and occlusal adjustment on mounted casts. The articulator should be well lubricated.

Materials for Mounting Casts

> Adjustable articulator
> A conventional face bow with bite fork
> Hard base plate wax and 28 gauge green sheet inlay wax
> Waxing instruments and a sharp knife
> Quick setting impression plaster
> Plaster bowl and spatula
> Flexible millimeter ruler and indelible pencil
> Water syringe and saliva ejector

The base plate wax should be very hard so that distortion will be minimized and can be readily observed if it occurs. Although soft wax is easier to work with than hard wax, it is more difficult to determine when distortion has occurred. The trimming of wax outside the mouth should be done with a very sharp knife to avoid distorting the wax impression. A Bard-Parker knife with a straight blade is useful for trimming the excess wax from the wax bite. The quick setting plaster is used for mounting the casts on the articulator. Impression plaster or stone with a very low dimensional setting change should be used.

Determining Hinge Axis

The conventional hinge axis is located by measuring with the flexible ruler from the middle of the tragus of the ear to the outer canthus of the eye and placing a mark with an indelible pencil 13 mm. in front of the border of the tragus (Fig. 10–1). The ruler should barely touch the tragus and the mark should be made as a right angle cross to make it easy for centering of the hollow arm of the face bow. Also palpate and make a mark on the skin for the infraorbital notch if the articulator has a device for recording of the axis-infraorbital plane (Fig. 10–2).

Use of Bite Fork

Wrap two to three layers of evenly heated base plate wax on the bite fork and place between the patient's teeth. The handle of the bite fork should be pointed 10 to 15° laterally in order to avoid conflict later (when mounting cast) with the incisal pin and table of the articulator. Have the patient bite slowly into the wax till imprints of the occlusal surfaces of both the mandibular and maxillary teeth provide steady support for the bite fork. Caution the patient against biting through the wax to the metal since the arms of the bite fork may bend and, being resilient, will bend back when taken out of the mouth. If this distortion occurs, the casts will not fit into the wax imprints accurately. The position of the mandible during this procedure is of no significance since the bite fork recording is done solely for the orientation of the maxillary models to the hinge axis and the infraorbital plane.

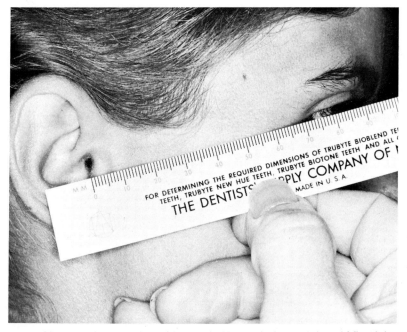

Figure 10–1.   Marking of conventional hinge axis 13 mm. in front of the middle of the tragus.

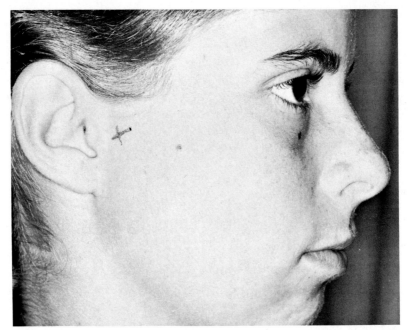

Figure 10-2. Infraorbital point and hinge axis marked with an indelible pencil.

With the bite fork in the mouth, chill the wax with cold water. After removal of the bite fork place the maxillary cast into the wax and check for possible contacts with soft oral tissues. If there is evidence of any such contacts, at least 1 mm. thickness of wax should be carved away in these areas since it may be assumed that the wax has displaced the soft tissues, and the casts made from anatomically true impressions would not seat properly into the wax bites. Also carve away wax from the buccal surfaces of the teeth so the cusp tips and incisal edges of the teeth on the cast seat properly in the wax bite. Make sure that the cast fits accurately into the wax bite. Discard the wax bite if there is any rock of the cast when it is fitted lightly into the wax bite and the described adjustment of the wax bite has been made.

Use of Face Bow

Chill the wax bite thoroughly and place the bite fork back into the patient's mouth and let him bite into the occlusal imprints to hold the bite fork steady while the face bow is brought into place and properly centered. The condylar tubes of the face bow should almost (but not quite) touch the skin over the center of the cross marks which have been made on the skin to designate the conventional hinge axis. The face bow should be so centered that the millimeter settings on both sides of the face bow are the same. Tighten the front set screw of the face bow, making sure there has been no change in position of the condylar tubes during this procedure. Some of the older face bows are entirely unsatisfactory because of poor mechanical construction of the screw that holds

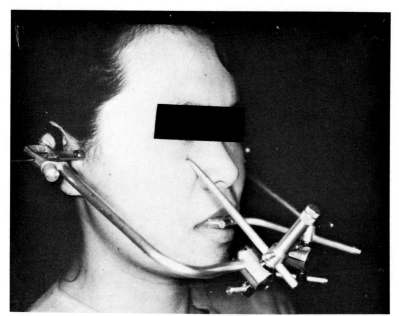

Figure 10–3.   Face bow with infraorbital pin in position.

the face bow to the bite fork. Place the infraorbital pin in position if the face bow has one (Fig. 10–3).

Mounting of Maxillary Cast

Set the condylar guidance of the articulator at 30° and the lateral guidance at 15°. Place the incisal pin at 0. Lock the condyles and be sure there is no "play" in the condylar lock before the face bow is centered in the articulator. Some articulators have adjustment screws to eliminate such play if present. If there is provision for recording of the infraorbital plane, this will determine the position of the bite fork (Fig. 10–4). If not, place the bite fork on an arbitrary level approximately in the vertical center of the articulator. This level is not related to the occlusal relationships,[3] but sufficient space for the mandibular cast should be allowed. The maxillary cast is placed in the wax bite on the bite fork and mounted with a thin flowing mix of quick setting impression plaster or quick setting stone.

Centric Relation Wax Bite

The next and most important step in the mounting of casts is to obtain a wax bite with the mandible in centric relation. Centric relation should first be located according to the method previously described (p. 204) and without wax in the mouth (Fig. 10–5). Heat evenly a strip of hard base plate wax about 4 inches long and 1 inch wide. The wax should preferably be heated in hot water and made as soft as it can and still be handled. Fold the strip of wax over to a

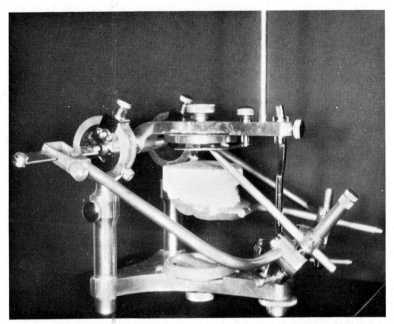

Figure 10–4. Face bow and maxillary cast in the articulator. Infraorbital pin determines level of cast in the articulator.

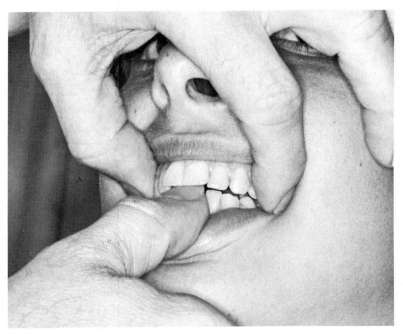

Figure 10–5. Location of centric relation. Apply mild guiding pressure on mandibular anterior teeth.

long double layer and rapidly place it on the patient's mandibular teeth. Hold the right hand on the patient's chin with the thumb on the mandibular incisors; with light pressure tap the patient's mandible up through the soft wax almost to the point of contact between the mandibular and maxillary teeth (Fig. 10–6). Before the wax is placed between the teeth it is advisable to have an orienting landmark established to indicate approximately the relationship between the maxillary and mandibular teeth, i.e., about 0.5 mm. opening in the posterior regions.

The operator should maintain a steady mild pressure on the patient's mandibular incisors while the excess of wax is carved away to expose the buccal cusp tips. The wax bite is then chilled with cold water. It is very important to maintain some distal pressure on the patient's mandible while the wax bite is being chilled, especially if he has teeth that are sensitive to cold. Under such circumstances cold water will precipitate immediately an increased contraction of the jaw muscles and possibly pull the mandible away from centric relation. After the buccal and labial surface of the wax has been chilled, have the patient open the mouth and chill the lingual aspect of the wax in the mouth, otherwise it may easily be distorted during removal. Any soft tissue contact made by the wax should be relieved by carving off about 1 mm. of wax.

If the thinnest layer of wax over the occlusal surfaces appears to be thicker

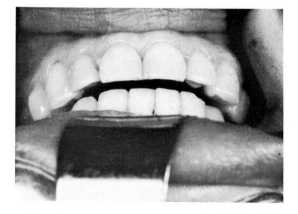

A

Figure 10–6. *A,* Centric relation with initial occlusal contact. *B,* Centric relation waxbite with a thin layer of wax between the teeth that made the initial contact. Wax properly carved to expose maxillary incisal edges and tips of cusps.

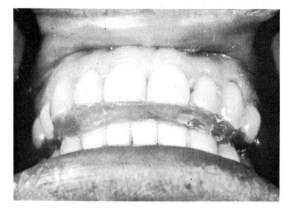

B

than about 0.5 mm., the bite should be retaken. If at any point the maxillary and mandibular teeth have made contact through the wax, the bite should also be retaken, since there is no sure way of knowing whether a slide in centric may have been initiated at that point.

By looking at the occlusal imprints in the wax bite against a source of light one can fairly well estimate what teeth will make initial contact in centric relation on the mounted casts. If these teeth happen to be the same teeth that were also shown to make contact using green inlay wax during location of the centric relation contacts prior to the mounting, this is some indication that the wax bite may be correct. However, such an observation does not prove that the mandible was equally retruded in both instances. Placing the bite back on the maxillary teeth and tapping the mandible carefully into the bite is also a fair check on the accuracy of the bite in centric relation.

Mounting Mandibular Cast

The centric wax bite is used for placement of the mandibular cast in the articulator. The incisal pin is dropped down about 2 mm. to compensate for the 0.5 mm. thickness of wax bite in the molar region. Inspect the wax bite and the casts carefully to see that they are free of wax shavings or other particles. Place the wax bite on the already mounted maxillary cast, and fit the mandibular cast carefully but firmly into the wax bite. Be sure that both casts fit completely into the imprints of the cusp tips and incisal edges in the wax bite. Make some notches on the sides of the base of the mandibular casts and tie the mandibular cast to the maxillary casts and the articulator as firmly as possible with a heavy cotton string. It is very important that the casts and the wax bite be held firmly together during the rest of the mounting. Mount the mandibular cast to the articulator with impression plaster or quick setting stone. Volume changes during setting of the plaster are very critical for this part of the mounting. For this reason, a small space between the mandibular cast and the mounting ring of the articulator is preferable to a large space. The greater the space the greater the potential volume change in setting of the plaster or stone.

The mounting in the articulator can now be checked against the occlusal relationship in the mouth with the mandible in centric relation by use of 28 gauge green inlay wax to locate the initial contacts in centric relation both in the mouth and in the articulator. The contact pattern should be identical in the mouth and the articulator for all the teeth. There should also be the same distance and direction of the slide in centric in the articulator as is present in the mouth. If findings are not identical, remount with a new centric relation wax bite is probably needed. Check also to see that opposing teeth are in contact in centric occlusion, especially in the molar regions.

Protrusive Wax Bite

A protrusive wax bite is needed for the setting of the condylar guidance. Let the patient look in a hand mirror and have him move the mandible 3 to 4 mm.

straight forward and down from centric relation.[11,12] Have the patient practice biting together in this protrusive position. It often helps the patient if guide marks are placed on the anterior teeth. A protrusive record of less than 3 mm. will not provide an accurate articular setting, and more than 5 mm. will cut off some of the curve of condylar guidance in the temporomandibular joint and the condylar guidance in the recommended articulators. It is also important to take a straight protrusive record with regards to avoiding the Bennett movement, since the indicated articulators have no provision for individual setting for Bennett movement. Depending on the amount of overbite, use two to four layers of well heated hard base plate wax for the protrusive bite. Have the patient bite into the agreed position without bringing the teeth into actual contact, i.e., stop about 0.5 to 1 mm. short of contact. Trim and chill the wax bite as described under centric relation bite.

Setting Condylar Guidance

Loosen the condylar screws on the articulator, open the centric locks, and remove the incisal pin. Place the protrusive wax bite on the mandibular cast, and move the upper part of the articulator back until the maxillary cast fits into the wax bite. Hold the two parts of the articulator firmly together and read off the condylar guidance on both sides of the articulator. Tighten the condylar screws. In most instances, with fairly normal temporomandibular joints, there will not be more than 2 to 5° of difference between the right and left condylar guidance, although differences may go up to 20° or more.[7] However, more than 10° difference should make one suspect that something had gone wrong during the mounting, and the procedures should be rechecked. After the setting of the condylar guidance, the case is ready for analysis in the articulator.

Other Mounting Procedures

A more precise mounting of casts may be necessary when extensive restorative procedures are necessary, especially those involving a change in vertical dimension. With such procedures a diagnostic wax-up and occlusal analysis are most helpful when a kinematic face bow or a pantograph is used and the casts are mounted in a fully adjustable articulator. One such method makes use of the Denar instrument system consisting of the D4-A articulator, pantograph, and accessories. The Denar pantograph can be transferred directly to the articulator, eliminating the necessity for additional procedures involving a mounting stand.

Only a brief outline of the mounting procedure using the Denar instrument system will be given since a detailed description of the system may be found elsewhere.[5] The first step in the mounting procedure is to make clutches using the Denar clutch former. This clutch device consists of a jig mechanism for locating and fabricating clutches directly in the mouth. Upper and lower frames of the clutch former are separated by a rubber die to allow ease of separation of the two members. Also, a center bearing screw facilitates gliding of

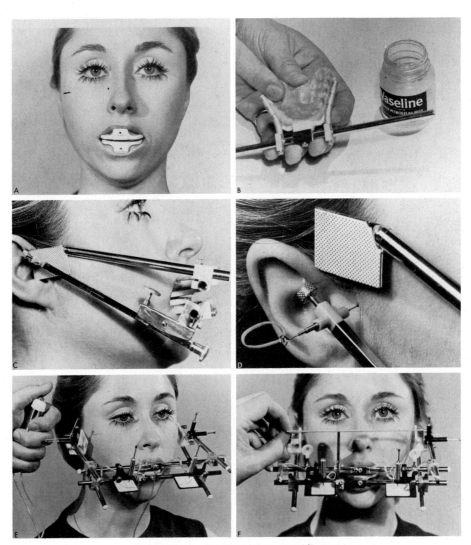

Figure 10–7.   See legend on opposite page.

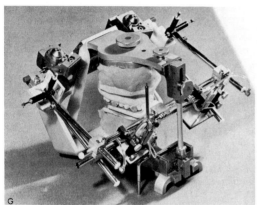
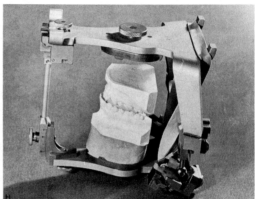
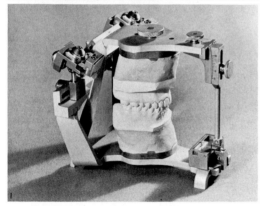

Figure 10–7. Mounting study casts on a fully adjustable articulator. *A,* Clutches inserted. Anterior reference line and point is shown. *B,* Vaseline being applied to prevent lutting material from sticking to clutch. *C,* Positioning of hinge axis locator. *D,* Transfer of hinge axis point to skin. *E,* Pantograph attached to clutches and survey being done. *F,* Alignment of reference point and two hinge axis points with articulator reference pin. *G,* Transfer of maxillary cast and pantograph to articulator as well as hinge axis transfer. *H,* Mounting of lower cast in centric relation with checkbite record. *I,* Study casts mounted and ready for analysis. (Photographs by courtesy of the Denar Corporation, Anaheim, California.)

the upper and lower clutches over each other during recording of excursive mandibular movements with the pantograph. The rubber die forms a concave bearing surface on the upper clutch and positions the central bearing screw in the lower clutch. Using quick-setting cold cure acrylic in the clutch forms, indentations of the maxillary and mandibular occlusal surfaces are obtained with the mandible guiding into terminal hinge closure. The clutch former and ease of adjustment provides a relatively simple, fast method for making clutches for most situations. When indicated, cast aluminum clutches may be keyed to the Denar pantograph.

After forming the clutches, the clutch assembly is anchored to anterior cross bars, and the occlusal surfaces are lubricated with mineral oil or a thin coating of vaseline (Figs. 10–7A, B). Prior to anchoring the clutch system to the teeth an anterior reference point is marked on the face. The anterior reference point is made on the skin 43 mm. superior to the incisal edge of a maxillary incisor with the point made in line with the inner canthus of the eye.

The clutches are inserted into the mouth and quick-setting plaster or hard-setting zinc oxide and eugenol impression paste is used to lock the edges of the clutch former arms (anchors) to the buccal surfaces of the teeth. After the clutches have been anchored to the teeth the Denar hinge axis analyzer is positioned on the maxillary cross bar so the flag is positioned in the sagitta plane (Fig. 10–7C). The stylus assembly of the hinge axis locator is secured to the mandibular cross bar. The mandible is guided into the terminal hinge position and the flag positioned until the stylus is over a dot on the flag coincident with the axis of pure rotational opening movement. When the dot, which is coincident to the terminal hinge axis, is located, the flag is moved to allow the inked stylus to be moved into contact with the skin (Fig. 10–7D). The right and left points of the terminal hinge axis are the posterior reference points. A horizontal reference plane line is made on the right side of the face in line with the anterior and posterior reference points. The anterior point and reference plane line can be made with a Denar reference plane locator and marker. Before the hinge axis is located and the pantograph used, the patient should be trained in movement to centric relation position, protrusive movement, and eccentric excursions of the mandible.

The pantograph is assembled on the patient (Figs. 10–7E, F), using the anterior and posterior reference points for orientation. Mandibular movements and centric relation position are recorded with a pneumatically activated stylus. The stylus should only be activated and recordings made when the patient makes the instructed and desired movements. Two records should be coincident for centric relation position, right and left lateral, and protrusive movements.

After obtaining the record desired, the pantograph and clutches are transferred to the Denar D4-A articulator (Fig. 10–7G). The anterior-posterior eminentia is set to 25 to 30° and the progressive side shift to 5 to 10°. The upper and lower members of the pantograph must be attached to the articulator through the clutches. The lower clutch is mounted directly to the lower member of the articulator. The lower member of the pantograph, mounted to the lower member of the articulator, is used to position and mount the upper member of the pantograph to the upper member of the articulator. The maxillary cast is positioned in the maxillary clutch and mounted to the upper member of the articulator. The maxillary clutch is then anchored to the maxillary mounted cast with wax or compound; it then moves with the upper member of the articulator. Thus the maxillary cast has been transferred to the articulator by facebow transfer using the pantograph (Figs. 10–7*H, I*).

At this time the articulator settings are made according to the lines of the

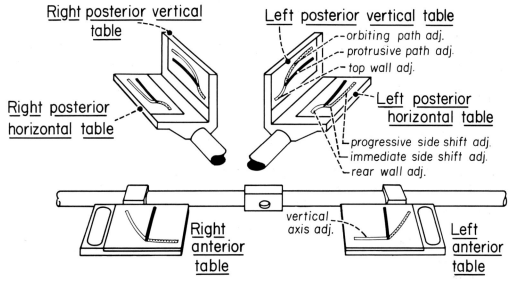

Figure 10–8. Diagram of tracings necessary to set articulator adjustments in Figure 10–7G.

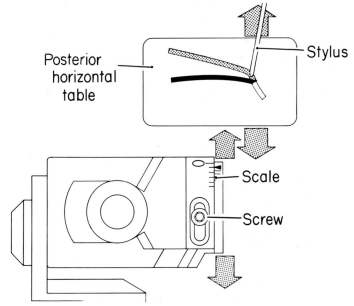

Figure 10–9. Close-up of screw adjustment and portion of line required to make adjustment for immediate side shift.

pantograph record (Fig. 10–8). Adjustments include protrusive, immediate side shift (Fig. 10–9), progressive side shift, rear wall, vertical axis, orbiting path, and top wall adjustment. Because of reciprocal influences, the adjustments must be made in proper sequence, observing concurrent and constructive requirements. Successive casts can be mounted on the articulator with its settings by the transfer facebow with the aid of the same three reference points.

When the articulator has been adjusted, a centric relation checkbite record must be obtained to relate the mandibular cast to the maxillary cast. This record may be obtained as outlined previously (p. 219).

A recent development is the Denar Centric Relator. This instrument provides for an accurate transfer of the mounting of casts on the office or school articulator to a laboratory instrument. In this way the dentist or student need not have several articulators or tie up a single articulator on which restorations are to be made.

Discussion of Mounting Procedures

There are a number of other acceptable procedures for mounting of models and an attempt will be made to answer some of the questions regarding why certain features of other techniques were not included here.

Why not determine the stationary hinge axis by a kinematic face bow? There is, of course, no objection to such a procedure, but for the diagnostic mounting of casts it is hardly worth the extra effort.[13,18] It has been found by experience that the initial contacts in centric relation can be accurately reproduced by the described method providing the wax bites are thin and major interferences that would require considerable closure in the articulator have been removed before the casts were made. Unquestionably, if any lowering or increase in occlusal vertical dimension is contemplated in the articulator, one has to use a kinematic face bow. If attempts are made to reproduce the individual Bennett movement, kinematic face bow recording is also essential,[9,16] but this is not even attempted by the average value articulators used in the described procedures.

Why not record the Bennett movement and take lateral check bites? Even with the most elaborate and complicated articulators and recording methods, the movement patterns of the mandible in the various functional excursions can be only approximately well duplicated.[17] It has never been shown by controlled experimentation that accuracy in reproduction of the Bennett movement beyond the average values built into a Hanau or Dentatus articulator is of clinical importance for comfortable function of the masticatory system. It must be admitted that the correct individual reproduction of the Bennett movement may be of great importance if attempts are made to reconstruct balanced occlusion in the classical sense of the word in far lateral excursions. However, in modern occlusal adjustment and reconstruction, the working side contacts are usually made heavier than the balancing side, and other contacts guide the lateral excursions rather than the balancing contacts.[14] This is done both for work in the articulator and directly in the mouth and, under these circumstances, an extremely accurate reproduction of Bennett movements and balancing side contacts loses most of its value. Lateral checkbites are not used for the reasons explained above and, furthermore, the recommended articulators do not always accept such bites since there is only limited possibility to adjust these articulators for such bites.

Why not use split cast techniques for control of the centric relation mounting? Experience has shown that the accuracy of the mounting procedures can be judged satisfactorily with the described wax techniques, and there is very little if anything to be gained from the more cumbersome split cast technique. Errors in determination of centric relation unfortunately can be duplicated with split cast technique[18] as well as with the wax technique, so the use of the split cast technique does not provide a reliable check for accuracy in the determination of centric relation.

Why not use some material other than hard wax for bites? Although a softer wax such as Aluwax has been used, distortions in the soft wax may occur during the mounting procedures and it seems that the hard wax, properly handled, assures the most accuracy. The reason for not using Johnson's bite rims or other paste techniques is that such bites cannot be trimmed accurately nor is there any assurance that the cusps of the casts fit perfectly into the bite.

Why not use an anterior guide of plastic or impression plaster to guide the mandible into centric relation during the wax bite technique? This method can be recommended when patients have a tendency to grasp for their anterior teeth when wax is placed between their teeth.[8] Providing this bite-block is constructed correctly for the jaw in centric relation, there is no objection to its use.

ANALYSIS OF MOUNTED CASTS

Initial contacts in centric relation can be recorded on the casts in the same manner as described for the oral examination (p. 208). Use carbon paper, dental tape (Madame Butterfly Red Dental Tape [20 or 30 inkings] is excellent for casts), green 28 to 32 gauge inlay wax, or very thin Cellophane strips. The latter is used to test whether the teeth actually make contact. One main advantage of mounted casts is the opportunity to observe by direct inspection the detailed relationship of the teeth during the slide from centric relation to centric occlusion.

An analysis of lateral excursions, although not very accurate using the mounting procedure just outlined, provides a fairly good opportunity to inspect the cusp and fossa relationship during simulated lateral function from the buccal and lingual aspects. Protrusive function is accurately duplicated for only a few millimeters forward from centric relation, but for that critical area it provides a good opportunity to study relationships between incisal guidance and the cusps of the posterior teeth.

Mounted casts are helpful in an analysis of occlusal function but their main value is in planning the occlusal adjustment and oral reconstruction, and as a teaching aid. However, the final diagnostic functional analysis of occlusion always has to be done in the patient's mouth and, as stated by Schweitzer,[15] "We must guard against evaluating occlusal therapy in terms of some rigid mechanical concepts."

REFERENCES

1. Bergström, G.: On the reproduction of dental articulation by means of articulators; A kinematic investigation. Acta odont. scandinav., 9:Suppl. 4, 1950.
2. Beyron, H. L.: Det adulta bettet ur funktionell synpunkt. Nordisk Klinish Odontologi. Kapitel, 8:3–11. Copenhagen, Forlaget for Faglitteratur, 1959.
3. Beyron, H. L.: Orienteringsproblem vid protetiska rekonstruktioner och bettstudier. Svensk Tandläk Tidsk., 35:1, 1942.
4. Granger, E. R.: Establishment of occlusion, The articulator and the patient. Dent. Clin. North America, 527, Nov., 1960.
5. Guichet, N. F.: Procedures for Occlusal Treatment. A teaching atlas. Anaheim, Calif., Denar Corporation, 1969.
6. Henrikson, O.: Registrering av gångjärnsaxeln. Exakthet uppnåd på patient. Odont. Tidsk., 68:125, 1960.
7. Isaacson, D.: A clinical study of the condyle path. J. Prosth. Dent., 9:927, 1959.
8. Lucia, V. O.: A technique for recording centric relation. J. Prosth. Dent., 14:492, 1964.
9. McCollum, B. B., and Stuart, C. E.: A Research Report (Gnathology). South Pasadena, Calif., Scientific Press, 1955.
10. Posselt, U.: The Physiology of Occlusion and Rehabilitation. Philadelphia, F. A. Davis Co., 1962.
11. Posselt, U., and Franzen, G.: Registration of the condyle path inclination by intraoral wax records: Variations in three instruments. J. Prosth. Dent., 10:441, 1960.
12. Posselt, U., and Nevstedt, P.: Registration of the condyle path inclination by intraoral wax records—its practical value. J. Prosth. Dent., 11:43, 1961.
13. Puff, A., and Krause, G.: Roentgenkinematographische Untersuchungen am Kiefergelenk unter funktioneller Belastung. Deutsche Zahnärztl. Ztschr., 20:189, 1965.
14. Schuyler, C. H.: An evaluation of incisal guidance and its influence in restorative dentistry. J. Prosth. Dent., 9:374, 1959.
15. Schweitzer, J. M.: A conservative approach to oral rehabilitation. J. Prosth. Dent., 11:119, 1961.
16. Stuart, C. E.: Accuracy in measuring functional dimensions and relations in oral prosthesis. J. Prosth. Dent., 9:220, 1959.
17. Weber, R.: Die Dreidimensionale Kondylenbahnregistrierung und ihre Konsequenzen. Schweiz. M. Zahnhk., 65:499, 1955.
18. Weinberg, L. A.: An evaluation of the face-bow mounting. J. Prosth. Dent., 11:32, 1961.

Films

1. "Examination of Occlusion"
2. "Mounting of Casts in a Semi-adjustable Articulator and Use of Bite Planes"
   May be loaned through:
   V. A. Central Office Film Library
   810 Vermont Avenue, N.W.
   Washington, D.C. 20420

   Film Library
   American Dental Association
   211 East Chicago Avenue
   Chicago, Ill. 60611

CHAPTER 11

DIAGNOSIS AND TREATMENT OF BRUXISM

DIAGNOSIS

The signs and symptoms of bruxism are not conspicuous in most instances;[39] however, certain signs and symptoms are indicative, although not pathognomonic or diagnostic. By careful observation of these signs and symptoms, severe cases of bruxism can usually be discovered. Since most of the patients with bruxism are unaware of the habit, a case history is usually unreliable.[11, 28] By informing a patient about the possibility of bruxism and having him inquire of family or friends, a positive history can often be obtained. In many instances, the habit of bruxism is brought from the subconscious to the conscious level by pointing out to the patient the possibility of the presence of such a habit. Although it has been suggested that such an inquiry can precipitate bruxism in patients who do not have this habit, from current knowledge of the neuromuscular mechanism of bruxism,[25, 38] this is very unlikely and so far it has not been proved that such a development can occur.

It is likely that almost every person occasionally when under stress will press or grind his teeth. However, this is not of much concern if there is no manifestation of trauma. Bruxism may lead to trauma from occlusion with manifestation in any of the various components of the masticatory system. Trauma to crowns and roots of teeth, trauma to the pulp, the periodontium, the masticatory neuromuscular complex, and to the oral mucosa are all possible; but only when there are signs and/or symptoms of trauma present in the masticatory system is bruxism a significant occlusal problem.

Signs and Symptoms

Nonfunctional Patterns of Occlusal Wear

Perhaps the most significant dental sign of bruxism is occlusal or incisal attrition patterns that do not conform to or coincide with normal masticatory

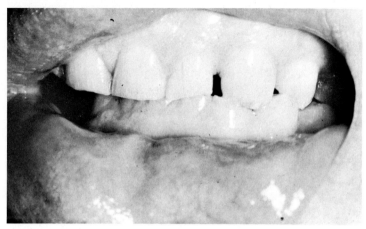

Figure 11–1. Extensive attrition extending outside the range of normal function is indicative of bruxism (male, age 31).

or swallowing wear patterns (Fig. 11–1). Such patterns of attrition or facets of wear are often seen out of the normal range for function at the incisal tip of a maxillary cuspid. These facets of wear are often rounded over to the labial surface of the cusp tip instead of blending into the lingual attrition facets that occur from mastication. Such facets may also be seen on maxillary bicuspids and incisors, as well as other teeth. Nonfunctional facets of wear may be so far removed from the normal functional range that it is painful for a patient to bring his jaw into a position where contact is established between maxillary and mandibular facets.

It is advisable to complete the oral examination without calling abnormal facets of wear to the patient's attention, since patients often go into extreme nonfunctional positions when difficult or touchy questions come up during the examination interview. Thus, the dentist may then have an opportunity to establish the diagnosis of bruxism through direct observation.

The mechanism of excessive wear associated with bruxism is, according to Uhlig,[52] based on the loosening and crushing of enamel prisms between contacting enamel surfaces, which provides the grit necessary for rapid wear of the enamel. Extensive occlusal or incisal wear (even within the normal pattern of jaw movements) in people living on a rather soft diet is usually the result of bruxism, especially when seen in young individuals. There is very little abrasive quality to foods commonly used and it seems reasonable to believe that marked occlusal wear is more apt to be the result of teeth contacting teeth than of teeth contacting food even when contacts during mastication and swallowing are considered.

Bruxism when combined with nervous regurgitation of acid stomach contents can lead to enamel erosion and to extremely rapid lingual incisive wear (Fig. 11–2). Since both bruxism and habitual regurgitation may result from nervous tension, the concomitant occurrence of these two disorders may occasionally be observed. The reason for "cupping" of the exposed dentin in severe wear from bruxism is not known (Fig. 11–3).

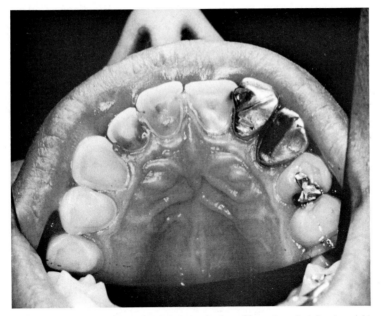

Figure 11–2. Bruxism combined with acid regurgitation. There is extensive loss of tooth substance on the palatal aspect—more on the teeth than on the gold crowns (male, age 46).

The wear pattern of longstanding bruxism is often very uneven and usually more severe on anterior than on posterior teeth in the natural dentition (Fig. 11–4). In patients who have dentures the wear may be more severe on the posterior teeth than the anterior teeth since the stability of the denture allows for the greatest pressure in the posterior regions (Fig. 11–5).

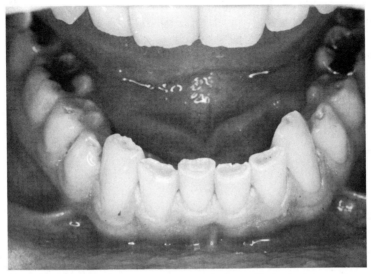

Figure 11–3. "Cuppings" and fracture of the enamel of mandibular incisors and associated bruxism (male, age 24).

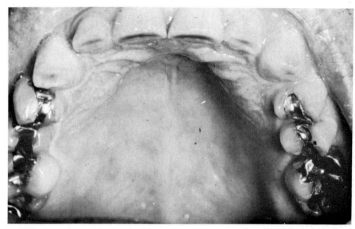

Figure 11–4. Wear from bruxism. The wear is much more extensive on the anterior than on the posterior teeth (male, age 31).

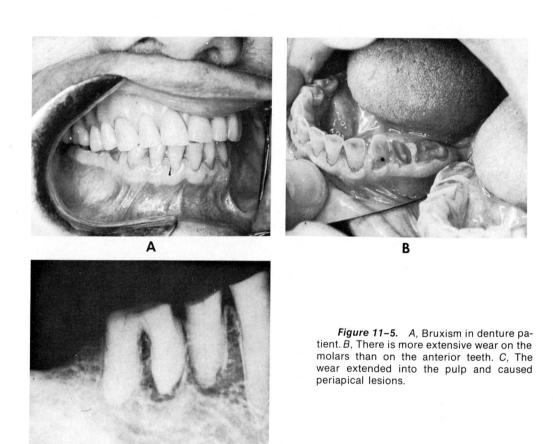

A

B

C

Figure 11–5. *A,* Bruxism in denture patient. *B,* There is more extensive wear on the molars than on the anterior teeth. *C,* The wear extended into the pulp and caused periapical lesions.

Unexpected Fractures of Teeth or Restorations

Splitting or fracturing of the teeth is another dental sign of bruxism (Fig. 11–6). Fractures may occur in intact teeth but are found mainly in association with occlusal wearing of the central fossa of soft restorations leaving hard cusp tips in occlusal interference. Fracturing of restorations and teeth may also occur outside the functional range of occlusion in patients with bruxism during episodes of extreme forced malposition of the jaws. Surgical dressings used following gingivectomy, for example, are often broken by occlusal contacts during bruxing movements at night, and such dressings should be checked for freedom of contacts both in masticatory and extramasticatory relations.

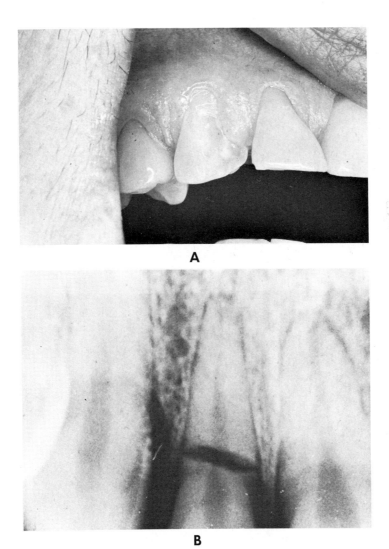

A

B

Figure 11–6. *A,* Fracture of intact cuspid by bruxism (female, age 66): *B,* Fracture of intact lateral incisor by bruxism (male, age 30).

Unexpected Mobility of Teeth

Increased mobility of teeth is often associated with bruxism and is especially significant when found in teeth with very little or no evidence of periodontal disease. Hirt and Mühlemann[19] showed that the teeth of patients with nocturnal bruxism have a measurably higher degree of mobility in the morning than later in the day. Such teeth often have a dull percussion sound[42] and may feel sore when the patient bites on them, especially in the morning.

Pulpal hyperemia with sensitivity, especially to cold, may be present in bruxism. Occasionally, necrosis of the pulp may also result from severe bruxism.[21]

Increased Tonus and Hypertrophy of Masticatory Muscles

Increased muscular tonus that is manifested as an uncontrolled resistance to the dentist's attempts to manipulate the patient's jaw to centric relation is very

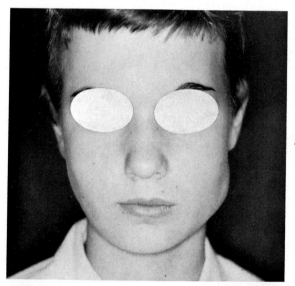

A

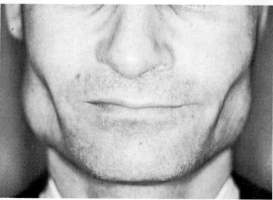

B

Figure 11–7. *A*, Unilateral hypertrophy of masseter muscle associated with bruxism. The bruxism and hypertrophy subsided almost completely over a period of 3 years after occlusal adjustment (female, age 13). *B*, Bilateral hypertrophy of masseter muscles associated with bruxism (male, age 37).

common in patients with bruxism. There is often unilateral or bilateral hypertrophy of the masticatory muscles, especially the masseter muscles (Fig. 11–7). Unilateral hypertrophy of the masseter is sometimes mistaken for a tumor of the parotid gland.[2, 20] The hypertrophy and hyperfunction of the masseter muscles may influence the development of the mandible during growth and lead to marked facial asymmetry.

While no laboratory tests can establish an unequivocal diagnosis of bruxism in borderline cases, electromyographic evidence of abnormally high muscle tonus in the jaw muscles, especially as an inability to relax between occlusal contacts, is highly indicative of bruxism.[38] A certain number of patients with severe bruxism can be taught to relax their jaw muscles to a normal state of tonus in spite of their tendency for bruxism. If conversation with such persons assumes an unpleasant character, a marked increase in muscle tension will appear immediately. A labile resting tonus of the masticatory muscles is often seen associated with bruxism. The increased muscular tonus with bruxism makes it very difficult, if not impossible, to locate occlusal interferences in the retrusive range between centric occlusion and centric relation.

Soreness of Masticatory Muscles

Sometimes the masticatory muscles are tender to palpation in patients with bruxism.[38, 43] The tender spots are most common along the anterior and lower border of the masseter and the medial pterygoid muscles but may also be found in the temporal region.

Sometimes patients with bruxism complain of a tired feeling in the jaws when they awaken in the morning, or they experience a "locking" of the jaw and the masseter and temporal muscles have to be massaged by the patient before the jaws can be opened.

Patients with hypertonicity of their jaw muscles and bruxism may bite their cheeks and lips and tongue accidentally as a result of sudden contraction of these muscles. Sometimes headaches of the type usually called tension or emotional headache are associated with abnormal muscle tension.[3, 32]

Temporomandibular Joint Discomfort and Pain

Patients with temporomandibular joint discomfort and pain of a traumatic nature usually grind their teeth,[40] but this aspect of bruxism will be discussed under temporomandibular joint disturbances.

Maxillary and Mandibular Exostoses

Exostoses of the mandible and maxilla may be the result of bruxism (Fig. 11–8). These bony overgrowths tend to recur if bruxism continues after their removal.

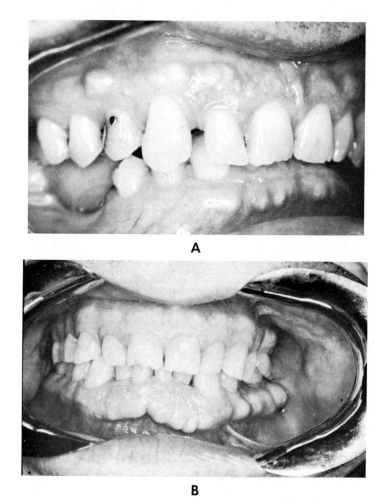

A

B

Figure 11-8. *A,* Beginning nodular exostosis in maxilla associated with bruxism (male, age 37). *B,* Extensive mandibular exostosis was removed surgically on one side but recurred in 2 years (male, age 65, with severe bruxism).

Audible Occlusal Sounds of Nonfunctional Grinding

The audible sound of bruxism is, of course, diagnostic when such a manifestation can be observed directly or recorded on a tape recorder during sleep. In many instances, the patient seeks advice for the bruxism because the noise of grinding the teeth during bouts of nocturnal bruxism has kept a spouse or roommate awake.

According to Uhlig,[52] the audibility of bruxism is determined by the tooth to tooth friction, the area in which the grinding occurs, and the force of grinding. He also observed that in 90 per cent or more of patients with bruxism there was no history of audible sounds associated with the bruxism. All investigators of the prevalence and incidence of bruxism stress the importance of having the patient alerted to the possible tendency for bruxism and suggest that he solicit information from family, friends or working associates.

Prevalence of Bruxism

A definite diagnosis of bruxism is often difficult to obtain because of the subconscious level of the habit; therefore, the figures in the literature indicating prevalence and incidence of bruxism vary over an extremely wide range. The most careful surveys of patients with periodontal disease indicate that a very high percentage of such patients have bruxism. Bundgaard-Jörgensen[8] found bruxism in 88 per cent of 496 patients regularly examined in his practice. Other prevalence figures vary between 20 and 80 per cent, depending upon the examination methods and the criteria used for diagnosis.[33, 35] Since only 8 per cent of Bundgaard-Jörgensen's[8] patients had audible bruxism, the prevalence figure obtained from his patients would have been very low if the sound of bruxism had been the only diagnostic criterion used.

The prevalence and incidence figures for bruxism will also depend upon what degree of nonfunctional occlusal contacts are diagnosed as bruxism. To be consistent with present knowledge, nonfunctional occlusal contacts of incidental nature or those associated with transient extreme stress should not be related to bruxism. The diagnosis of bruxism should be based on an established habit pattern which has led to one or more of the previously discussed signs and symptoms.

Nervous System Involvement

Discomfort from occlusal interference or pain may also affect the central nervous system. A statement sometimes heard from a patient is "This new filling is driving me crazy." In such instances, there is a lowering of the irritability thresholds for the neurons associated with the reflex-controlled jaw movements as well as an increase in the muscle tonus by direct stimulus of the fusimotor nervous system.[41] Overfatigue and subsequent pain from sustained contractions within the jaw muscles will also lower the irritability threshold in the neurons controlling the reflex action and become a part of this "feedback" mechanism. This vicious cycle of self-perpetuating increase in muscle tension related to functional disturbances in the teeth, periodontium, other oral tissues, temporomandibular joints and the masticatory muscles is the basis for bruxism in persons under psychic or emotional stress. The hypertonic, sometimes painful, status of the jaw muscles in bruxism is of the same nature as the occupational myalgias in the arm and neck muscles of typists under mental stress, or postural myalgias manifested as backache in persons under psychic tension with postural anomalies.[38]

Centric Relation and Centric Occlusion

Since a discrepancy between centric relation and centric occlusion has been found to be the most common trigger factor for bruxism,[38] it is essential that such a discrepancy be located during diagnostic procedures. However, the increased tonus in the masticatory muscles makes it very difficult, if not impossible, to locate occlusal interferences in the retrusive range. Various acrylic splints or bite plates may have to be used to induce muscle relaxation before occlusal disharmony can be diagnosed. Tranquilizing drugs, if not found dangerous, or psychotherapy may also provide the needed muscle relaxation.[1, 9, 16]

In addition to a discrepancy between centric occlusion and centric relation, balancing side and working side interferences may also trigger bruxism. Furthermore, local factors other than occlusal interferences may contribute to hypertonicity of the jaw muscles and initiate abnormal jaw movements. Such conditions are gingival flaps of third molars, gingival hyperplasia, any type of periodontal disease with pain,[10] surface irregularities of the lip, cheek and tongue, and pain or discomfort in the temporomandibular joint and jaw muscles.[40]

Significance of Diagnosis

Bruxism is of extreme clinical importance since the presence or absence of bruxism indicates a patient's individual reaction to his occlusal imperfections. A patient with very little occlusal interference and marked bruxism is difficult to treat by any procedure that involves occlusal relations. The presence of bruxism documents the low tolerance level of occlusal interference. On the other hand, a person with considerable occlusal interference and no bruxism does not tend to develop trauma from occlusion or other functional disturbances even if restorative or prosthetic procedures should end up slightly short of perfection.

Discomfort from soreness in teeth, muscles, and temporomandibular joints associated with bruxism will often increase with psychic tension and irritability which, in turn, will increase muscle tonus and bruxism. It is essential, therefore, that this condition be diagnosed and treated before this vicious cycle of "feedback" has resulted in permanent damage to the masticatory system.

Summary

The diagnosis of bruxism is based on suggestive clinical signs and symptoms followed by a confirmatory history from the patient or other sources. Various recording devices for sound, tooth mobility and muscle action are helpful in establishing the diagnosis of bruxism.

Bruxism is the best available indicator of a patient's tolerance or intolerance to occlusal disharmony. Occlusal analysis is difficult and often provides unreliable results in patients with active bruxism. The use of temporary bite planes, occlusal splints, drugs or psychotherapy may be necessary to achieve the muscle relaxation needed for diagnosis of the occlusal trigger factors of bruxism.

TREATMENT

Bruxism is of extreme clinical importance in treatment planning. It is essential to successful treatment of any disorder of a dysfunctional nature that the etiologic factors be recognized under the diagnostic procedures and that the causative factors be eliminated. The complexity of the etiology of bruxism and the diagnostic problems already discussed make it easy to understand the current state of confusion and controversy that exists about the treatment of bruxism. Because of a lack of conclusive diagnostic criteria it is also very difficult to prove satisfactorily whether bruxism has been eliminated by any given treatment procedure.

From a clinical and practical standpoint bruxism should be reduced below the level at which it is capable of producing recognizable harm to the teeth, the periodontium or any other part of the masticatory system. This result does not necessarily mean that the individual never clenches or grinds his teeth; it does indicate that the vicious cycle between habitual bruxism and increasing muscle tension (the neuromuscular 'feedback' mechanism) has been broken and bruxism eliminated as a pernicious habit.

Since bruxism has a dual cause that includes psychic and local occlusal factors,[4] a rational treatment should include the elimination of both disturbing etiologic factors. And, since both psychic tension and a local trigger factor have to be present to initiate bruxism,[38] this dysfunctional habit can be eliminated by either psychic or local therapy. It has been shown conclusively that this is true for grinding or eccentric bruxism, but it is not entirely clear whether local therapy has the same degree of importance in the elimination of clenching or centric bruxism as does psychic therapy.

Another confusing aspect of bruxism is related to the threshold values for tolerance of occlusal interference. Depending on variations in the patient's state of psychic stress, the same occlusal interference that acts as a very potent trigger factor for bruxism one week may or may not bother the patient or precipitate bruxism the next week. The identical occlusal interferences may trigger bruxism in one individual and be of no consequence in another, again depending on the degree of psychic stress. In order to eliminate bruxism, one has either to lower the threshold for neuromuscular irritability below the point where the patient's occlusal interference does not act as a trigger for bruxism, or enough occlusal interference has to be removed to get within the tolerance limit for the patient's neuromuscular mechanism. The very best treatment of bruxism is to influence both the psychic and occlusal factors in a favorable way. An outline of possible methods for the treatment of bruxism follows.

Adjunctive Therapy

Psychotherapy

Psychotherapy aimed at lowering emotional or psychic tension of the patient has been suggested and occasionally used successfully by several investigators.[28] However, a number of patients with bruxism have deep-seated emotional or psychic disturbances which the dentist is not trained to evaluate or to treat. The dentist should, therefore, be very careful about getting involved in any kind of psychotherapy beyond general counseling. Suicides have occurred during the time that treatment for bruxism was being performed. Bundgaard-Jörgensen[8] reported three suicides in a group of 50 adult patients being treated for bruxism. Twenty of these 50 patients sought psychiatric treatment and half were treated successfully. Psychoanalysis has also been recommended for patients with bruxism.

There is no doubt that psychotherapy properly executed may reduce tension and at least temporarily eliminate bruxism. However, this is a complex and time-consuming therapy which should be reserved for patients who are in obvious need of such treatment. These patients should be told firmly that they need help from somebody who is better qualified to help them with their problems than the dentist. Probably less than 1 per cent of all individuals with bruxism need psychotherapy, but the dentist can save himself and the patient from unnecessary disappointment and even harassment if he, during the examination and diagnostic procedures, can single out such patients.

The overwhelming majority of patients with bruxism do not need complex psychotherapy. Thus, in the majority of cases such therapy is impractical and of dubious value since a large number of patients can be helped through simple counseling by the dentist. An attempt should be made to explain to the patient the relationship between the bruxism and his emotional or nervous tension. The idea that the bruxism is an outlet for nervous tension is usually rejected vehemently by the patient and should never be argued. However, when the patient has had time and opportunity to think it over, he usually states during subsequent appointments that what was said about the bruxism was probably correct and has helped him to understand his own problems better. A dentist should be very careful not to probe too deeply into a patient's emotional problems since this approach may aggravate the instability of the psychoneurotic individual.

Systemic drug therapy (to lower psychic tension and thereby reduce bruxism) may be temporarily effective but is not advisable. Tranquilizing drugs may temporarily alleviate muscle tension and lower the threshold for neuromuscular response to occlusal interference enough to stop bruxism, but as soon as the drug is withdrawn the bruxism will return.[16] Furthermore, patients with bruxism may have psychic problems which make them likely to welcome tranquilizers as a means of escaping tension; this may predispose to addiction. The only permissible (although not advisable) use of such drugs in patients with bruxism is for the purpose of temporarily eliminating painful muscle spasms to give the dentist an opportunity to diagnose and eliminate occlusal interferences.

Autosuggestion and Hypnosis

Autosuggestion has been a favorite therapy for bruxism over many years and is recommended by several authors.[5, 12, 27, 31] If the precipitating factors of bruxism are left unrecognized and untreated, autosuggestion will in most instances be of very little or no value unless there is an intentional or unintentional substitution of another habit for bruxism. Recently, hyponosis has been recommended as a means to break the habit of bruxism;[15] however, this type of treatment may be dangerous under certain conditions. If both the psychic tension and the occlusal trigger for bruxism are left untreated, and the patient through posthypnotic suggestion is forbidden to avail himself of his established outlet for emotional tension, it is conceivable that a serious psychoneurotic reaction may be precipitated. Such a reaction may follow the frustration of touching the occlusal trigger spots without being allowed to follow this contact with the established muscle reaction. In most instances, of course, the posthypnotic suggestion will be overpowered rapidly and the patient will resume his bruxism without a serious psychic reaction.

Relaxing Exercises and Physiotherapy

Relaxing exercises, both of general and local nature, may serve to decrease muscle tension and bruxism.[8, 50] Postural exercise, often related to the Mensendieck system, has been recommended for patients with bruxism.[30] Other authors have recommended local exercises of the masticatory muscles.[44] Although these exercises may eliminate temporarily the discomfort of muscle tension associated with bruxism, this represents a treatment aimed at alleviation of symptoms rather than elimination of the cause, and the bruxism will return any time psychic tension lowers the tolerance level for the occlusal disharmony below the bruxism level again. Exercises, massage, heat and other forms of physiotherapy will provide the same relief for bruxism as for myalgias of postural or other nature, but since it does not cure the bruxism it should be used only to support other forms of therapy.

Elimination of Oral Pain and Discomfort

Elimination of oral pain and discomfort associated with periodontal disease or pathologic conditions in the lip, cheek and tongue as well as pain or irritation elsewhere in the masticatory system will lower the muscle tonus and have a favorable effect upon bruxism both from the standpoint of local factors and from the standpoint of the central nervous system.

Occlusal Therapy

Occlusal Adjustment

Occlusal therapy in the form of occlusal adjustment, bite raising gold crowns on molars, and vulcanite splints covering the occlusal surfaces of all teeth were all procedures recommended by Karolyi at the beginning of this century.[22, 23] In principle, these are still the most successful methods for treatment of bruxism, although many variants and refinements of the techniques for occlusal adjustment, splints and occlusal rehabilitation have been introduced since Karolyi's time.

It appears that elimination of the occlusal trigger areas (occlusal interferences) is the treatment of first choice, at least as far as the dentist is concerned.[51] Combined clinical and electromyographic studies have also shown that bruxism may be eliminated, or at least controlled beyond the stage where it poses a clinically recognizable problem, by precise occlusal adjustment.[38] This therapy is, of course, dependent on an adequate number of occluding teeth with good periodontal support whereby it is possible to establish a stable well-balanced occlusion after the adjustment. About 75 patients have been observed over various periods of time up to 5 years, and the results have confirmed the conclusions of previously published observations.[38] A few of the patients have experienced temporary relapses to bruxism associated with reoccurrence of occlusal interference, in most instances as a result of new dental restorations. Minor occlusal adjustment has again alleviated their bruxism.

Although occlusal adjustment seems like an easy treatment for bruxism, it is in many instances time-consuming and difficult to carry the occlusal adjustment to the degree of perfection that is required in order to eliminate all occlusal interferences that may trigger bruxism. Even more difficult and often impossible is the establishment of a stable occlusal relationship following the elimination of the interferences.

The high degree of muscle tonus that is commonly found in patients with bruxism often makes it extremely difficult, if not impossible, to achieve the complete relaxation of patients' jaw muscles that is required for location of centric relation or the stationary hinge position of the mandible. It has been a common experience that what in error was considered to be centric relation at the first session of an occlusal adjustment has changed several times during subsequent adjustments. Such apparent changes in centric relation continue to occur until a relaxed stable terminal hinge position can be located following elimination of most of the occlusal interferences or following the use of an acrylic bite plate.

An occlusal adjustment should be performed in detail as described in Chapter 13. The perception level for interocclusal interference for patients with bruxism is apparently even keener than the average 0.02 mm. level for average individuals.[7] One can hardly touch an occlusal contact area with a fine stone before such a patient notices the difference. Although it is of essential importance to establish a stable centric relation, it is also important that no premature contacts or occlusal interferences be left between centric relation and the patient's centric occlusion. An uneven contact relationship in closure from rest position to occlusal contact (centric position) often acts as a trigger for clenching or small bruxing movements. Such slight occlusal instability in habitual closure is best detected when the patient taps his teeth lightly together while he is sitting in an upright position with his head unsupported.

All possible effort should also be made to detect and eliminate balancing side interferences. Many patients with bruxism move their mandible way outside the normal masticatory range in search for occlusal interferences. The adjustment should, therefore, be carried beyond the field of normal functional movements. Ledges on anterior teeth between normal attrition facets and bruxism facets should be carefully eliminated since such ledges may act as triggers for bruxism. Several sessions of occlusal adjustment are usually needed to eliminate bruxism, even when done by the most experienced operator.

Bite Plates and Splints

Many types of bite plates and occlusal splints have been recommended for the treatment of bruxism since Karolyi introduced the vulcanite occlusal splints.[23] The purposes of bite plates and splints have been (1) to stop the bruxism by elimination of the occlusal interferences; (2) to let the patient grind the teeth against acrylic or two occlusal splints and thereby avoid occlusal wear; and (3) to restrict the jaw movements and break the habit of bruxism. The terms "bite plates" and "occlusal splints" are often used interchangeably, but the term "bite plate" should be used only for Hawley[18] type of appliances and the term "occlusal splints" for those appliances that brace and hold together several teeth.

The main requirements for both bite plates and splints are that they should (1) eliminate the occlusal interferences with a minimal amount of bite opening; and (2) maintain a stable position of the teeth while the appliance is used. An attempt will be made to describe and evaluate various bite plates and splints on the basis of how they satisfy these two requirements.

Bite Plates. Bite plates in their simplest form have an acrylic plate with one retaining clasp on each side of the arch in the molar area. The acrylic has been built up behind the anterior teeth to a flat plateau against which the lower incisor teeth contact. The plateau of acrylic raises the bite enough that the posterior teeth cannot make contact. Another modification incorporates a labial arch wire as a Hawley retainer. These types of appliances tend to traumatize the gingival tissues (Fig. 11–9). The third, and the best, modification of the bite plate has been suggested by Sved.[48] In this modification the acrylic is extended from the plateau of acrylic over the incisor edge of the maxillary front teeth (Fig. 11–10).

Bite plates are all very easy to make with a heat or cold cure type of acrylic on a maxillary cast.[14, 17, 37] The plate is fitted directly into the mouth and adjusted, and self-curing acrylic is added to the palatal plateau area if needed to make even contact with the mandibular incisors. The bite should be raised only enough to provide freedom of contact between the posterior teeth. Following adjustment, the biting pressure should be even on the mandibular anterior teeth against the palatal acrylic. These bite plates eliminate occlusal interferences in centric and balancing interferences in lateral excursions. Protrusive interference is usually not eliminated by any of these bite plates, but this seems in

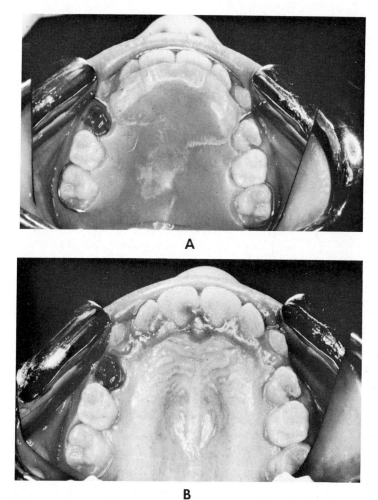

A

B

Figure 11–9.   *A,* Hawley appliance with bite raising anterior plateau. *B,* Trauma to the gingival tissues from such an appliance.

most instances to be of less significance than centric and balancing interferences. The esthetic result may be fairly good, and the bite plate is well accepted by the patient because of the common relief of symptoms provided by this simple appliance.

The main drawback of all bite plates is that they allow for movement of teeth. This drawback is most serious with the simple bite plate since it does not have a labial arch wire and allows both the anterior and the posterior teeth to move. In the modified Hawley bite plate the labial arch wire is supposed to hold the maxillary anterior teeth in position; however, some jiggling of these teeth may ensue and, of course, the posterior teeth may extrude. The splinting action over the maxillary anterior teeth achieved with the Sved[48, 49] bite plate provides much better stability in the anterior region than the other two types because the forces are applied to the anterior teeth in an axial direction.[36] However, the tendency for extrusion of the posterior teeth when this appliance is used over a

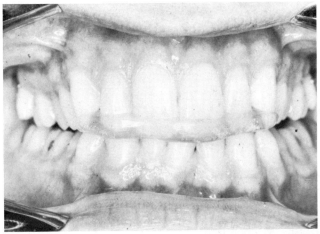

A

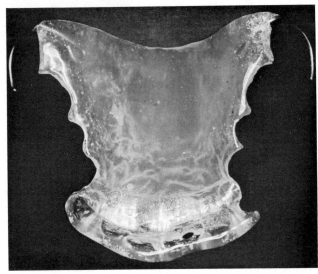

B

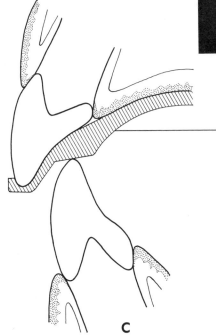

C

Figure 11–10. *A*, Sved bite plate with minimal bite raising. *B*, Sved bite plate. *C*, Schematic profile drawings of Sved bite plate. Note slight slant of palatal plateau so that impact of mandibular incisors meets perpendicular to the flat surface. All mandibular incisors and cuspids should contact this plateau evenly. S—Sved bite plate.

prolonged period of time makes it unsuitable for long term usage. Another shortcoming is that incisal guidance of the bite plate may interfere with Bennett movement; the appliance provides relief for about 50 per cent of patients with long-term temporomandibular joint symptoms of dysfunction.

Bite plates are of some value as an adjunct to occlusal adjustment and oral reconstruction since they may provide muscle relaxation and comfort to the patients, thereby allowing the dentist to record true centric relation. It is usually sufficient to have the patient use the bite plate for one or two weeks while sleeping in order to obtain muscle relaxation. If relief of symptoms cannot be achieved over two to three weeks with a bite plate, one should change to the use of occlusal splints.

Occlusal Splints. By far the best appliance for patients with dysfunctional symptoms is the occlusal splint, which covers all of the teeth either in the mandible or the maxilla.[37] However, it is usually easier to fit in the maxilla than in the mandible (Fig. 11–11). The splint should have a flat occlusal surface, with occlusal contact in centric for all of the opposing teeth, and be absolutely free of occlusal interference in any excursion. There should be sufficient cuspid rise

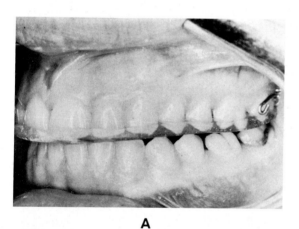

A

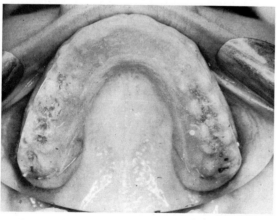

B

Figure 11–11. *A*, Occlusal splint in maxilla with centric stops for all of the opposing teeth. *B*, The middle part of the palate should not be covered by acrylic.

in the acrylic to avoid balancing interferences (Fig. 11–12). Such a splint can either be made following mounting of casts in an adjustable articulator or with only a maxillary cast without mounting. If the splint is made from casts mounted on an articulator and the acrylic is heat cured, it is fairly easy to fit the splint in the mouth. If an acrylic splint is made on one cast without any attempt to fit the occlusion, the occlusal surface of the splint can be ground off almost to the teeth and then a layer of self-curing acrylic can be added to the occlusal surface. Before the acrylic sets the patient is instructed to bite together in centric and to make lateral and protrusive movements so that imprints of all of the opposing teeth are obtained and lateral and protrusive paths are registered. After the acrylic is hard the occlusal surface is ground flat in such a way that occlusal stops are maintained for all of the opposing teeth. These splints can be worn both day and night, but in most instances satisfactory results are obtained by wearing them at night only.

If the complete coverage type of acrylic splint just described has been properly made, there is an immediate decrease in muscle tonus which can be recognized both clinically and electromyographically.[13] The tendency for bruxism is usually greatly diminished or eliminated by the splint and there is, therefore, very little or no evidence of wear on the surface of the acrylic even after prolonged use. The complete coverage splint can be used for any length of time

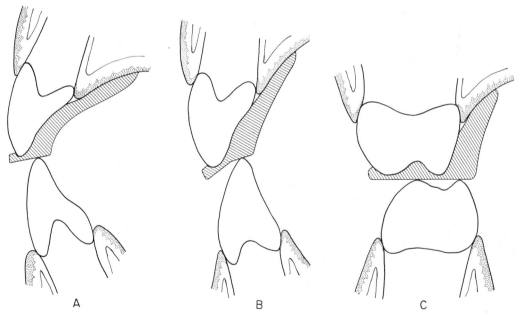

Figure 11–12. Schematic drawings of an occlusal splint. *A,* The anterior part should be slanted to allow a perpendicular impact of the mandibular front teeth. The bite has to be raised sufficiently to allow free passage of the mandibular anterior teeth over the acrylic-covered incisal edges of the maxillary front teeth. *B,* About 1 or 2 mm. from centric there should be a slight "cuspid raise" in the acrylic in the cuspid area to avoid balancing contacts. *C,* Both buccal and lingual cusps of bicuspids and molars in the mandible should preferably make contacts with the splint when the mandible is close to centric relation. However, with lingual tipping of the mandibular molars it is often enough to have contact on the disto-buccal mandibular cusps.

since it does not allow the teeth to move. It also stabilizes the teeth and prevents occlusal wear of the teeth. It has been found that after the patient has worn the splint for two to three weeks the muscles are usually relaxed and occlusal adjustment can be refined to the point where the splint is no longer needed. If the bruxism has not been eliminated after the occlusal adjustment, and there is extensive occlusal wear, or mobile teeth, the complete coverage splint can be used at night indefinitely, provided periodic evaluations of the splint are made.

Another type of occlusal splint is the bilateral posterior onlay which usually covers the mandibular molars and bicuspids (Fig. 11–13). These splints are made either for the purpose of increasing the occlusal vertical dimension, or for providing bilateral pivot contacts in the first molar area.[45] Years ago such onlay splints were usually made of metal and often cemented to the teeth. Now they are made either of acrylic or of metal and they may either be removable, or be temporarily cemented to the teeth. Bilateral posterior onlays may provide temporary relief from symptoms in patients with bruxism and muscle or temporomandibular joint pain since such relief is experienced from any therapy that eliminates the trigger factors (occlusal interferences). However, onlay splints are unacceptable since they usually lead to intrusion of molars and bicuspids and extrusion of the front teeth, with subsequent occlusal interferences and recurrent symptoms.

There is no scientific evidence to indicate that increased muscle tonus and bruxism are related to abnormally increased interocclusal space. However, it does appear that the sensitivity of the neuromuscular mechanism to occlusal interferences is increased if the occlusal vertical dimension is increased, and there is a decrease in the interocclusal space. This observation corresponds to clinical experience in complete denture prosthesis in that the tendency for decubital ulcers and denture instability increases with an increase in occlusal vertical dimension.

A third type of occlusal splint is made of soft acrylic or latex rubber.[29] Some of these splints, like the Kesling appliance,[26] are intended to hold the mandible in a certain relationship to the maxilla by grasping both the mandibular and maxillary teeth in the same appliance.[47, 49] Such an appliance is usually not successful for patients with bruxism; they either bite the appliance into pieces or dislodge it during sleep. Less bulky than the bite guards and serving the same purpose are splints made by adding soft acrylic on the occlusal surfaces of the regular hard acrylic splints previously described. These splints may feel comfortable to patients with a clenching habit at the time of insertion because the soft acrylic provides an even pressure on the teeth when they bite into it. But there is a tendency for patients to "play" with these appliances by biting on the resilient surface. Furthermore, such surfaces cannot be finished so accurately as the hard acrylic so there will be more trigger areas for bruxism.

The best device for a patient with bruxism is still the well fitted hard acrylic splint covering all occlusal and incisal surfaces either in the maxilla or the mandible, with centric stops for all opposing teeth and completely devoid of occlusal interferences.

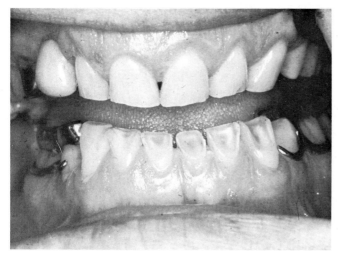

A

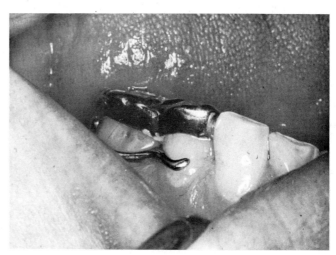

Figure 11-13. A and B, Onlay splint for "bite opening" and to avoid future incisal wear. C, After 3 months the worn front teeth were again making contact with the splint in place. The posterior teeth covered by the splint had been intruded and the front teeth extruded so that the posterior teeth did not make contact when the splint was removed and the patient was biting hard.

B

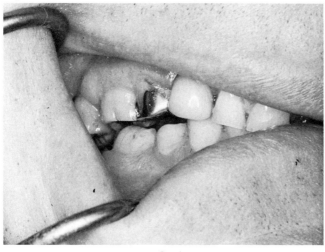

C

Occlusal Reconstruction and Prostheses

Restorative dentistry is indicated in the treatment of bruxism when a stable, well-balanced occlusion cannot be established through occlusal adjustment alone. Occlusal restorations may also be indicated in order to substitute for or prevent excessive loss of tooth substance by bruxism (Fig. 11–14). When for esthetic and technical reasons the occlusal vertical dimension has to be raised, the increase in vertical dimension should be kept to a minimum. Also, in centric the restorations should have occlusal contact with all of the teeth in the opposing dental arch in order to maintain a stable result. It is essential that the occlusal pattern in such restorations be as ideal as possible in order to minimize the tendency for bruxism and to prevent future occlusal wear. The restorations should also be of the same degree of hardness to prevent uneven wear. It is advisable to let the patient wear an occlusal splint (p. 248) for 2 to 3 months before the final recording of centric relation is made. There is often a very marked change in jaw relations following the use of an occlusal splint as seen

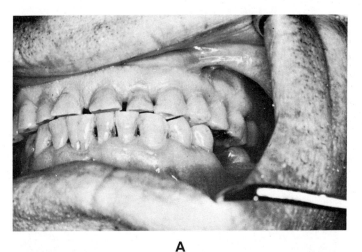

A

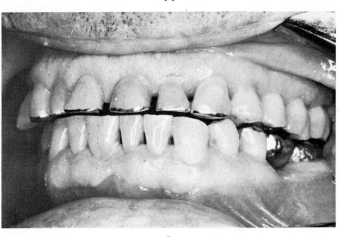

B

Figure 11–14. A, Severe attrition associated with bruxism. B, Gold inlays attached with pins to ''shoe'' the areas of most severe attrition. This type of therapy does not stop bruxism and is usually followed by continued wear of teeth and restorations (male, age 45).

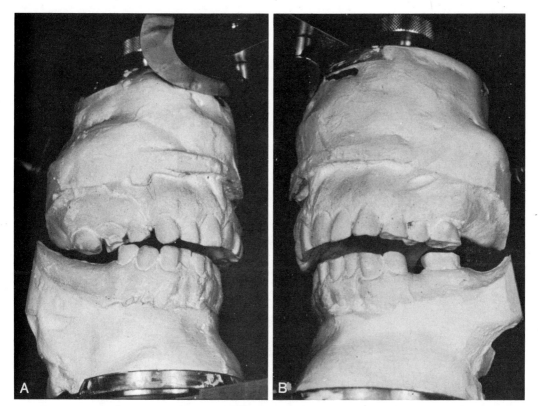

Figure 11–15. Casts mounted in centric relation after two months' use of maxillary bite plane.

in Figure 11–15 following two months on an occlusal splint. Reconstruction done after such repositioning of the mandible is usually successful because the discrepancy between centric relation and the abnormal position associated with bruxism has been eliminated. If the patient's occlusal wear pattern from bruxism is simply duplicated in the restorations, as has been recommended,[6] the bruxism and excessive wear will continue. A faulty occlusal pattern in oral reconstruction for patients with bruxism may lead to increased bruxism, destruction of the restorations, and temporomandibular joint and muscle pain.

To raise the bite by placing restorations only on bicuspids and molars is an unsatisfactory and potentially harmful procedure for reasons already discussed under onlay type of temporary occlusal splints.

What has been said about bruxism in individuals with natural teeth also applies to patients with removable partial and complete dentures. Instead of adapting to a less than perfect denture occlusion by establishing learned convenience patterns for the masticatory movements, patients will seek out occlusal interferences and start playing with their appliances as an expression of bruxism. The results may be "denture sore mouth,"[33] excessive wear of both dentures and opposing teeth, breakage of appliances, and temporomandibular joint and muscle discomfort or pain.

Several patients with bruxism have been seen in whom good natural teeth have been extracted and complete maxillary dentures made with the hope of improving the bruxism and providing relief for oral or temporomandibular joint discomfort. Unfortunately, such patients usually end up with a series of ill-fitting dentures and increasing discomfort and occlusal problems that could have been handled much more satisfactorily if the natural teeth had not been extracted.

When a patient has complete dentures and severe bruxism, it is very difficult to assure a correct centric relationship unless the dentures are left out of the mouth for some days or a temporary flat acrylic splint is made on top of the occlusal surface of the teeth. The splint is then adjusted and worn for 2 or 3 weeks until muscle relaxation can be obtained and a reliable recording of centric relation secured.

Occlusal adjustment of dentures for patients with bruxism can usually be done better with a good mounting in an articulator than in the mouth. The presence of tense jaw muscles and poor coordination of jaw movement, combined with the resiliency of the mucosa, makes intraoral adjustment highly problematic for such individuals.

Biting Habits Related to Bruxism

A habitual tendency to bite on various objects brought into the mouth[45] or biting on the oral soft tissues represents an outlet for emotional or psychic tension and is, therefore, related to bruxism. In several patients with bruxism it has been noted that when their occlusal interferences have been removed they have substituted for bruxism such habits as biting the fingernails or the mounting of their eyeglasses, biting on the lip or tongue, pushing the teeth with the fingers, or pressing or rubbing the tongue against the teeth. In extreme or serious cases of sore tongue or cheek, a patient may need psychiatric help, but in the overwhelming majority of cases these habits are of little clinical significance. Often the habits can be controlled by explaining the matter to the patient. However, when it comes to well-established habits of tongue and lip biting in adults, these habits are very difficult to break even if conditioning "reminder" types of appliances are used. It is often advisable to leave such habits alone if no recognizable harm has resulted. Hypnosis should not be used to stop such habits since this may precipitate a psychoneurotic crisis.

Occupational habits of holding building nails in the mouth or biting thread and other habits such as chewing pencils can often be eliminated by conscious efforts of the patient.

Spastic Disorders Accompanied by Bruxism

Bruxism arising from spastic disorders is very rare. Inasmuch as such disorders are related to the abnormal neuromuscular mechanism of the patient the treatment is mostly within the domain of the physician. However, it has been found that, for example, patients with chorea have been helped to a certain extent (as far as their bruxism is concerned) by occlusal adjustment or by use of acrylic occlusal splints for reducing the hypertonicity of the jaw muscles that is related to occlusal interferences.

REFERENCES

1. Amols, W.: Clinical experience with a new muscle relaxant, zoxazolamine. J. Am. Dent. A., *163*:742, 1956.
2. Barton, R. T.: Benign masseteric hypertrophy; a syndrome of importance in the differential diagnosis of parotid tumors. J.A.M.A., *164*:1646, 1957.
3. Berlin, R., and Dessner, L.: Bruxism and chronic headache. Odont. Tskr., 68:261, 1960.
4. Bober, H.: Grundlagen der Therapie der Hauptformen des nächtlichen Zähneknirchens. Oesterr. Ztschr. Stomatol., *52*:449, 1955.
5. Boyens, P. J.: Value of autosuggestion in the therapy of "bruxism" and other biting habits. J. Am. Dent. A., *27*:1773, 1940.
6. Brecker, S. C.: A clinical approach to occlusion. Dent. Clin. North America, 163, March, 1962.
7. Brill, N., Schübeler, S., and Tryde, G.: Aspects of occlusal sense in natural and artificial teeth. J. Prosth. Dent., *12*:123, 1962.
8. Bundgaard-Jörgensen, F.: Afslapningsovelser som led i behandlingen af habituelle dysfunktioner i mastikationsapparatet. Odont. Tidsk., *58*:448, 1950.
9. Chasins, A. I.: Methocarbamal (Robaxin) as an adjunct in the treatment of bruxism. J. Dent. Med., *14*:166, 1959.
10. Eschler, J.: Bruxism and function of the masticatory muscles. Paradontologie, *15*:109, 1961.
11. Forsberg, A.: Parodontalsjukdom som led i ett psykomotorik syndrom. Sv. Tandl. Tidskr., *49*:681, 1956.
12. Frohman, B.: The application of psychotherapy to dental problems. Dent. Cosmos, *73*:1117, 1931.
13. Fuchs, P.: Neue Untersuchungen über die Kaumuskeltätigkeit während des Nachtschlafes. D. Z. Z., *24*:563, 1969.
14. Gecker, L. M., and Weil, R. B.: Bruxism—a rationale of therapy. J. Am. Dent. A., *66*:14, 1963.
15. Gelbred, M. B.: Treatment of bruxism. A case report. J. Hypnos. & Psychol. Dent., *1*:18, 1958.
16. Goldstein, M.: A clinical investigation of mephate in dentistry. Dent. Digest, *62*:454, 498–501, 1956.
17. Grupe, H. E., and Gromek, J. J.: Bruxism splint. Technique using quick cure acrylic. J. Periodont., *30*:156, 1959.
18. Hawley, C. A.: Removable retainer. Internat. J. Orthodont., 5:291, 1919.
19. Hirt, H. A., and Mühlemann, H. R.: Diagnosis of bruxism by means of tooth mobility measurements. Paradontologie, *9*:47, 1955.
20. Hultin, M.: Hypertrofi av musculus masseter. Sv. Tandl. Tidsk., *53*:549, 1960.
21. Ingle, J. I.: Alveolar osteoporosis and pulpal death associated with compulsive bruxism. Oral Surg., *13*:1371, 1960.
22. Karolyi, M.: Beobachtungen über Pyorrhoea alveolaris. (Ref. from 40 Jahresversammlung des Centralvereines deutscher Zahnärtze, Leipzig, 1901.) Oesterr. ungar Vrtljschr. Zahnh. *17*:279, 1901.
23. Karolyi, M.: Über Alveolarpyorrhoe. (Ref. Jahresversammlung des Standesvereines Berliner Zahnärzte, Berlin, 1904.) Oesterr. ungar. Vrtljschr. Zahnh., *21*:85, 1905.
24. Karolyi, M.: Zur Therapie der Erkrankungen der Mundschleimhaut. Oesterr. ungar. Vtjschr. Zahnh. 22:226, 1906.
25. Kawamura, Y., Tsukamoto, S., and Miyoshi, K.: Experimental studies on neural mechanisms of bruxism. J. Dent. Res., *40*:217, 1961.
26. Kesling, H. D.: Co-ordinating the predetermined pattern and tooth positioner with conventional treatment. Am. J. Orthodont. & Oral Surg., *32*:285, 1946.
27. Leof, M.: Clamping and grinding habits; Their relation to periodontal disease. J. Am. Dent. A., *31*:184, 1944.

28. Lipke, D., and Posselt, U.: Parafunctions of the masticatory system (bruxism). West. Soc. Periodont. J., *8*:133, 1960.
29. Matthews, E.: A treatment for the teeth-grinding habit. Dent. Rec., *62*:154, 1942.
30. Mensendieck, B. M.: The Mensendieck System of Functional Exercises. Portland, Maine, 1937.
31. Miller, S. C., and Firestone, J. M.: Psychosomatic factors in the etiology of periodontal disease. Am. J. Orthodont & Oral Surg., *33*:675, 1947.
32. Monica, W. S.: Headaches caused by bruxism. Am. Otology, *68*:1159, 1959.
33. Moore, D. S.: Bruxism, diagnosis and treatment. J. Periodont., *27*:277, 1956.
34. Nyquist, G.: A study of denture sore mouth; An investigation of traumatic, allergic and toxic lesions of the oral mucosa arising from the use of full dentures. Acta odont. scandinav., *10*: Suppl. 9, 1952.
35. Peterson, L. N., and Dunkin, R. T.: The incidence of bruxism in adults. Acad. Rev., *4*:79, 1956.
36. Posselt, U., and Wolff, I. B.: Bite Guards and Bite Plates: Follow-Up Examination of Their Effect on Bruxism and Temporomandibular Joint Systems. Paradontopath., 17th Congrès, 326, 1963.
37. Posselt, U.: Physiology of Occlusion and Rehabilitation. Philadelphia, F. A. Davis Co., 1962.
38. Ramfjord, S. P.: Bruxism, a clinical and electromyographic study. J. Am. Dent. A., *62*:21, 1961.
39. Ramfjord, S. P.: Diagnosis of Bruxism. Paradontopath., 17th Congrès, 53, 1963.
40. Ramfjord, S. P.: Dysfunctional temporomandibular joint and muscle pain. J. Prosth. Dent., *11*:353, 1961.
41. Ramfjord, S. P.: Significance of recent research on occlusion for the teaching and practice of dentistry. J. Prosth. Dent. *16*:96–105, Jan.-Feb., 1966.
42. Reichborn-Kjennerud, I.: Tennenes Fysiologiske og pathologiske Mobilitet. Odont. Tidsk., *62*:154, 1954.
43. Schaps, P.: Schmerzhafte, isolierte Crampi im Bereich der Kaumuskulatur. D. Zahn-, Mund- und Kieferhk., *34*:120, 1960.
44. Schwarz, L. L.: Temporomandibular joint syndromes. J. Prosth. Dent., *7*:489, 1957.
45. Sears, V. H.: Occlusal pivots. J. Prosth. Dent., *6*:332, 1956.
46. Sorrin, S.: Habit: An etiologic factor of periodontal disease. Dent. Digest, *41*:290, 1935.
47. Strother, E. W., and Mitchell, G. E.: Bruxism: A review and a case report. J. Dent. Med., *9*:189, 1954.
48. Sved, A.: Changing the occlusal level and a new method of retention. Am. J. Orthodont. & Oral Surg., *30*:527, 1944.
49. Sved, A.: The problem of retention. Am. J. Orthodont., *39*:659, 1953.
50. Seyffart, H., and Steen-Johnson, S.: Belastnings sykdommer i tyggeapparatet hos barn. Norsk. Tandl. Tidsk., *66*:295, 1956.
51. Tishler, B.: Occlusal habit neuroses. Dent. Cosmos, *70*:690, 1928.
52. Uhlig, H.: Sollen Metallkronen "abriebfest" sein? Deutsch Zahn-, Mund- und Kieferhk., *25:* 276, 1957.

Films

1. "Examination of Occlusion"
2. "Mounting of Casts in a Semi-adjustable Articulator and use of Bite Plates"

> May be loaned through:
> V. A. Central Office Film Library
> 810 Vermont Avenue, N.W.
> Washington, D.C. 20420
>
> Film Library
> American Dental Association
> 211 East Chicago Avenue
> Chicago, Ill. 60611

CHAPTER 12

SIGNS AND SYMPTOMS OF TRAUMA FROM OCCLUSION

The diagnosis of trauma from occlusion is based on a functional analysis of occlusal relations, the investing and supporting structures of the teeth, the muscles of mastication, and the teeth. The analysis combines both a clinical and radiographic examination.[10] A positive diagnosis can be made only if an injury can be located in some part of the masticatory system and that injury is related to the occlusion.[31]

The etiology of trauma from occlusion has been presented in Chapter 5 and diagnostic techniques in Chapters 9 and 10. The present chapter will be devoted to the signs and symptoms of trauma from occlusion.

DIAGNOSIS

The clinical manifestations of trauma from occlusion are often inconspicuous unless an acute traumatic condition exists. None of the clinical signs is in itself diagnostic; to be meaningful signs have to be related to a close examination of the occlusal relations, history, and roentgenographic findings. A discussion of the signs of trauma from occlusion follows.

Signs of Trauma From Occlusion

Increased Tooth Mobility

By far the most common clinical sign of trauma from occlusion is an increase in tooth mobility.[3,9,16,26] The initial increase in mobility is the result of a thickening of the periodontal membrane associated with resorption of the alveolar bone and replacement of the dense collagenous fibers of the periodontal membrane by soft granulation tissue. In trauma from occlusion of long standing, the granulation tissue may be changed to collagenous fiber connective tissue, but the increased width of the periodontal membrane will still allow for the hypermobility of the tooth. Root resorption and lowering of the alveolar crest may also contribute to the clinical manifestation of hypermobility associated with trauma from occlusion.

The degree of mobility of a tooth depends on the forces placed upon it and the resistance of the supporting structures. It is necessary to consider the origin of the force, the direction, the magnitude, and the frequency; resistance involves the extent of the supporting areas and the integrity of the supporting tissues.[19] The integrity of the supporting tissues can be changed by trauma from occlusion, by loss of support from periodontal disease, by blastomatoid and neoplastic conditions, and by systemic conditions or disease altering the polymerization of the ground substance and affecting the integrity of the collagen fibers of the periodontal membrane.

Tooth mobility can be tested in a scientific way by various devices or by a commonly used method of clinical assessment carried out by rocking the tooth between two instruments, or between the tip of one instrument and the fingertip of the examiner. Increased tooth mobility may be of systemic or local origin. For example, it has been shown by exacting methods of measurement that tooth mobility is increased during pregnancy.[17] It has also been shown that tooth mobility in persons with nocturnal bruxism is greater in the morning than later in the day.[8] In the first instance the cause of the mobility is of systemic origin; in the second instance it is local in nature. Increased tooth mobility associated with trauma from occlusion suggests mobility that can be recognized by a simple attempt to rock or move the tooth.

It is extremely important that the mobility of teeth be related to the amount of periodontal support present, since in advanced periodontal disease hypermobility is commonly observed in association with pocket formation and loss of support. Any test of mobility should, therefore, be combined with an examination of pocket depth and radiographs.

Attention should also be paid to the periapical tissues, since pulpal disease may also induce hypermobility of teeth. The direction of the greatest amplitude of mobility may give some clue to the direction of the traumatic force; however, contact relations between the teeth may obscure or alter the impact of the traumatic forces upon the periodontal tissues. When a tooth with a fairly normal amount of periodontal support has an increased mobility, trauma from occlusion should definitely be considered as the most likely cause. Teeth that have been rocked back and forth over a long period of time may have increased mobility from compensatory widening of the periodontal space, and there may be actually no evidence of trauma at the time of examination.

Changes in Percussion Sounds

A tooth in trauma from occlusion will have a dull percussion sound in contrast to the relatively sharp percussion sound heard in a tooth with a normal periodontium. This change in percussion sound is probably the result of the partial resorption of the lamina dura and the altered width and consistency of the periodontal membrane.

Migration of Teeth

Loss of interproximal contacts and migration of teeth may be the sequelae of traumatic occlusal relations. It should be realized that unusual habit patterns may cause migration of teeth and trauma from occlusion beyond the functional range of normal occlusal contacts. Often there may be an indication of an abnormal occlusal wear pattern. However, in some instances, the teeth may be pressed out of their normal contact relationship without any indication of occlusal wear.

Atypical Pattern of Occlusal Wear

Wear facets that do not conform to the masticatory pattern of the individual are indicative of bruxism and the presence of abnormal occlusal forces. Such wear facets should, therefore, alert the examiner to look for possible evidence of traumatic injury to the periodontal structures, although it should be understood that a large number of individuals with bruxism do not have any indication of traumatic injury to the periodontal structures. In many instances the trauma is confined to the hard structures of the teeth and does not involve the periodontium.

Hypertonicity of the Masticatory Muscles

In persons with bruxism and hypertonicity of the masticatory muscles there is an increased hazard for trauma to the periodontal structures, and in any person with bruxism there is an increased potential for trauma from occlusion because of abnormal muscle activity. The trauma from occlusion may also be manifest in the muscles and muscle attachments in relation to bruxism as explained in Chapter 11.

Periodontal Abscesses

If a person has deep periodontal pockets, especially the intrabony type or pocket involving bi- and trifurcations, trauma from occlusion may easily precipitate abscess formation in such pockets (Fig. 12–1). Bacteria from the pocket may be pressed into tissues being traumatized and having a lowered metabolism and resistance, thus increasing the possibility of bacterial infection in these weakened tissues with subsequent abscess formation.

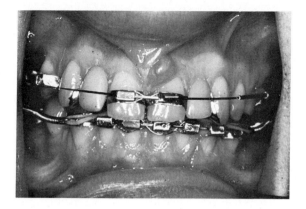

Figure 12-1. Periodontal abscess associated with an attempt to move a tooth orthodontically into a deep intrabony pocket without prior scaling and curettage.

Gingival Changes

Since the description of McCall's festoons and Stillman's[28] clefts (Fig. 12–2), there have always been great interest and considerable controversy with regard to the possible gingival changes associated with trauma from occlusion. It has been well established that traumatic occlusion does not produce gingival inflammation. It has also been established that traumatic occlusion does not initiate periodontal pockets in the absence of local surface irritants. No gingival changes have been produced by experimental trauma from occlusion in animals, and cases of gingival atrophy can usually be traced to faulty toothbrushing or other gingival irritations. There is no clear-cut evidence to indicate that such manifestations are caused by trauma from occlusion. On the basis of current knowledge of the common vascular supply of the gingival tissues,[5] it is hard to see how trauma from occlusion can interfere with this vascular supply to the extent that edema, cyanosis or even atrophy could result from trauma from occlusion. However, a deviation of this average pattern of vascular supply might conceivably be present in a few instances, increasing the significance of traumatic occlusion to the vascular supply of the gingiva in the case of some of the

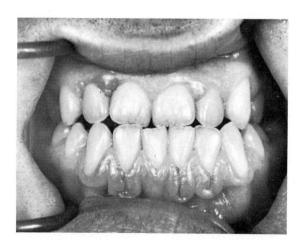

Figure 12-2. Stillman's clefts on mandibular incisors and McCall's festoons on mandibular cusps. Also present are subgingival calculus and gingivitis.

vessels entering the gingiva through the periodontal membrane in an area of trauma. Of all the listed signs, the increase in tooth mobility and soreness to pressure are by far the most significant clinical indications of trauma from occlusion in the periodontium.

Temporomandibular Joint Changes

Signs of trauma from occlusion manifested in the temporomandibular joints will be discussed in Chapter 17.

SYMPTOMS OF TRAUMATIC OCCLUSION

Traumatic occlusion is often asymptomatic unless an acute traumatic situation exists. Sometimes the patient complains of vague or poorly defined symptoms of discomfort in regions of the jaws without any apparent relationship to the teeth. Although these symptoms may have their origin in trauma from occlusion, there are many other sources of similar diffuse pains to be considered in differential diagnosis. A discussion of the symptoms of trauma from occlusion follows.

As with the signs of trauma from occlusion, one or more of the symptoms may be present in any given case. Each symptom should also be evaluated for its relationship to disturbances other than trauma from occlusion.

Periodontal Pain

In cases of severe trauma from occlusion of fairly short duration the tooth may be very sore to bite on and sore to percussion. In such instances, the traumatic occlusion is usually associated with the recent insertion of dental appliances or restorations; or it is related to an injury to the jaw or teeth. However, in the common causes of chronic, longstanding trauma from occlusion there is little or no pain on biting on the tooth or to percussion; the symptoms, if present, are of the nature of a vague, regional discomfort, rather than a distinctly localized area of pain.

Pulpal Pain

Sensitivity of the teeth, especially to cold, is commonly found in association with trauma from occlusion. Presumably this sensitivity is the result of passive congestion or venous hyperemia and increased blood pressure within the pulp, since traumatic pressures on the tooth interfere less with the arterial blood supply to the pulp than the venous return through the apical foramen. Strangulation with death of the pulp has occasionally been observed with severe bruxism. The common pulpal hypersensitivity following insertion of occlusal dental restorations can often be made to disappear almost immediately following adjustment of the occlusal relations of such restorations. Generalized sensitivity of the teeth associated with severe bruxism is usually associated with both periodontal and pulpal sensitivity and will often disappear following proper occlusal therapy.

Referred Pain

Pain referred from periodontal injury can be felt in the area of the maxillary sinuses or spread anywhere in the jaw and face region. However, muscle pain directly related to muscular hypertonicity and spasm is more commonly the source of such diffuse pain than the pain being referred from the periodontal structures.[30]

Food Impaction

Plunger cusp effect of occlusal interferences may produce a functional opening of contact between the teeth and lead to food impaction[7] in areas where the contacts appear normal when tested with the jaws separated and the teeth not occluding (Fig. 12–3). The history of food impaction without apparent abnormal contact relationship indicates a disturbance in the functional relations between the teeth. Such disturbance is often associated with traumatic occlusion. The wedging effect of a plunger cusp is most significant when the interproximal contact relationships have been disturbed as a result of loss of teeth, or when wear has resulted in loss of marginal ridges.

Traumatic Temporomandibular Joint Arthritis and Muscle Pain

In the presence of signs and symptoms of traumatic temporomandibular joint arthritis and related pain there is practically always an occlusal disharmony present which might have led to injury to the periodontium. However, in many

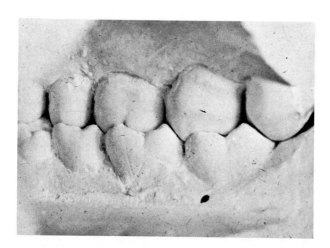

Figure 12–3. Plunger cusps, lingual view. Deep overbite and extensive lateral function had worn off the marginal ridges and made the cusps steeper in the mesiodistal direction. With tough food between the teeth, these cusps now wedge contacts open and force food into the opened interproximal spaces.

patients such injuries may be manifested in the temporomandibular joint and adjacent muscles rather than in the teeth and their supporting structures.

Loose Teeth and Other Symptoms

In instances of severe trauma from occlusion, especially associated with loss of periodontal support, the patient may have noticed that his teeth are loose and his complaint may be an annoying hypermobility of the teeth.

A patient with trauma from occlusion will occasionally experience an itching sensation in the periodontium, which makes him press or grind his teeth.

RADIOGRAPHIC SIGNS OF TRAUMA FROM OCCLUSION

The radiographic signs of trauma from occlusion are often inconspicuous and can be observed only by careful examination of technically excellent radiographs.[32] The pathological changes in trauma from occlusion that can be seen roentgenographically are primarily present on the surface of the root of the tooth or on the surface of the socket of the tooth. The width of the periodontal membrane (radiographically, the periodontal space[11]) is also altered by trauma from occlusion. However, trauma from occlusion is often manifest in the buccolingual direction, and alterations on the surface of the alveolar bone on the buccal or lingual side of a tooth are not clearly recognizable in roentgenograms.[6] By variation in angulation from one roentgenogram to another, at least the mesiobuccal, mesiolingual, distobuccal and distolingual aspects of a tooth can be studied better than when the central x-ray beam goes through the tooth in a straight buccolingual direction.[1]

It is very important that all of several radiographs of each area be studied in a complete mouth series so that every exposure of a tooth is carefully examined. If the trauma is on the mesial or distal side of the tooth, the radiographic findings are easy to observe. Attention should be given to the continuity of the lamina dura or alveolar bone plate, the width of the periodontal space, and the outline of the root surface. One should also look for pulpal calcification and resorption or condensation in the supporting bone surrounding the socket of the tooth. A discussion of the radiographic signs of trauma from occlusion follows.

One or more of the radiographic signs of trauma from occlusion may be present in any given case. None of the radiographic signs associated with trauma from occlusion is specific and diagnostic in itself; diagnosis of trauma from occlusion can be made only on the basis of the combined information from history, clinical and roentgenographic examination.

Alteration of Lamina Dura

Changes in the lamina dura may vary from an uneven thickening,[22] to loss of continuity, to complete loss around teeth in severe trauma from occlusion (Fig. 12–4).

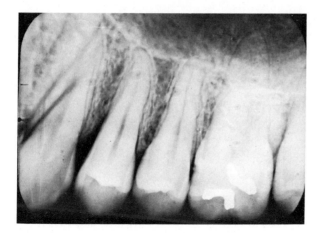

Figure 12–4. Partial loss of lamina dura on mesial aspects of bicuspids involved in trauma from occlusion.

The thickness is, in many instances, an unreliable sign, since it may be the result of superimposition of the buccolingual aspects of the lamina dura due to concave mesial or distal root surfaces of bicuspids or molar teeth. In such instances, the lamina dura appears radiographically much thicker than normal.

Much more important than the thickness of the lamina dura is the loss of its continuity, which indicates a resorptive process on the surface that is characteristic of traumatic occlusion. Resorption is most commonly seen in association with trauma from pressure, while an increase in the thickness of the lamina dura is usually associated with tension.[13] The location of the area of resorption is dependent upon the direction of the traumatic force upon the tooth. If these forces were directed mainly in a horizontal direction, the bone resorption would be evident mainly in the areas around the neck of the tooth and around the apex. If the traumatic force is in an axial direction, the resorption would be mainly in the bifurcation areas (Fig. 12–5) or around the apex of the teeth. However, in most instances the traumatic forces have a combined axial and lateral component, with evidence of resorption around the apex and around the cervical area of the tooth. In cases of severe trauma from occlusion, there may be almost complete loss of the lamina dura.

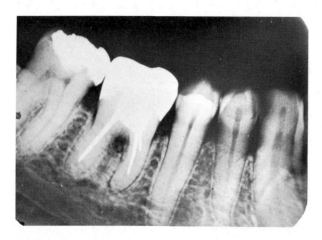

Figure 12–5. Resorption of lamina dura in bifurcation area of first molar without pocket involvement of bifurcation that was related to trauma from occlusion.

Bone resorption may also extend beyond the lamina dura and involve the supporting bone. Radiographically, this is manifest mainly in the cervical area of the tooth as so-called "funnel-shaped" resorption of both alveolar and supporting bone.[29]

Alteration of Periodontal Space

Close attention should be paid to the width of the periodontal space between the tooth and the surrounding bone (Fig. 12–6), a slight variation in this space being normal.[11] According to Coolidge,[4] this physiologic variation, associated with normal occlusal function, is about 0.05 mm. The distance from the tooth to the alveolar bone is shortest between the apical one-third and the middle of the root, and is slightly wider at the cervical and apical areas. This small variation cannot be readily recognized in radiographs by the naked eye. If a clearly visible variation in the width of the periodonta space is present, it has to be assumed that the tooth has been exposed to forces that are in excess of normal functional forces. However, such a widening of the periodontal space may be part of a compensatory hypertrophy of such periodontal structures as the alveolar bone and the periodontal fibers in association with bruxism. In such instances, the lamina dura is thick and intact. It is of much greater significance in the diagnosis of traumatic occlusion if the widening of the periodontal space is accompanied by some resorption of the lamina dura.[15, 16, 25, 27]

It is difficult to explain the widening of the periodontal space mesially and distally in teeth with good interproximal contact, since one might assume that the widening of the periodontal space from trauma in such teeth would be mainly on the buccal and lingual side of the teeth. Such interproximal widening, however, is quite often seen associated with severe trauma from occlusion; it must be the result of the combined effect of pressure and tension upon the alveolar bone.

Figure 12–6. Widened periodontal space on mesial aspect of teeth with trauma from occlusion involving a maxillary fixed bridge.

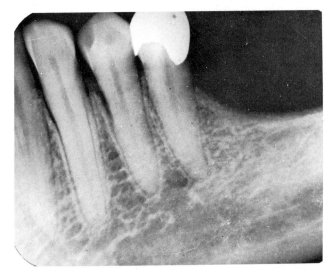

Root Resorption

The first radiographic evidence of root resorption may be observed as a loss of the continuity of the root surface and a slight scalloping or fuzziness of the outline of the root surface around the apex of teeth. This loss of a distinct outline of the surface of the root is best observed by a magnifying glass and good illumination of the radiographs. It is very important to discover these early signs of root resorption in cases of orthodontic therapy or when abutment teeth are receiving heavy occlusal loads in association with oral reconstruction. This early stage of root resorption is reversible by cemental repair; but when a definite shorting of the root appears, the loss of root length is permanent.[14] Extensive root resorption may be seen associated with dysfunctional occlusal stresses resulting from traumatic orthodontic therapy (Fig. 12–7), bruxism, or dental restorations and should be differentiated from hypoplasia or inadequate development of root structures.

Radiographic evidence of so-called "internal resorption" may also appear in association with abnormal occlusal stresses (Fig. 12–8). In many such instances the resorption has had its origin in the periodontal membrane rather than in the pulp, and the reparative processes have resulted in replacement of some of the resorbed cementum and dentin by osteodentin, osteocementum, or regular bone surrounded by granulation tissue. Sometimes during repair, a tooth may undergo ankyiosis. If the area of resorption is not open to the oral cavity and there is a normal vital reaction of the pulp, the only treatment for such teeth should be elimination of the traumatic occlusal forces.

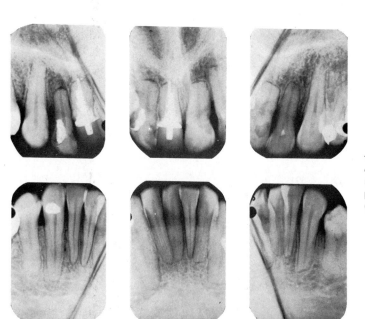

Figure 12–7. Root resorption associated with rapid orthodontic movement. The roots were normal 4 months prior to these roentgenograms (male, age 26).

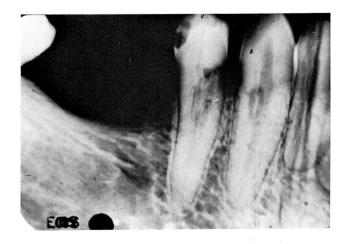

Figure 12-8. "Internal resorption" of mandibular cuspid and first bicuspid. Both teeth traumatized severely by bruxism. The bicuspid was lost subsequent to extensive attempts at therapy. The cuspid was not treated except for occlusal adjustment. The areas of resorption calcified, and 13 years later, the tooth has a normal vitality reaction and functions well.

Hypercementosis

The so-called clubbing of the apical areas of teeth from hypercementosis may be found in association with excessive occlusal forces (Fig. 12–9). It is not unusual to see a combination of hypercementosis and resorption in the apical area of teeth in heavy occlusion.[15, 16, 24, 27] The hypercementosis will increase the surface area of the root and allow for the attachment of an increased number of periodontal fibers, enabling the tooth to withstand an increase in functional load, and will decrease the potential for future periodontal trauma.

Osteosclerosis

A condensation or sclerosis of bone around the apices of teeth in trauma from occlusion can occasionally be observed. The sclerosis is usually seen as a delayed reaction to previous periodontal trauma and is of little or no clinical significance (Fig. 12–10).

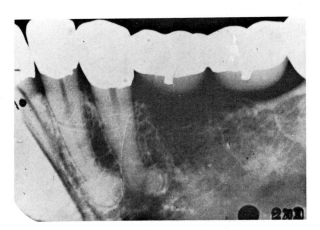

Figure 12-9. Hypercementosis on abutments from "high" fixed bridge.

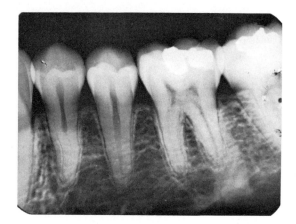

Figure 12–10. Osteosclerosis and shorter than normal roots on first molar after 4 years of extensive orthodontic treatment with first molars as main areas of anchorage.

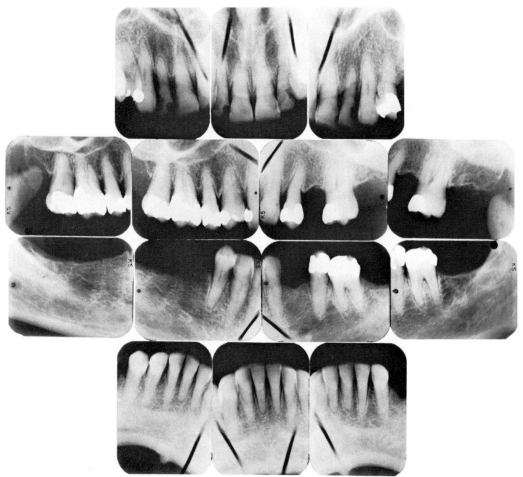

Figure 12–11. Pulpal calcification and widening of periodontal spaces around the necks of the teeth and in the bifurcation areas. Extremely severe bruxism resulted in splitting of some of the teeth and their subsequent extraction (female, age 36).

Pulpal Calcification

Circulatory disturbances of the pulp with dystrophic calcification of pulpal tissue (Fig. 12–11) or secondary dentin formation may be caused by traumatic occlusion.[24] Complete calcification of the pulpal canal may occur in cases of longstanding, severe trauma or may also be seen following a single serious traumatic accident to the tooth during which a gross disturbance of the circulation has occurred. The association between traumatic occlusion and denticles has not been adequately studied. Denticles have been observed in unerupted teeth and in teeth that have never functioned, so they are certainly not diagnostic of trauma from occlusion.

Fractures of Roots

A few cases have been observed in which the roots of intact teeth have been fractured during episodes of bruxism (Fig. 11–6, *B*). Transverse fractures can be readily seen radiographically; however, longitudinal splits of the root associated with trauma are almost impossible to see radiographically.

Temporomandibular Joint Roentgenograms

The value of roentgenograms of the temporomandibular joints in the diagnosis of trauma from occlusion will be discussed in Chapter 17.

REFERENCES

1. Berghagen, N., and Hjelström, P.: Three-dimensional intra-oral radiography. Acta odont. scandinav., *14*:189, 1956.
2. Beyeler, K., and Dreyfus, J.: Prinzip einer Elektro-dynamischen Apparatus zur Messung des Lockerungsgrades der Zahne. Paradontolgie, *1*:113, 1947.
3. Bonis, Franz, Jr.: Etiologische Faktoren der sogenannten Alveolar-Pyorrhoe mit besonderer Berücksichtigung der Uberlastungslehre. Ztschr. Stomatol., *21*:527, 1923.
4. Coolidge, E.: The thickness of the periodontal membrane. J. Am. Dent. A., *24*:1260, 1937.
5. Goldman, H. M.: Gingival vascular supply in induced occlusal traumatism. Oral Surg., *9*:939, 1956.
6. Goldman, H. M., Millsap, J. S., and Brenman, H. S.: Origin of registration of the architectural pattern, the lamina dura, and the alveolar crest in the dental radiograph. Oral Surg., *10*:749, 1957.
7. Hirschfeld, I.: Food impaction. J. Am. Dent. A., *17*:1504, 1930.
8. Hirt, H. A., and Mühlemann, H. R.: Diagnosis of bruxism by means of tooth mobility measurements. Paradontologie, *9*:47, 1955.
9. Karolyi, M.: Beobachtungen über Pyorrhoe alveolaris. Oesterr. ungar Vrtljschr. Zahnh., *17*:279–283, 1901.
10. Lindblom, G.: The significance of "bite-analysis" in modern dentistry. Dent. Rec., *68*:254, 1948.
11. Lonberg, P.: Om periodontal rummet i rontgenbilden. Sv. Tandl. Tidsk., *53*:477, 1960.
12. Manly, R. S., Yurkstas, A., and Reswick, J. B.: An instrument for measuring tooth mobility. J. Periodont., *22*:148, 1951.
13. Massler, M.: Changes in the lamina dura during tooth movement. Am. J. Orthodont., *40*:364, 1954.

14. Massler, M., and Malone, A. J.: Root resorption in human permanent teeth. Am. J. Orthodont., *40*:619, 1954.
15. McCall, J. O.: The radiogram as an aid in the diagnosis and prognosis of periodontal lesions. J. Am. Dent. A., *14*:2073, 1927.
16. McCall, J. O.: Traumatic occlusion. J. Am. Dent. A., *26*:519, 1939.
17. Mühlemann, H. R.: Ten years of tooth mobility measurements. J. Periodont., *31*:110, 1960.
18. Mühlemann, H. R.: Tooth mobility. The measuring method, initial and secondary tooth mobility. J. Periodont., *25*:22, 1954.
19. Mühlemann, H. R., Wartmann, P., Marthaler, T. M.: Zahnbeweglichkeit, intra-alveoläre Wurtzellänge, biologischer Faktor. Paradontologie, *9*:24, 1955.
20. O'Leary, T. J., and Rudd, K. D.: An instrument for measuring horizontal tooth mobility. Periodont, *1*:249, 1963.
21. Parfitt, G. J.: Measurement of the physiological mobility of individual teeth in an axial direction. J. Dent. Res., *39*:608, 1960.
22. Pollia, J.: Fundamental principles of alveolo-dental radiology. Dental Items of Interest. Brooklyn, N. Y., Brooklyn Publishing Co., 1930.
23. Ramfjord, S. P.: Dysfunctional temporomandibular joint and muscle pain. J. Prosth. Dent., *11*:353, 1961.
24. Reichborn-Kjennerud, I.: Funktionell prothestische Behandlung und Prophylaxe der Zahnlockerung und der Dysgnathien. *In* Häupl, K.: Die Zahn-, Mund-, und Kieferheilkunde. Vol. 4. Munchen, Urban and Schwartzenberg, 1956.
25. Smith, T.: Traumatic occlusion and its correction in the treatment of pyorrhea alveolaris. Nat. Dent. A. J., *8*:971, 1921.
26. Stillman, P. R.: Occlusion—The fundamental element in dental science. Internat. J. Orthodont. & Oral Surg., *11*:822, 1925.
27. Stillman, P. R.: Traumatic occlusion. Nat. Dent. A. J., *6*:691, 1919.
28. Stillman, P. R., and McCall, J. O.: A Textbook of Clinical Periodontia. New York, The Macmillan Co., 1922.
29. Thielemann, K.: Biomechanik der Paradentose. Leipzig, Herman Meusser, 1938.
30. Travell, J., and Rinzler, S. H.: The Myofacial Genesis of Pain. Postgrad. Med., *11*:425, 1952.
31. World Workshop in Periodontics, 1966. Ramfjord, S. P., Kerr, D. A., and Ash, M. M. (Eds.) Ann Arbor, University of Michigan, 1966.
32. Worth, H. M.: Principles and Practice of Oral Radiographic Interpretation. Chicago, Year Book Medical Publishers, Inc., 1963.

CHAPTER 13

OCCLUSAL ADJUSTMENT OF NATURAL TEETH

Occlusal adjustment has had a long and tumultuous history; this is because occlusal adjustment has often not been based on acceptable biologic principles. For example, if a tooth that feels sore to bite on is reduced in height there will be an obvious temporary relief of symptoms. Also if a tooth or a "high spot" on the restoration of a tooth disturbs the neuromuscular mechanism, the logical step towards relief has been to grind off the high spot. So-called "spot grinding" has therefore been practiced since instruments become available for such procedures. However, the grinding has usually been done without understanding and regard for the total function of the masticatory system and the temporary relief of pain has often ended in compounded occlusal problems due to shifting of the position of the teeth.

Another irrational approach to occlusal adjustment was to "equilibrate" the natural dentition to resemble as much as possible a fictive ideal occlusion or "balanced" denture occlusion. These ideas were introduced by Bonwill,[6] but gained real momentum following Gysi's[14, 15] work on balanced occlusion in dentures. Following the introduction of this concept, there was senseless mutilation of the teeth of numerous patients with functionally normal occlusion. During the last decade, however, such a misguided concept has been replaced because of our present-day understanding of the physiology and dynamics of the individual occlusion which is characterized by variations and adaptive capacities.

OBJECTIVES

It may be of interest to list some of the indications for occlusal adjustment that have been suggested in the dental literature: existence of traumatic occlusion,[31, 36] existence of bruxism,[5, 25] existence of some form of TMJ pathosis,[5,26] hypertonicity of masticatory, head and neck muscles,[26,43] limited mandibular movements,[5] mesial positioning of the mandible,[5,43] when functional relations and relations at rest are not harmonious,[11,29,31,36,41,43,45] unilateral mastication,[5] nonocclusion that can be corrected by grinding,[5,29] and to improve functional relations, increase masticatory efficiency and produce an even distribution of occlusal stresses.[5,11,27,37] Still other indications have been suggested, such as when teeth are impinging on soft tissues,[5] when teeth have migrated,[5] existence of food impaction,[5,29,36,41,45] presence of tooth mobility,[37] to reduce torque on specific teeth,[5] the presence of dental pain associated with occlusion,[5,43] when marginal ridges are not level,[5,29,41] prior to occlusal reconstruction,[43] for restorations or insertion of dental appliances, in the presence of fractured cusps or repeated fractures of jacket crowns,[43] the existence of some form of periodontal disease,[5,11,27,37] the presence of excessive amounts of calculus,[5,37] after orthodontic therapy,[43] and speech defects.[5] It is sometimes advocated that occlusal adjustment should be done only if one or more of the listed conditions are present,[5] but some authorities recommend a prophylactic adjustment in order to eliminate the potential for future pathologic conditions.[34,36,45]

The rationale for doing an occlusal adjustment can be grouped into the following categories: (1) the improvement of functional relations and to induce physiologic stimulation of the entire masticatory system, (2) the elimination of trauma from occlusion, (3) the elimination of abnormal muscle tension, bruxism, and associated discomfort or pain, (4) the elimination of dysfunctional temporomandibular joint discomfort or pain, (5) the establishment of an optimal occlusal pattern prior to extensive restorative procedures, (6) the reshaping and contouring of the teeth for masticatory efficiency and gingival protection, (7) to aid in the stabilization of orthodontic results, and (8) the reconditioning of some abnormal swallowing habits.[25]

A primary objective of occlusal adjustment is improvement of the functional relations of the dentition in such a way that the teeth and the periodontium will receive uniform functional stimulation and the occlusal surfaces of the teeth will be exposed to an even physiologic wear. The masticatory system is a functional unit, and proper functional stimuli are of the utmost importance for the development and maintenance of a strong and healthy periodontium with high functional capacity and optimal resistance to injury. The functional self-cleansing of the surfaces of the teeth, with prevention of marginal gingivitis from plaque retention, is also enhanced by normal multidirectional occlusal function. Such function is induced as a necessity for survival under primitive living conditions, but with the soft food of modern civilization, convenience patterns of restricted occlusal pathways from slight cuspal disharmony may persist and become exaggerated as a result of uneven occlusal wear.

It has been shown that occlusal adjustment may induce multidirectional functional pathways if the adjustment results in equally convenient and efficient functional relations in the various directions.[3]

Occlusal adjustment is logically the first consideration for treatment of trauma from occlusion and associated signs and symptoms. However, all cases of trauma from occlusion cannot be cured by occlusal adjustment. Other procedures such as orthodontic therapy, splinting of teeth, restorative dentistry, etc., may be needed. It is not advisable to carry out occlusal adjustment as a routine procedure to prevent potential trauma from occlusion in the absence of other indication for occlusal adjustment.

The role of occlusal adjustment in patients with bruxism has been discussed under treatment of bruxism (p. 243), and occlusal adjustment in the management of functional temporomandibular joint disturbances is given detailed coverage under treatment of temporomandibular joint disorders (p. 401). The need for occlusal adjustment in relation to restorative dentistry (Chapter 15) and orthodontic procedures (Chapter 14) is also covered in the chapters devoted to these procedures.

An objective of occlusal adjustment that should not be overlooked is the shaping and recontouring of teeth for maximal masticatory efficiency and gingival protection. Such an objective is not directed toward flattening of cusps or simply reducing occlusal surfaces, but it is directed toward cutting effectiveness and the elimination of food impaction.

It was observed during a study of bruxism that some individuals with a tooth-apart swallow developed a normal tooth-together swallow following occlusal adjustment of centric relation.[25] These findings have been reconfirmed in other patients also, mainly when orthodontic therapy has induced a marked discrepancy between centric relation and centric occlusion.

REQUIREMENTS OF AN ACCEPTABLE TECHNIQUE

Many techniques have been recommended for occlusal adjustment or "equilibration."[1,7-9,12,17-19,21,23,24,28,30,31,33-36,38,42,44,46] Such techniques should be accepted or rejected on the basis of their adherence to the physiologic principles of the masticatory system. The most important requirements for these techniques of occlusal adjustment are discussed below.

Elimination of Premature Contacts and Occlusal Interferences

The elimination of premature contacts in the field between centric relation and centric occlusion is especially important for individuals with evidence of bruxism, muscle, temporomandibular joint and swallowing disorders. Also important are occlusal interferences that hamper or hinder smooth gliding occlusal jaw movements in other excursions and constitute obstacles to harmonious function of the entire masticatory system. Even the earliest attempts at "spot grinding" were aimed at elimination of occlusal interferences; and if this were the only concern, the goal could easily be reached by use of "milling paste" or vibrating devices. However, it was discovered a long time ago that the indiscriminate removal of occlusal interferences often leads to an uncomfortable occlusion for mastication, and recurrence of interferences.

Establishment of Optimal Masticatory Effectiveness

The functional principles involved in the procedure for occlusal adjustment were introduced about 30 years ago by Schuyler.[31] He based his very logical rules for occlusal adjustment upon a combined consideration of removal of premature contacts or occlusal interferences and the creation of an optimal number of functional occlusal contacts. Most subsequent writers have to a greater or lesser extent paraphrased Schuyler's principles as will also be done here.

Most early rules for occlusal adjustment suffered from two major short-comings or misleading concepts: (1) experience from prosthetics was applied directly to the natural dentition without due regard to the dynamics of the single tooth and its tendency to move when occlusal stresses are changed, and (2) the principle of balanced occlusion with three point contacts was unjustifiedly given the same significance in the natural as in an artificial dentition. Consequently, because of these shortcomings, teeth often moved into new occlusal interferences following occlusal adjustment. In addition, the adjustment turned into a much too radical "equilibration" in attempts to achieve balanced occlusion in a denture sense. Bilateral balance of occlusal contacts is not a desirable objective in the normal dentition for it has been established both clinically and electromyographically that balancing side contacts, if present, should be lighter than the working side contacts to allow for optimal working function.

Establishment of Stable Occlusal Relationships

Establishment of stable occlusal relationships following occlusal adjustment is by far the most neglected and the most difficult principle to satisfy. Very little attention has been given to this important phase of occlusal adjustment in the extensive dental literature, although occlusal adjustment becomes a meaningless procedure if occlusal relations cannot be stabilized after the adjustment. Sometimes it may be impossible to provide occlusal stability by grinding alone, and restorative dental procedures may be needed to stabilize the teeth. Even so, one should make certain that every procedure in occlusal adjustment is directed as much as possible toward stability of the occlusal relations of the teeth.

Several factors should be included under stability of occlusion: functional and positional stability of the teeth,[40] reproduceable stability of the terminal hinge axis,[16] and maintenance of an undisturbed harmonious neuromuscular pattern for functional movements.[25]

Direction of Main Occlusal Forces

Another important consideration is to bring the occlusal forces within the physiologic tolerance level of the individual teeth by a judiciously planned occlusal adjustment. It is a well established principle that axial forces are better tolerated than lateral forces, so in cases where the teeth have poor periodontal support it is especially important to reduce lateral forces to a minimum. However, lateral forces in a normal dentition are physiologic and desirable from the standpoint of development and maintenance of strong periodontal support for the teeth. It should also be realized that the magnitude of lateral forces is not necessarily in proportion to the steepness of the cusp or the incisal guidance since these forces under normal circumstances are controlled by the neuromuscular mechanism and the protective proprioception in the periodontal membrane. On the other hand, the lateral forces in bruxism may be excessive even with flat occlusal surfaces. The most effective control of lateral forces is achieved by grinding certain teeth with weak support (such as bicuspids) out of lateral function so that a cuspid or well supported molar can carry the entire load of the lateral function. Whenever stability of teeth is a problem, the occlusal forces should be directed as much as possible in an axial direction.

It is especially important that there are no palpable horizontally directed impacts on any tooth when the patient closes firmly into centric occlusion.

Establishment of Efficient Multidirectional Patterns

Multidirectional function is induced by equal convenience and masticatory efficiency in the various directions. This means about equal cuspal inclination and cutting sharpness of the occlusal surfaces bilaterally. Equal effectiveness is also dependent on the presence of complete maxillary and mandibular functional units, and the absence of pain or food impaction.

PROCEDURES FOR OCCLUSAL ADJUSTMENT

The occlusal adjustment technique should adhere as closely as technically possible to the previously listed principles or requirements, and it should also follow a logical sequence of procedures since the steps in the technique should facilitate each succeeding step. A technique for comprehensive occlusal adjustment will be outlined first. Modifications of these procedures will be discussed later.

Goals for Adjustment of Centric

The objectives for adjustment of centric include: (1) Elimination of premature contacts in centric relation and centric occlusion, (2) establishment of freedom in centric in the horizontal plane with centric occlusion slightly anterior in jaw position to centric relation and with even pressure on all posterior teeth, and (3) elimination of all horizontal-lateral impact in centric closure.

Locations of Premature Contacts in Centric Relation

A detailed discussion on location of premature contacts in centric relation can be found in Chapter 9.

It is very important to spend sufficient time and effort to accurately determine premature contacts. Lacquer is probably the most accurate medium,[39] but it is cumbersome to use and clinically not very practical. The use of green inlay wax (28 or 32 gauge) and carbon paper will provide clinically acceptable accuracy.

Besides marking of the initial premature contact in centric relation, the pathways of the slide from centric relation to centric occlusion and the holding contacts in centric occlusion should be recorded. This can usually be achieved by having the patient squeeze his teeth together from centric relation to centric occlusion with thin carbon paper between the teeth. It is recommended that wax be used to determine which teeth make premature occlusal contacts, and the carbon paper to determine where on the teeth the premature contacts occur, where interfering sliding contacts are located, and where the holding contacts or centric stops, which are essential for occlusal stability, are located.

The mandibular closure to centric relation should always be guided by the operator, and it should never be left to the patient to relocate centric relation since proprioceptive signals from the teeth may change during the various steps of occlusal adjustment while the contact relationships are being changed.

Rules for Adjustment of Centric

The individual variations in contact relationships between cusps and fossae in the natural dentition make it virtually impossible to formulate foolproof, generally applicable rules for occlusal contact relations in individuals with "normal" intercuspidation; however, it is possible to make some generalizations in a rational approach to occlusal adjustment based on careful correlation of the previously listed requirements for techniques of occlusal adjustment. It should be emphasized that before any grinding is done according to memorized rules, the operator should have a definite answer to the overwhelmingly important question of what will happen, not only to the tooth to be ground but to the entire dentition after the contemplated grinding has been performed. Will the grinding eliminate the premature contact or interference? Will it improve function? Will it promote a stable occlusion and a lasting good result? Will the stress distribution be favorable after the grinding? Will the grinding facilitate neuromuscular selection of multidirectional functional movements? Is the tooth proposed for the grinding a more favorable choice than the opposite tooth on the basis of the previously listed considerations?

When the premature contacts in centric relation have been located, it should be determined by visual observation in what direction these contacts guide the mandible during slow complete closure to centric occlusion. Because of the horseshoe shape of the dental arches, modified by a posterior widening, a distal positioning of the mandible (relative to centric occlusion) will bring into contact the mesially and bucally directed surfaces of the lingual cusps of the maxillary molars and bicuspids against the distally and lingually directed surfaces of the buccal cusps of the mandibular molars and bicuspids. The tips of the lingual maxillary cusps and the buccal mandibular cusps may also be involved in this contact relationship. Furthermore, the lingual maxillary cusps and their mesial and buccal inclines may make contacts prematurely against distally and lingually directed surfaces (marginal and transverse ridges) in the mandibular central fossa and make the mandible glide forward from centric relation to centric occlusion.

Since it has been found both clinically and electromyographically[24] that optimal relaxation of the jaw muscles and harmonious muscle activity in swallowing are best achieved by elimination of the slide from centric relation to centric occlusion, the first step toward comprehensive occlusal adjustment is elimination of the slide. This will necessitate grinding on some of the cusps or inclines involved in contact relationship during the slide. Occlusal stability and function is to a great extent based on the mandibular buccal cusps fitting into the central fossae and embrasures of the maxillary teeth and the lingual maxillary cusps fitting into the central fossae and embrasures of mandibular teeth.

In the occlusal adjustment of "slide in centric" or "eccentric slide" one should try to stabilize the occlusion and maintain cuspal function by fitting the buccal cusps of the mandibular teeth into the central fossae of the maxilla and the lingual cusps of the maxillary teeth into central fossae of the mandibular teeth. This is achieved mainly by grinding on the involved inclines toward the fossae in such a way that a seat is ground for the buccal cusp of the mandibular teeth in the maxillary central fossa. The seat for the cusp should be ground down to the same level as the seat for the cusp in centric occlusion. Such grinding provides a horizontal or flat area of "centric" between centric relation and centric occlusion. This flat area provides for so-called "long centric" (Mann and Pankey[22]) or "freedom in centric."[32] Similar provision is made for the lingual maxillary cusp in the mandibular central fossae. In order to follow this principle, the grinding will be done mainly on mesial and buccal surfaces of lingual maxillary cusps and on the distal aspect of marginal and transverse ridges in the mandible, and sometimes on distolingual surfaces of buccal mandibular cusps. The buccal mandibular cusps and the lingual maxillary cusps should make contact anywhere between centric relation and centric occlusion on a flat surface so the impact of this contact is directed axially on the teeth, thus avoiding any tipping force as a result of the adjustment.

There are, however, certain anatomic problems that may complicate the implementation of these general principles. The buccal cusps of the mandibular bicuspids and the mesiobuccal cusps of the molars fit into an opposite embrasure area as do the lingual cusps of the maxillary bicuspids and distolingual cusps of the molars. In the unworn dentition the slopes of the cusps may make contacts on approximating marginal ridges rather than the tip of the cusp making contact at the bottom of the embrasure. In this event, the cusp tip may extend slightly beyond the marginal ridge contact area into the embrasure area (Fig. 13–1, *A*). If a seat is provided for such a cusp tip on a level with the previous centric stop on the surface of the marginal ridge, the cusp will appear

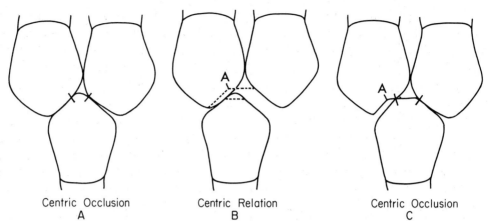

Centric Occlusion
A

Centric Relation
B

Centric Occlusion
C

Figure 13–1.   Schematic illustration of correction of premature contacts and slide in centric where tip of supporting cusp fits into embrasure in centric occlusion. *A,* Occlusal contacts in centric occlusion. *B,* Premature contact at A on maxillary second premolar in centric relation. Dotted line on maxillary premolar indicates grinding to provide a seat for the cusp of the mandibular second premolar. The dotted line on the cusp tip of the mandibular premolar indicates grinding to prevent "tripping" of the cusp in the embrasure between the marginal ridges of the maxillary premolars. *C,* After grinding, centric stops are still present in centric occlusion and there is freedom and stability between centric relation and centric occlusion.

too high when the mandible is in centric relation. Such a cusp tip can be reduced slightly to the upper level of the centric occlusion contact on the cusp against the marginal ridge (Fig. 13–1, *B, C*). It would be incorrect to grind off the distal surface of the buccal mandibular cusps since this would jeopardize some centric stops in centric occlusion and alter the impact of the chewing force on the teeth and create a potential for migration of the teeth (Fig. 13–2). It has to be assumed from recent evidence that a person continues to chew into his

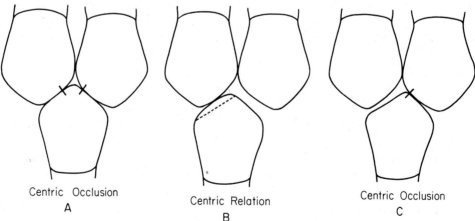

Centric Occlusion
A

Centric Relation
B

Centric Occlusion
C

Figure 13–2.   Incorrect grinding in circumstance illustrated in Figure 13–1. *A,* Occlusal contacts on marginal ridges in centric occlusion. *B,* Premature contact in centric relation. Dotted line indicates incorrect grinding. *C,* Result of incorrect grinding; in centric occlusion a centric stop has been lost as well as loss of lateral working contact.

previous centric occlusion even if the occlusion is adjusted to centric relation as outlined in this description.[13] It is, therefore, essential that occlusal stability and full functional capacity be maintained for centric occlusion after the occlusal adjustment.

A lateral slide of the mandible from centric relation to centric occlusion is corrected according to the same principle as the forward slide. This means occlusal seats should be provided for the mandibular buccal cusps in the maxillary fossae and for the lingual maxillary cusps in the central mandibular fossae. The fossae should be widened to the deepest level of the centric stop in centric occlusion (Fig. 13–3). A combination of interferences may necessitate simultaneous widening of both the maxillary and mandibular fossae.

If the centric stop in centric occlusion is on buccal and lingual inclines instead of being at the base of the fossa, one should still widen the fossa from the deepest level of the centric stop and reduce the tip of the opposing cusp slightly if it protrudes into the central fossa deeper than the level of the centric stops in centric occlusion (Fig. 13–4).

If an extensive lateral slide is the result of contacts between the buccal cusps of the mandibular teeth with their lingual inclines and the lingual cusps of the maxillary teeth with their buccal inclines and it is severe enough that it cannot be eliminated unless a cusp is sacrificed, the lingual maxillary cusp should usually be reduced rather than the buccal mandibular cusp (Fig. 13–5). However, in some instances, a little off both cusps is permissible provided the mandibular buccal cusp contact in centric and working is not lost. This choice is made in the best interest of both stability and function.

If the lateral slide is caused by contacts between the buccal inclines of a lingual mandibular cusp against a lingual maxillary cusp, the correction should be made on the buccal incline of the lingual mandibular cusp with widening of

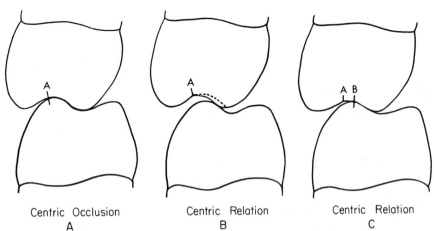

Centric Occlusion
A

Centric Relation
B

Centric Relation
C

Figure 13–3. Correction of lateral slide of mandible from centric relation to centric occlusion. *A,* Contact relation of buccal cusp and fossa at A in centric occlusion. *B,* Contact relation in centric relation. Dotted line indicates necessary grinding to widen fossa to eliminate lateral slide. *C,* After grinding, contact at B in centric relation is on same level as contact A in centric occlusion.

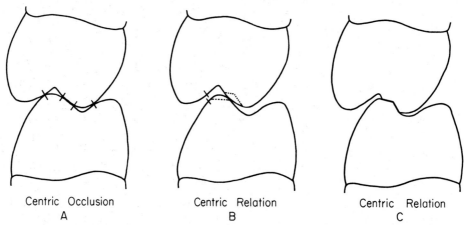

Centric Occlusion   Centric Relation   Centric Relation
A   B   C

Figure 13–4. Correction of lateral slide when centric stops are present on buccal and lingual in-clines rather than at bottom of fossa. A, Centric stops in centric occlusion. B, Premature contact in cen-tric relation. Dotted lines show indicated grinding to eliminate lateral slide. The tip of the buccal cusp of mandibular molar should be reduced slightly as indicated by the dotted line if the cusp protrudes into the maxillary fossa and "trips" on the seat prepared in the maxillary molar when the mandible moves from centric relation to centric occlusion. C, Centric relation with occlusal seat in maxillary molar on the same level as the centric stop in centric occlusion, providing "freedom in centric" and functional stability.

the central fossa at the deepest level of the centric occlusion stops (Fig. 13–6). If in this situation a cusp tip has to be reduced to eliminate the slide, the re-duction should be on the lingual mandibular cusp since this cusp does not maintain a stabilizing or supportive function either in centric relation or centric occlusion. A flat area of "freedom in centric" or "play in centric," combined with the "long centric" anteriorly and posteriorly, is the common result of such occlusal adjustment.

Correct Grinding   Incorrect Grinding — and — Result

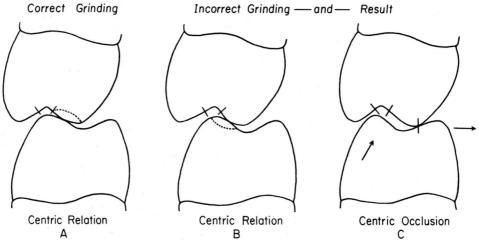

Centric Relation   Centric Relation   Centric Occlusion
A   B   C

Figure 13–5. Correction of extensive lateral slide as a result of premature contact of lingual incline of mandibular buccal cusp and buccal incline of maxillary lingual cusp. A, Dotted line on maxillary molar indicates correct grinding. Note avoidance of grinding centric stop of centric occlusion. B, Shows incor-rect grinding of mandibular buccal cusp incline. C, Result of incorrect grinding with loss of centric stop of buccal mandibular cusp in centric occlusion and tipping of mandibular molar in the direction of the arrows.

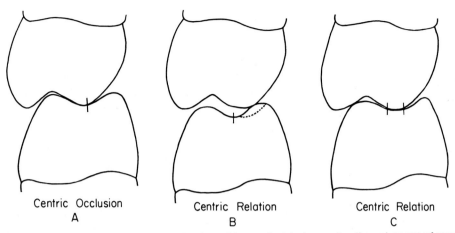

Figure 13–6. Correction of lateral slide caused by contact between the lingual cusps of maxillary and mandibular teeth. *A*, Position of centric stop in centric occlusion. *B*, Dotted line indicates correct grinding for correction of slide. *C*, Contact relationship in centric relation after correct grinding.

A premature contact either in centric relation or centric occlusion, or an interference with a smooth easy glide between centric relation and centric occlusion, may be disturbing to occlusal harmony without producing a slide when the patient bites together. Such "high spots" should be eliminated according to Schuyler's well established functional principle for adjustment of premature contacts in centric.[31] If a cusp is making premature contact in centric and does not make contact in the lateral excursions, the grinding for adjustment should be done in the fossa opposing the high cusp (Fig. 13–7). Only when the cusp is making a premature contact in centric and lateral excursions should the cusp be reduced (Fig. 13–8). Such grinding should also provide centric stops with axially directed impact of the occlusal forces in centric.

At the completion of the adjustment of centric relation, the opposing molars

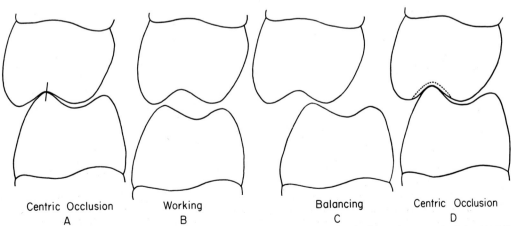

Figure 13–7. Correction for premature contact in centric only. *A*, Premature contact in centric occlusion. *B* and *C*, Absence of contact in working and balancing relations. *D*, Dotted line indicates correct grinding in the fossa opposing the high mandibular cusp.

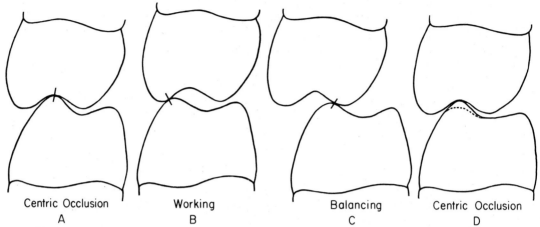

Centric Occlusion	Working	Balancing	Centric Occlusion
A	B	C	D

Figure 13–8. Correction for premature contact of a cusp in centric and lateral excursions. *A,* Contact relation in centric occlusion. *B* and *C,* Cusp contact in working and balancing relations. *D,* Dotted line on mandibular buccal cusp indicates correct grinding.

and bicuspids should make simultaneous occlusal contact when the mandible is tapped into centric relation (p. 204), and the mandible should not slide or tip when the patient bites hard together following this light contact. There should also be even contacts in centric occlusion and maintained contacts without any interference when the mandible moves between centric relation and centric occlusion. The adjusted centric occlusion should be straight in front of centric relation (relative to mandibular movement) and parallel to the midsagittal plane. This stable occlusion in the field of "long centric" or "freedom of movements in centric" should not represent either loss or gain of occlusal vertical dimension. The anterior teeth will usually be out of contact in centric relation but may touch lightly in centric occlusion.

The most important rule for adjustment of centric is never to leave the impact of the occlusal forces in centric relation or centric occlusion on unbalanced slanting inclines that may induce tooth movement. The seats for the supporting cusps ("centric stops") have to be either on a flat surface perpendicular to the long axis of the teeth or on opposing balancing inclines (Fig.

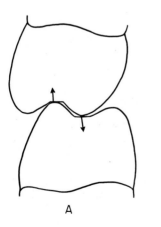

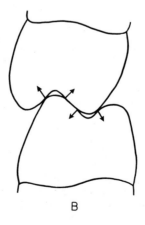

Figure 13–9. The adjustment of centric should result in flat "centric stops" or stops on opposing balanced inclines. *A,* Seats for supporting cusps should be on a flat surface perpendicular to the long axis of the teeth. *B,* Seats for supporting cusps on opposing balanced inclines.

A   B

13–9). If such a relationship cannot be achieved, it is often indicated that the occlusion be stabilized with occlusal and marginal restorations, especially in patients with temporomandibular joint dysfunction or bruxism.

RULES FOR ADJUSTMENT OF WORKING SIDE AND PROTRUSIVE INTERFERENCES

The goals for adjustment of eccentric excursions are: (1) to provide multidirectional unrestricted smooth gliding contact patterns, (2) to provide similar incisal and cuspid guidance for both sides, and (3) to eliminate interferences or provide guidance on the balancing or nonfunctioning side.

The location of working side and protrusive interferences has also been discussed in Chapter 9. These interferences are much easier to determine than centric interferences since both carbon paper and dental tapes provide relatively good markings from rubbing occlusal contacts together with light pressure. Green inlay wax or lacquer can also be used for fine corrections at the finishing stage of the adjustment.[39]

Although patients may not chew farther posteriorly than lateral to centric occlusion,[2] they may go sufficiently posteriorly to catch interferences during bruxism. It is therefore recommended to go as far posteriorly in diagnosis and adjustment of lateral excursions as the mandible can be moved in a gothic arch tracing. This may cover a slightly larger area than needed for some patients, but it provides the assurance that the patient cannot reach posteriorly and laterally for occlusal interferences that might have been left if the adjustment had not been carried out to include the retrusive lateral excursions. Lateral and protrusive adjustment should cover the entire field within the functional boundaries of the jaws in combined lateral and protrusive as well as straight protrusive excursions.

The elimination of occlusal interferences on the working side of the lateral excursion should be done according to Schuyler's[31] time-honored "BULL" rule (Buccal of Upper, Lingual of Lower). This rule means grinding on the bucco-occlusal inclines (the lingual inclines of the buccal cusps) of the maxillary teeth and the linguo-occlusal inclines (the buccal inclines of the lingual cusps) of the mandibular teeth (Fig. 13–10). This method of grinding maintains the centric contacts and the occlusal stability undisturbed and provides maximum functional contact around centric where most of the masticatory function is carried out. At the same time the method provides for elimination of interferences and for restriction of the functional occlusal field of teeth with poor periodontal support (Fig. 13–11).

A serious warning should be given against grinding on the buccal aspect of the buccal mandibular cusps and the lingual aspect of the maxillary lingual cusps, since such grinding may jeopardize both occlusal stability and function in the area where functional contacts are most important (Fig. 13–12).

In a study of buccolingual sections of a number of occluded casts of denti-

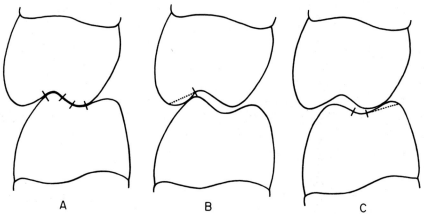

Figure 13–10. Correction of occlusal interferences on the working side of lateral excursions. *A*, Contact relation in centric occlusion. *B*, Dotted line on lingual incline of maxillary buccal cusp indicates correct grinding of occlusal interference. *C*, Dotted line on buccal incline of mandibular lingual cusp indicates correct grinding for removal of occlusal interference.

tions with various degrees of occlusal wear up to almost flat occlusal surfaces, it was never observed that the buccal mandibular cusps were too large for the maxillary central fossa or the lingual maxillary cusps too large for the mandibular central fossa in a way that would merit narrowing of these cusps.

It is important to establish a bilateral smooth gliding movement pattern with approximately equal cuspal inclination and cutting efficiency of occlusal anatomy since bilateral function is dependent on equal ease of movements and masticatory effectiveness on both sides.

Unrestricted smooth occlusal paths are more important than the number of contacts that can be brought into lateral function and, in cases of posterior

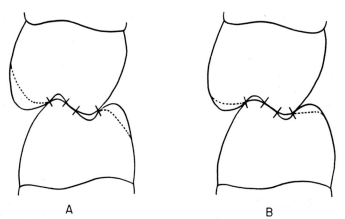

Figure 13–11. Grinding to restrict the functional contacts in the presence of poor periodontal support. *A*, Correct grinding on the lingual cusp of the mandibular molar. Excessive grinding of the buccal surfaces of the maxillary cusp leads to cheek biting. *B*, Correct grinding of the maxillary buccal cusp shown by dotted line. Where restriction of the occlusal field is not desired for the mandibular teeth, the grinding may be limited to that shown by the dotted line on the lingual cusp. Note that maximum functional contact is maintained around centric.

Incorrect   Grinding

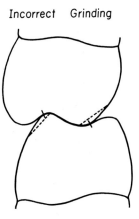

Figure 13–12. Incorrect grinding for elimination of occlusal inter-ferences. Grinding as indicated by the dotted lines results in loss of functional contact in working excursions and loss of centric stops and stability.

teeth with minimal periodontal support, it may be advisable to end up with a very narrow field of occlusal contacts close to centric and to utilize "cuspid rise"[10] for lateral excursions if the cuspids have a good periodontal support.

Interferences between the maxillary and mandibular anterior teeth either in lateral or protrusive excursions should be corrected by grinding on the lingual aspect of the maxillary incisors and cuspids along the path of the interference.

The grinding should be extended incisally from the point of initial contact in lateral or protrusive excursion, leaving this point itself undisturbed. This often will mean that the grinding is done on an area several mm. away from the centric occlusion stop mark on the maxillary teeth, since the functional incisal guidance does not always follow the entire contour of the lingual surfaces of the maxillary anterior teeth (Fig. 13–13).

In some instances, there is no functional centric stop or contact between the maxillary and mandibular front teeth. The position of the teeth is then main-tained either by tongue or lip habits, or by contacts in lateral and protrusive excursions, especially in patients with bruxism. However, if the incisal edges of the mandibular incisors or cuspids are ground off to reduce excessive over-bite or protrusive interferences, these teeth usually erupt back to their previous incisal relationship with recurrence of overbite and protrusive interference — unless the patient in the meantime develops an undesirable tongue habit or bruxism and thereby maintains the open bite.

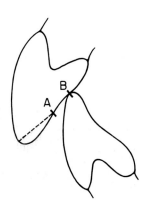

Figure 13–13. Correction of interferences between maxillary and mandibular anterior teeth during lateral or pro-trusive excursions. Point A indicates initial contact in protru-sive excursion. Point B indicates centric occlusion stop. Dotted line indicates grinding incisally from point of initial contact to remove interference.

Esthetics and variance in tooth position impose fairly narrow restrictions on what can be accomplished by occlusal adjustment in the correction of malocclusion or occlusal interferences in the region of the anterior teeth. However, from the standpoint of function, muscle harmony and comfort, it does not seem very important how steep incisal guidance or deep overbite may be as long as freedom of lateral movements can be established. Even with impinging overbite, where occlusal adjustment certainly cannot correct the gross malocclusion, a reduction in steepness of the incisal guidance on the lingual surface of the maxillary teeth may provide great improvement in function if such grinding provides an opportunity for lateral functional movements that were previously blocked by the steep incisal guidance. Such patients may develop a two-phased chewing cycle during which, in the first phase, incision of food is made with the front teeth without complete posterior closure and, in the second phase, food is brought back to the posterior teeth with complete posterior closure and mastication is made without impinging food against the palate or the labial mandibular gingiva.

In most instances, no attempt is made to harmonize the protrusive guidance with the cuspal inclination in the molar and bicuspid regions since such harmony is not essential for good function and muscle comfort. However, according to Beyron's[3] observations, a deep overbite with restricted protrusive function may induce an unfavorable occlusal wear pattern. For this reason, it is desirable to establish as a compromise a combined lateral and protrusive pattern with simultaneous functional contacts or group function on the cuspid, lateral and central incisors on each side.

Under no circumstances should there be established heavy contact in the posterior regions during protrusive contact excursions. Furthermore, there is no evidence to indicate that even light posterior contacts are desirable in protrusive excursions. The incisal guidance is therefore not reduced for the purpose of establishing posterior contacts in the protrusive range of function. If there are interferences in the posterior regions during protrusive excursions, this should be relieved on the bucco-occlusal surfaces (the lingual surfaces of the buccal cusps) of the maxillary teeth and the linguo-occlusal surfaces (buccal surfaces of the lingual cusp) of the mandibular teeth, as in the correction of working side interferences.

Adjustment of Balancing Side Interferences

The determination of balancing side interferences can be made with techniques similar to the ones used for the detection of centric and working side interferences. Balancing side interferences are those which occur between maxillary and mandibular supporting cusps and their occlusal inclines. Since these cusps maintain centric stops and thus are essential to the stability of the position of the teeth, the removal of interferences has to be done with great care, so that as many and as widely diversified centric stops as possible are retained after the adjustment. The main rule, as pointed out by Schuyler,[31] is to do the whole grinding on only one or two interfering cusps or inclines if they both serve as centric stops for the teeth. However, by careful analysis it will be found that centric stops can often be partially maintained by precision grinding which involves widening of sulcular pathways for the interfering cusps rather than by radical cuspal reduction.

Some centric stops may have to be sacrificed in order to eliminate the interferences, but all of the centric contact points or stops should never be ground away for any particular tooth. It is extremely important to analyze carefully the future consequences with regard to occlusal stability and function before it is decided whether the grinding should be done on the lingual cusps (including their buccal inclines in the maxilla) or on the buccal cusps (including their lingual inclines in the mandible) when centric stops have to be sacrificed. The decision on where to grind should be made after due consideration is given to: (1) the tendency for drifting or tipping of the teeth following the grinding; (2) the resulting direction of the forces in centric occlusion related to the periodontal support of the teeth; (3) the effect on working side function of the teeth following the grinding; and (4) the possibility for maintaining part of the centric stops involved in the interference. These considerations are especially important for patients with a tendency for clenching and grinding their teeth since the heavy contacting forces in bruxism will readily tip the teeth if given an opportunity, and occlusal interferences are then bound to reappear (Fig. 13–14).

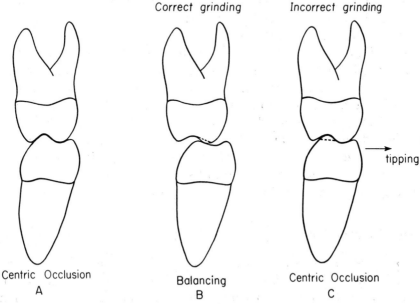

Figure 13–14. Correction of balancing side interferences. *A,* Contact relations in centric occlusion. *B,* Occlusal interference in balancing. Dotted line indicates correct grinding to remove interference and preserve stability. *C,* Grinding of the buccal mandibular cusp as indicated by the dotted line may cause the molar to tip lingually and the balancing side interference to recur.

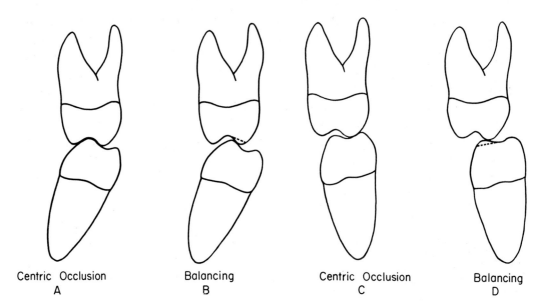

Centric Occlusion
A

Balancing
B

Centric Occlusion
C

Balancing
D

Figure 13–15. *A* and *B*, Correction of balancing side interference when posterior mandibular tooth is tipped lingually. *A*, Contact relations in centric occlusion. *B*, Correct grinding to remove the interference is indicated by dotted line on the buccal incline of the maxillary lingual cusp. *C* and *D*, Correction of balancing side interference when posterior mandibular tooth is tipped buccally. *C*, Contact relations in centric occlusion. *D*, Correct grinding of the buccal cusp of the mandibular molar is indicated by the dotted line.

If a posterior tooth is tipped or occlusal irregularities exist so the cusp or incline which is making interfering contact in balancing excursion is out of contact in centric, grind on that cusp or incline. Stability is then maintained by the contacting cusp that is not ground (Fig. 13–15).

The balancing side contacts, if present, should be ground off so that in empty occlusal movements they are slightly out of contact or at least they touch more lightly than the contacts on the working side. No attempts should be made to grind down guiding inclines on the working side for the sole purpose of bringing in balancing side contacts. A good way to check the balancing side contacts is to place a strip of 28 gauge green inlay wax over the occlusal surfaces on one side at a time and have the patient move the mandible with the teeth in contact over to the side opposite to the wax strip without biting together in centric. The wax should not be completely penetrated by this procedure if the balancing side contacts are as light as they should be.

Rules for Adjustment of Crossbite

Although the same basic principles apply to occlusal adjustment of crossbite as to the normal occlusion, the previously outlined rules for adjustment have to be modified for the particular occlusal relationship and dynamics of the crossbite.

In crossbite the buccal cusps of the maxillary teeth and the lingual cusps of the mandibular teeth act as supporting cusps for the occlusal vertical dimension. A forward slide from centric relation to centric occlusion from premature contacts in the bicuspid and molar regions should be adjusted by grinding on the distal or distolingual incline of the buccal mandibular cusps. Such grinding provides a centric relation stop more mesially or buccally in the mandibular central fossa than the previous centric occlusion contact. The "long centric" or "freedom in centric" (area of occlusion between centric occlusion and the centric relation) should be on a horizontal flat level. If premature contact is made by the lingual mandibular cusp against a mesially directed incline in the maxillary central fossa and toward the lingual maxillary cusps, the grinding should be done on the maxillary teeth to provide a stable seat for the supporting lingual mandibular cusp.

Lateral slides are corrected in a similar way by widening the mandibular central fossa to provide a seat in centric relation for the buccal maxillary cusps and widening the maxillary central fossa to provide a seat for the lingual mandibular cusps. If a posterior tooth is too high (without a slide in closure) the grinding is done according to the same rule as for the high tooth in normal occlusion. Grind the high cusp only if it is high both in centric and lateral excursions, otherwise deepen the fossa opposing the higher cusp.

Anterior crossbite of a functional type may sometimes be corrected by a distal repositioning of the mandible to centric relation as determined by the temporomandibular joints. This may involve grinding not only on the front teeth, but on all the contact areas that participate in the forward slide of the mandible all the way to centric occlusion. Before such grinding is executed, one has to be sure that the mandibular front teeth will catch inside the labial edge of the maxillary front teeth with the jaw in centric relation after the adjustment. Without previous mounting and correction of casts mounted in an articulator in the stationary posterior hinge position (centric relation), it is difficult to visualize directly in the patient's mouth whether such an incisal catch can be established. Generally speaking, if the crowns of the maxillary anterior teeth are pointing lingually and the mandibular anterior teeth are pointing labially, the chances for a successful correction of the crossbite by grinding are good (Fig. 13–16). However, if the patient has an Angle Class III malocclusion, in which the crowns of the maxillary incisors point labially and the mandibular incisors lingually, grinding would move the incisal edges of these teeth farther apart (Fig. 13–17). If contact in centric relation can be established in an anterior crossbite, the incisal edges should be slanted so the impact of the centric contact tends to push the maxillary front teeth forward and the mandibular incisors lingually (Fig. 13–16, *B, C*).

The principle of guiding or moving teeth by deliberately placing the centric stops on slanting inclines is commonly used for interceptive guidance of occlusal relations in children (Fig. 13–18). Sometimes a very dramatic effect may be gained in functional posterior crossbites or disturbed eruption patterns.

The correction of working side interferences in crossbite has to be done either on the lingual incline of the buccal maxillary cusps (may also have to include these cusps), or on the buccal incline of the lingual mandibular cusps

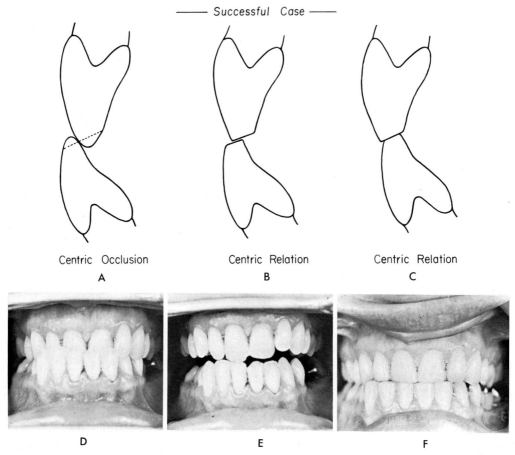

Figure 13–16. Adjustment of anterior crossbite. *A*, Incisal relations in centric occlusion. Dotted lines on maxillary and mandibular teeth indicate angle of grinding. *B*, After grinding with incisal contacts in centric relation. *C*, Incisal contacts in centric relation 1 year after grinding. *D*, Clinical view of anterior crossbite with mandible in centric occlusion. *E*, Contact relations in centric relation. *F*, Contact relations in centric relation 1 year after occlusal adjustment and posterior reconstruction.

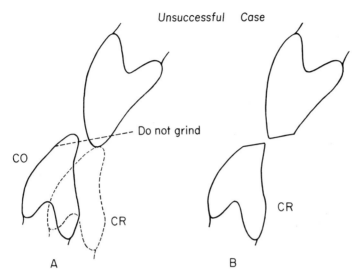

Figure 13–17. Unsuccessful case of correction of anterior crossbite complicated by Angle Class III malocclusion. *A,* Incisal relations of anterior teeth in centric occlusion (CO) and centric relation (CR). Because of the labial inclination of the maxillary and lingual inclination of the mandibular teeth, it is advisable not to grind as indicated by the dotted line. *B,* If grinding is done, the incisal edges will not make functional contact.

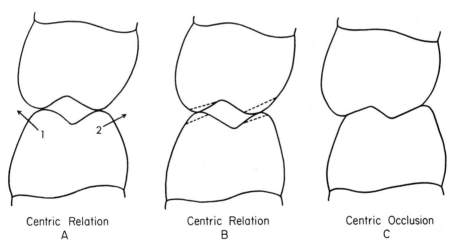

Figure 13–18. Grinding for interceptive guidance of occlusal relations in children. *A,* Contact relations in centric relation. Arrow 1 indicates the possibility of gliding into crossbite in centric occlusion. Arrow 2 indicates possibility for gliding into normal occlusal relationship in centric occlusion. *B,* Dotted lines indicate grinding to secure glide into normal occlusal relationship. *C,* Occlusal relationship in centric occlusion after grinding as indicated. Readjustment will be required after the teeth reach their final position. It is best if guidance is gained without grinding on the mandibular buccal and maxillary lingual cusps.

(possibly including the cusps). These cusps are supporting cusps in crossbite and are important for stability. In case a cusp with a centric stop has to be sacrificed, grind on the cusp that is least important for stability and function.

Interferences on the balancing side in crossbite should be removed on the buccal inclines of the lingual maxillary cusps and/or the lingual incline of the buccal mandibular cusps, including these cusps when necessary for smooth unhindered function.

Completion of Adjustment

After centric, lateral and protrusive excursions have been adjusted the entire field of occlusal function should be examined by letting the patient perform occlusal contact movements in various directions. While this is done, the operator should hold his hand on the patient's chin to feel whether all movements are smooth and unrestricted. Small interferences to smooth movements are best located by placing green inlay wax on the occlusal surfaces and having the patient bite lightly together, then moving the mandible with light occlusal force in the direction of the interference. The high spot will then wear through the wax so it can be located and marked with a soft lead pencil before the wax is removed. The high spot is then relieved according to the previously discussed principles and rules.

Following the elimination of all premature contacts and occlusal interferences, the occlusal surfaces, incisal edges and cusps should be reshaped for optimal functional efficiency and esthetics. The occlusal anatomy of teeth and fillings can usually be activated or sharpened without loss of centric stops or contacts. The pressure required to masticate tough food can be reduced appreciably by such grinding and the gingival tissues may be protected against food impaction or impingement.

The buccolingual width of the occlusal table of molars and bicuspids may also be reduced by grinding on the buccal surfaces of the maxillary teeth and lingual surfaces of the crowns of mandibular teeth (Fig. 13–19). This may reduce the lateral functional load and be of some significance for teeth

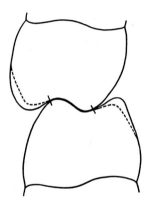

Figure 13–19. Reduction of buccolingual width of occlusal table of posterior teeth. Grinding should be done as indicated by dotted lines. Excessive grinding of the maxillary buccal surface should be avoided because of loss of overjet and resulting cheek biting.

with bruxism. Excessive grinding of the buccal cusp may result in cheek biting in the molar area.

Routine reshaping of wear facets is not indicated if the adjustment has followed the outlined principles. There is no scientific evidence to support routine elimination of wear facets. Grinding for elimination of such facets has a common tendency to result in rearrangement of the teeth and impaired occlusal function until the wear facets reappear after some time. Extensive wear of teeth is usually the result of bruxism, and the masticatory effectiveness of these dentitions is usually good in spite of, or because of, the wear of the teeth. Provided the occlusal adjustment has been carried out properly, bruxism usually will be markedly reduced following the adjustment. Thus, the significance of the functional contact along the surfaces of the wear facets is also reduced.

Esthetics can often be improved greatly by grinding jagged incisal edges even and softening sharp corners of the teeth. During such procedures one has to be careful not to remove centric stops or functional contacts for the teeth involved.

After the grinding has been completed, it is important to polish all the ground surfaces since roughness may act as a "trigger" for bruxism and thus induce abnormal occlusal stresses. Milling paste should never be used in any phase of adjustment of the natural dentition, since the indiscriminatory abrasion that results from the use of such abrasives will eliminate centric contacts and thereby predispose to an uncontrollable resetting of the teeth with possible reappearance of occlusal interferences. Functional contacts around centric may also be lost if such paste is used. Even if metal foil is used to protect the cusp tips of one arch from wear,[4] the use of milling paste is not recommended since the presence of the foil alters the occlusal relationships of the teeth.

If rather extensive grinding has been performed or sensitive surfaces have been encountered, it is advisable to apply a desensitizing solution before the patient is dismissed (2 per cent sodium fluoride, 8 per cent stannous fluoride, or other desensitizing agents). It should also be indicated to the patient that postgrinding sensitivity does not indicate any weakening of the teeth and that the sensitivity will subside.

The patients should be re-examined 4 to 6 weeks following occlusal adjustment for control of the results. It is impossible to avoid completely some repositioning of the teeth following occlusal adjustment. Some resetting of the teeth may be desirable since it may close contacts that had been opened by traumatic occlusion (Fig. 13–20). However, any movement of the teeth may lead to reappearance of slight occlusal interferences which should then be eliminated at the control visit. Another disturbing phenomenon is that centric relation or the terminal hinge position of the mandible may change considerably after occlusal adjustment in patients with tense jaw muscles and/or temporomandibular joint pain or dysfunction. The occlusions of these patients have to be readjusted till the mandible assumes a stable terminal hinge position, which may involve several appointments over a period of several months.

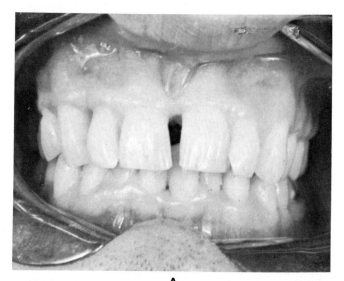

A

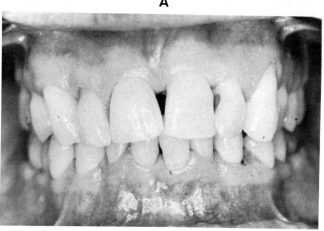

B

Figure 13–20. Closing of space between maxillary incisors following occlusal adjustment. *A*, Opening between maxillary incisors prior to occlusal adjustment. *B*, Closure of space (1 year follow-up).

The most challenging phase of occlusal adjustment is to achieve occlusal stability after the adjustment. This may not always be accomplished by grinding alone, and the placement of restorations, orthodontic therapy, or splinting of teeth may be needed to stabilize the occlusion. If such measures are needed, this should be explained to the patient before the occlusal adjustment is started. The most common cause of reoccurrence of temporomandibular joint and muscle pain accompanied by bruxism after occlusal adjustment is lack of occlusal stability, and this factor merits the most careful analysis before, during and after adjustment.

Special Equipment and Procedures

Properly mounted casts are helpful for analysis of occlusion and for planning of the occlusal adjustment (p. 229).[20] However, after an operator has gained some experience, the occlusal adjustment can be performed with accuracy directly in the patient's mouth without going through a trial adjustment on mounted casts. It is recommended that casts be mounted and trial adjustments be done in any case in which the operator cannot fully visualize or anticipate the result that should follow the occlusal adjustment (such as in the case of anterior functional crossbites). Items needed for the location of interferences include carbon paper, 28 or 32 gauge green inlay wax, occlusal indicator wax and a soft lead pencil.

For the actual removal of tooth substance by grinding, various suitable stones can be used. It is important that the stones used for adjustment of centric be small enough to allow for detailed access to the anatomic features of the occlusal surfaces. A small knife-edge stone for the handpiece is useful for grinding on facets engaged in "slide in centric." The seats for the cusp tips and the "long centric" have to be established by very small inverted cone-diamond points in the contra angle handpiece. The adjustment for lateral and protrusive excursions can be done with small or medium sized wheel-type stones. A waterspray should be used and the operator should press a finger against the buccal surface of the tooth to be ground. The stone should rotate in the direction of the adjacent teeth to minimize the vibration and discomfort of the patient. A slightly abrasive rubber wheel dipped in 2 per cent sodium fluoride should be used for finishing of the adjustment in the lateral and protrusive excursions and for polishing. For rounding the sharp corners of anterior teeth, use 1/2- to 3/4-inch sandpaper discs of various grits.

INDICATIONS FOR OCCLUSAL ADJUSTMENT

1. *Primary Trauma from Occlusion*
   A. Periodontal
   B. Dental
   C. Pulpal
   D. T.M.J.
   E. Neuromuscular
   F. Oral soft tissues
2. *Secondary Trauma from Occlusion*
   Tooth mobility associated with loss of support
3. *Prior to Extensive Restorative Dental Treatment*
4. *Restricted Functional Movements*
5. *Instability of Occlusion following Orthodontic and Other Dental Treatment*

It is extremely important that both the dentist and the patient know definitely why the contemplated occlusal adjustment should be done before the teeth are touched by any stones. As indicated at the beginning of this chapter, many objectives for occlusal adjustment have been suggested, and some of these are very controversial. Many patients have had occlusal prob ems created by occlusal adjustment procedures, and the percentage of iatrogenic disease has been disturbingly high in this field. The main reasons are: (1) faulty initial diagnosis, (2) faulty indications or premises for occlusal adjustment, (3) faulty or inadequate technical principles, and (4) technical shortcomings of the operator in performing occlusal adjustment. It is, therefore, in the best interest both of the patient and the dentist that occlusal adjustment be attempted only for valid reasons and be done to the minimal extent required for the desired result in the individual patient.

As discussed under physiology of occlusion, it is essential for the comfort of the masticatory system of some individuals that they have an ideal occlusion. However, most patients have a physiologically normal occlusion within an adaptive range of imperfections in occlusal relations. Equally or more important than the occlusal relations is how the patient adapts or reacts to occlusal interferences. This adaptability or reaction has to be considered under indications for occlusal adjustment since occlusal interferences that definitely should be eliminated for one patient do not need to be removed for another patient who may be able to tolerate the interferences since they are within his adaptive range.

With due regard to individual occlusal requirements, a complete occlusal adjustment (as described in this chapter) is indicated in the conditions described below.

Evidence of Trauma From Occlusion.   If there is evidence of traumatic occlusion, there is usually a lack of neuromuscular coordination that cannot be corrected unless the occlusion is adjusted completely. Merely taking off a bothersome high spot on one tooth may reorient the patient to another interference which eventually may be as troublesome as the initial one that was removed. Not all cases of trauma from occlusion can be cured by occlusal adjustment since splinting, or even extraction of teeth with far advanced periodontal disease may be indicated. However, occlusal adjustment should be the first consideration for the elimination of trauma from occlusion.

In order to obtain a good result it is conceivable that in many instances it would not be necessary to adjust the retrusive range from centric occlusion to centric relation down to a flat plane provided the forward "slide in centric" could be made even on all of the involved teeth and directed straight forward. No well documented study is available based on this premise. The reason it is recommended that the slide be eliminated and a flat "long centric' created is that this has been documented to be effective in elimination of functional disturbances. Furthermore, the establishment of an even forward slide strictly confined to the midsagittal plane would be more difficult to achieve and less conducive to occlusal stability than the recommended method.

Bruxism.   The importance of occlusal interferences as trigger factors in patients with high muscle tonus is well known. For these patients the premature contacts in centric relation are especially important as triggers to muscle spasms associated with swa lowing. These patients need ideal occlusion in all of the various functional ranges and are the most difficult patients for occlusal adjustment. In most instances it is advisable to use an occlusal splint for mandibular repositioning and muscle relaxation prior to occlusal adjustment.

Dysfunctional Pain. The same remarks apply to patients with dysfunctional temporomandibular joint pain or muscle discomfort. Such patients usually need several adjustments before their true centric relation can be established, unless occlusal splints or other aids are used for proper positioning of the jaws prior to the adjustment.

Advanced Loss of Periodontal Support. Occlusal relations become more and more important with a decrease in the support of the teeth, and occlusal stability is harder to achieve in such patients than in patients with normal periodontal support. It is therefore a rational procedure to establish as ideal an occlusal relation for the teeth as possible in order to avoid trauma from occlusion without splinting of the teeth. In advanced cases of periodontal tissue loss it may be impossible to eliminate traumatic occlusion unless the teeth are splinted.

Extensive Occlusal Reconstruction. The role of occlusal adjustment in oral rehabilitation is discussed in the separate chapters on restorative dentistry and splinting of teeth.

Tooth-apart Swallow. A few patients with abnormal habits of tooth-apart or "infantile" swallow can be helped to assume a normal tooth-together swallow after occlusal adjustment. The most important factor for these patients seems to be elimination of the "slide in centric."

Partial Adjustment

The majority of patients in a dental practice have premature contacts and occlusal interferences without indications for complete occlusal adjustment. There is considerable disagreement in the literature about "prophylactic" occlusal adjustment for such patients,[28] and the prevailing opinion is that nothing should be done to the occlusion unless there are signs or symptoms of traumatic occlusion or neuromuscular disturbances. One of the problems in this controversy is related to definitions of health and disease. If health is defined as the absence of clinically recognizable disease, one may say that an occlusion without recognizable signs or symptoms of trauma is compatible with health. On the other hand, if the definition of health is based on an optimal cellular state as well as on clinical comfort and well-being, the recognition of deviations from health becomes difficult. In this respect the health of the masticatory system would include neuromuscular harmony, of which the more subtle aspects can be evaluated only by electromyography. Muscle sensitivity to occlusal interferences goes far beyond clinically recognizable signs or symptoms.

Metabolic activity and self-cleansing of the teeth also is enhanced by normal function, and it has been shown by Beyron[3] that multidirectional masticatory function, when compared with restricted or unilateral function, has a favorable effect on the prognosis for health of the dentition. It therefore appears logical that multidirectional functional movements should be encouraged, and this is possible by elimination of occlusal interferences which act as obstacles to such function.

When it comes to the more subtle effects of a slide in centric upon clinically unrecognized muscle tension and bruxism, it would be a questionable practice on the basis of current knowledge to adjust the occlusion routinely if there are no obvious neuromuscular, swallowing or periodontal disturbances present. Therefore, it is recommended that gross interferences restricting lateral and protrusive mandibular movements be removed routinely if this can be accomplished without extensive grinding or where such grinding is not detrimental to esthetics. This can usually be accomplished in 5 to 10 minutes, since the only objective is to allow for unrestricted smooth gliding occlusal movements in various directions so physiologic wear can be induced later by normal function. If the patient has adapted well to bilateral restriction of jaw movements by the cuspid teeth, this situation is usually left without any attempt at occlusal adjustment. The "slide in centric" from centric relation to centric occlusion is not altered if there is no horizontal impact in centric occlusion closure and no neuromuscular and/or temporomandibular joint disturbances.

A removal of gross interferences in lateral and protrusive excursion for patients who will benefit functionally in an obvious way from such grinding or partial occlusal adjustment is not directly "prophylactic" against either periodontal disease or traumatic occlusion; but this will enhance the functional comfort of the masticatory system and improve the long term prognosis for the entire masticatory system.

The often expressed fear of creation of "occlusal neurotics" from grinding on teeth is attributable to faulty grinding and a wrong approach in the presentation of occlusal adjustment to the patient. Nobody has proved in a scientifically acceptable manner that any harm has resulted from properly conducted occlusal adjustment according to the principles outlined in this chapter.

If only a partial adjustment is contemplated for improvement of function, the patient should be told in definite terms that this is done to make it easier for him to chew on both sides, that it will not feel completely even at first, that it will take some time for him to get used to it, etc. The patients who are apt to develop "occlusal neurosis" after faulty occlusal adjustment were probably also unconscious bruxers before the adjustment. Patients with bruxism should have either the very best occlusal adjustment, or no adjustment unless a competent adjustment is available.

One last bit of advice concerning occlusal adjustment is to be conservative regarding tooth substance. When in doubt about how much tooth substance to remove, be on the cautious side.

Demonstration Case

The following pictorial series (Figs. 13–21 to 13–32) is the account of an actual occlusal adjustment of a patient with chronic temporomandibular joint

(*Text continued on page 311.*)

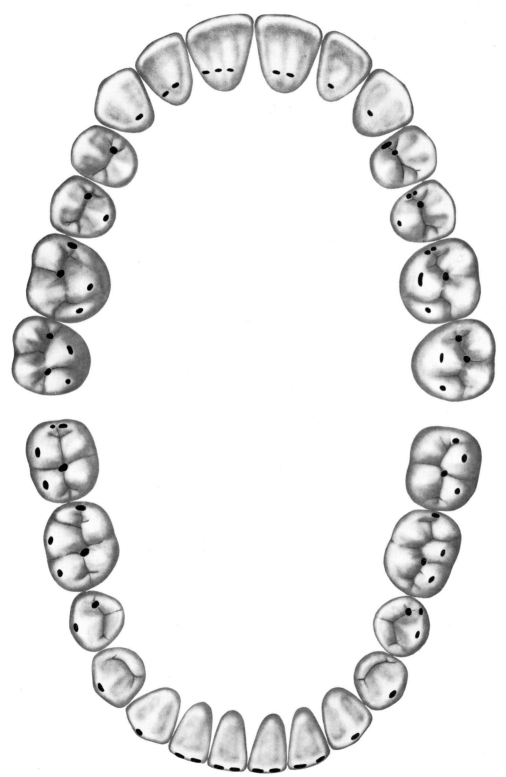

Figure 13–21.   Occlusal and incisal stops in centric occlusion. The centric stops are indicated by the black areas.

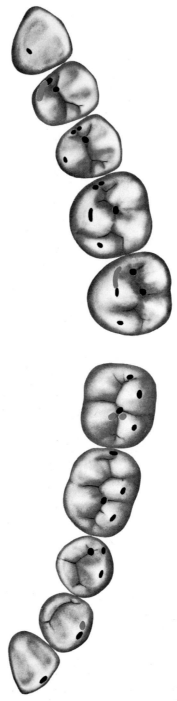

Figure 13–22. Premature contacts in centric relation are indicated by the red areas.

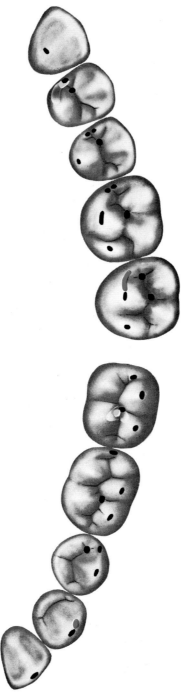

Figure 13–23. Removal of premature contacts illustrated in Figure 13–22 is accomplished by grinding according to principles previously outlined whereby centric stops and supporting cusps are maintained. Thus, grinding is done on the mesiolingual line angle of the maxillary first premolar and on the distal inclines of the transverse ridges of the mesial, lingual and buccal cusps of the mandibular second molar.

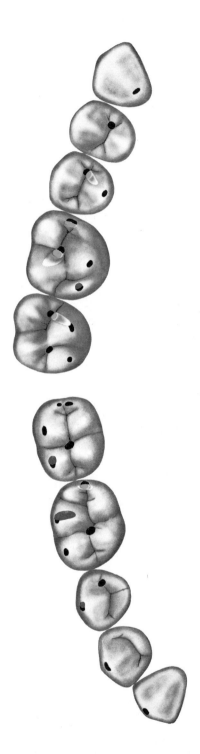

Figure 13–24. Removal of premature contacts on the right side of the arches is illustrated. Green areas represent occlusal stops in centric relation. The green areas, as well as areas distal to them in the maxilla indicate areas which have been ground to eliminate premature contacts and to provide seats for supporting cusps that are at the same level as stops (black areas) in centric occlusion. Areas which have been ground are: the mesial incline of the buccal aspect of the mesiolingual cusp of the maxillary second molar; the mesiolingual aspect of the distal buccal cusp and oblique ridge of the maxillary first molar; the mesial aspect of the transverse ridge of the lingual cusp of the maxillary second premolar; and the distal marginal ridge of the mandibular first molar.

Figure 13–25. Correction of premature contacts causing a lateral slide in centric. *A,* Premature contacts are indicated by red areas on the buccal cusps of the mandibular second molar and on the lingual aspect of the inclines and ridges of the mesial and distal cusps of the maxillary second molar. *B,* Green areas on maxillary second molar indicate new seats for buccal cusps of mandibular second molar. Grinding has been extended distally and buccally from these seats on the maxillary second molar to provide for curvature of the buccal cusps of the mandibular molar. Centric stops (black areas) have been maintained and new seats (green areas) for supporting cusps in centric relation are on the same level as the stops in centric occlusion.

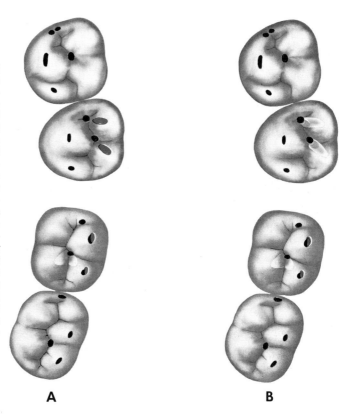

A   B

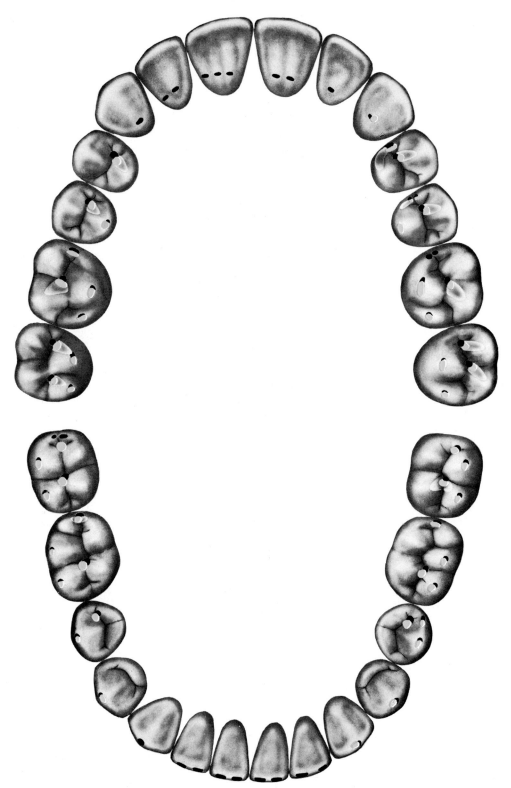

Figure 13--26. Completion of occlusal adjustment in centric. Green areas indicate stops in centric relation and black areas indicate stops in centric occlusion. The anterior and lateral slide has been eliminated and the horizontal contact area between centric relation and centric occlusion allows for a "long centric."

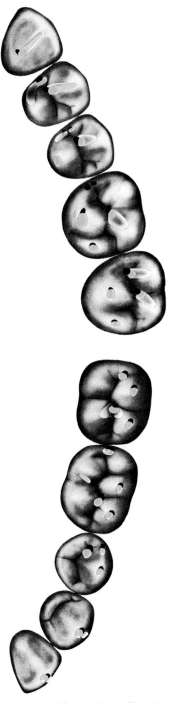

Figure 13–27. Correction for working side relations. The blue areas indicate contacts in lateral excursion. In accordance with the B.U.L.L. rule, grinding is done on the buccal cusp of the maxillary first premolar and the lingual cusp of the mandibular molar. In order to maintain centric stops and working relation contact, grinding is done on the maxillary rather than mandibular cuspid.

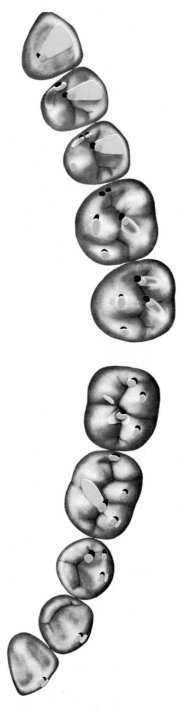

Figure 13–28. After additional grinding, occlusal interferences are removed and greater functional contact is obtained in working relation. Grinding is done on the lingual aspects of the maxillary cuspid, and buccal cusps of the first and second premolars, mesiobuccal cusp of the maxillary first and second molars, and on the incisal ridges of the maxillary incisors and lingual cusps of mandibular molars. See text for principles governing amount of grinding to be done in working relation.

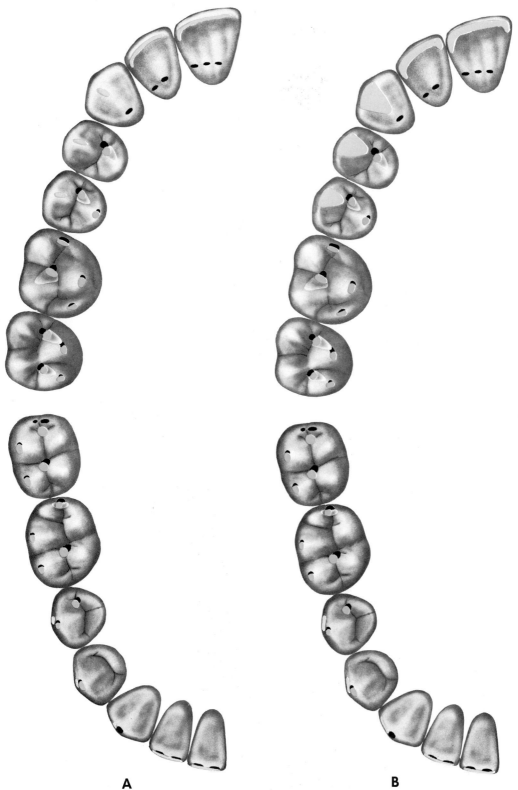

Figure 13–29. Correction for working side opposite to that shown in Figures 13–27 and 28. *A,* Blue areas indicate working side contact prior to grinding. Grinding is limited to the areas of blue on the maxillary teeth. *B,* After additional grinding, the area of functional contact in working relation is increased and occlusal interferences are removed; however, balancing interferences as indicated in Figure 13–30 prevent unrestricted gliding movements.

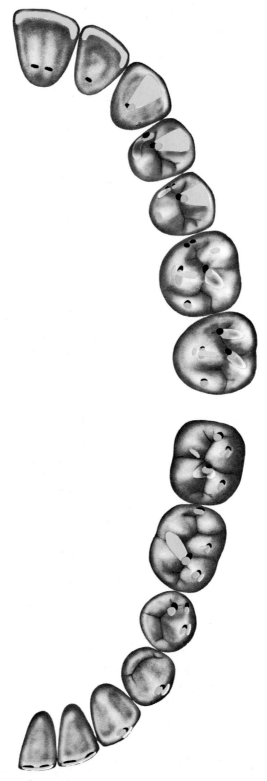

Figure 13–30. Correction of balancing side interferences. Yellow areas on lingual cusps of the maxillary molars indicate balancing interferences to be ground.

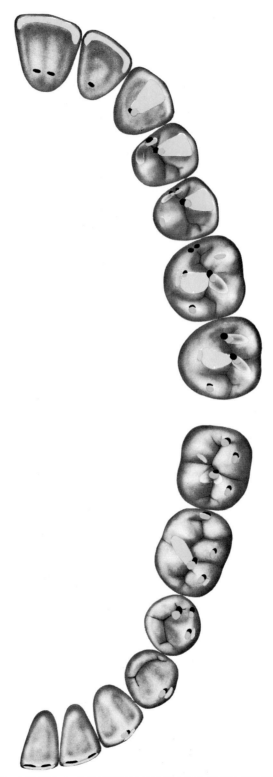

Figure 13–31. After grinding as indicated by yellow areas on the maxillary molars only very light contact (or no contact) should be present on the balancing side. As ba ancing side interferences are removed, greater functional contact on the working side may be anticipated, as indicated in Figure 13–32. Note that some of the stops on the lingual cusp of the maxillary first molar and all of the centric stop on the lingual cusp of the maxillary second molar had to be removed.

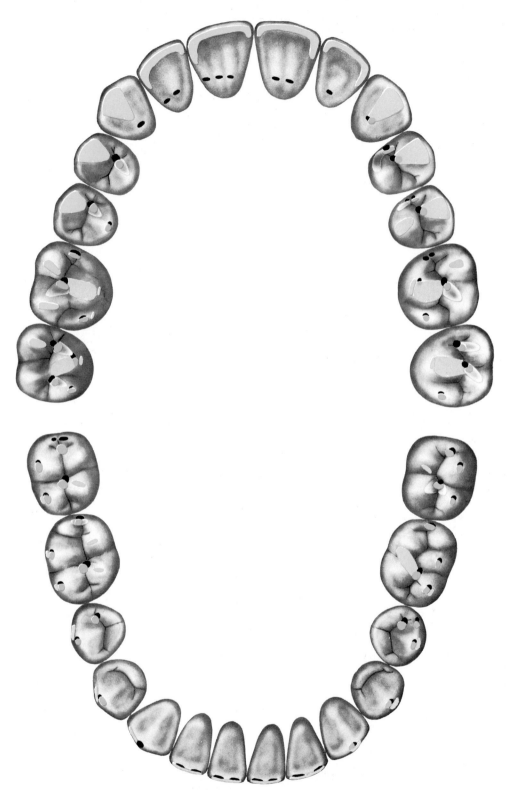

Figure 13–32. After completion of the grinding. Black areas indicate stops in centric occlusion; green areas, stops in centric relation; blue areas, contacts in working relations; and yellow areas, where balancing interferences have been removed. With additional grinding in working relation, working contact has been established on the mesial buccal cusp of the maxillary second molar (patient's right side). Note also that it was necessary to remove the centric stop on the maxillary second premolar (patient's left side) to remove a balancing interference.

arthritis and muscle pain. The patient had premature contacts in centric relation leading to a forward, as well as a lateral, "slide in centric." Although the artist's rendition of the dentition is relatively normal, the subject's occlusion was not, insofar as the occlusal relations were concerned. This aspect can be seen readily in the figure representing occlusal stops in centric occlusion (Fig. 13–21). For a comparison with what is considered to be most representative of the positions of occlusal stops in centric occlusion, refer to Figure 4–1 in Chapter 4, Physiology of Occlusion.

REFERENCES

1. Ackermann, F.: Équilibre-Déséquilibre, Les équilibrations occluso-articulées Meulages fonctionnels. Schweiz. Mschr. Zahnk., 62:49, 1952.
2. Adams, S. H., and Zander, H. A.: Functional tooth contacts in lateral and in centric occlusion. J. Am. Dent. A., 69:465, 1964.
3. Beyron, H. L.: Characteristics of functionally optimal occlusion and principles of occlusal rehabilitation. J. Am. Dent. A., 48:648, 1954.
4. Blass, J. L.: Controlled use of an abrasive in occlusal surface adjustment. J. Am. Dent. A., 29: 259, 1942.
5. Blass, J. L.: Occlusal equilibration in periodontal treatment. New York Dent. J., 22:121, 1956.
6. Bonwill, W. G. A.: The geometrical and mechanical laws of the articulation of the human teeth. The anatomical articulator. In Litch, W. F.: The American System of Dentistry. Vol. 2. Philadelphia, Lea Brothers, 1887, pp. 486–498.
7. Brown, S. W.: Disharmony between centric relation and centric occlusion as a factor in producing improper tooth wear and trauma. Dent. Digest, 52:434, 1946.
8. Cerveris, A. R.: Vibracentric equilibration of centric occlusion. J. Am. Dent. A., 63:476, 1961.
9. Cripps, S.: Occlusal equilibration of the natural dentition. Brit. Dent. J., 88:90, 1950.
10. D'Amico, A.: Canine teeth—normal functional relation of the natural teeth of man. South. Calif. Dent. A. J., 26:6; 49; 127; 175; 194; 239; 1958.
11. Emslie, R. D.: Malocclusion and periodontal health. A periodontologist's viewpoint. Europ. Orth. Soc., 254:265, 1954.
12. Engelberger, A., et al.: Diagnostik und Therapie der funktionellen Störungen im Kausystem. Schweiz. Mschr. Zahnk., 70:586, 1960.
13. Graf, H., and Zander, H. A.: Tooth contact patterns in mastication. J. Prosth. Dent., 13:1055, 1963.
14. Gysi, A.: Der Wert der seitlichen Kaubewegungen. Schw. Vtjschr. Zahnh., 29:1, 33, 1919.
15. Gysi, A.: Masticating efficiency in natural and artificial teeth. Dent. Digest, 21:1; 69; 139; 207; 275; 431; 694; 1915.
16. Hughes, H. J.: The terminal hinge-axis of the mandible. Typed thesis, University of Michigan, 1963.
17. Jankelson, B.: A technique for obtaining optimum functional relationship for the natural dentition. Dent. Clin. North America, 131, 1960.
18. Karolyi, M.: Beobachtungen über Pyorrhea Alveolaris und Caries dentium. Oesterr.-ungar. Vtjschr. Zahnh., 18:520, 1902.
19. Lauritzen, A. G.: Function, prime object of restorative dentistry; a definite procedure to obtain it. J. Am. Dent. A., 42:523, 1951.
20. Lindblom, G.: The significance of "bite analysis" in modern dentistry. Dent. Rec., 68:254, 1948.
21. Madsen, B. C.: Occlusion: A cardinal consideration. J. Am. Dent. A., 41:691, 1950.
22. Mann, A. W., and Pankey, L. D.: Oral rehabilitation utilizing the Pankey-Mann instrument and functional bite technique. Dent. Clin. North America, 215, March, 1959.
23. Maunsbach, O., and Posselt, U.: Bettslipning som funktionskorrigerande hjälpmedel. Odont. Rev., 6:163, 1955.

24. McLean, D. W.: Diagnosis and correction of pathologic occlusion. J. Am. Dent. A., *29*:1202, 1942.
25. Ramfjord, S. P.: Bruxism, a clinical and electromyographic study. J. Am. Dent. A., *62*:21, 1961.
26. Ramfjord, S. P.: Dysfunctional temporomandibular joint and muscle pain. J. Prosth. Dent., *11*:353, 1961.
27. Reeves, R. L.: Occlusal traumatism—Its pathological effects and diagnosis. J. Am. Dent. A., *59*:439, 1959.
28. Schireson, S.: Grinding teeth for masticatory efficiency and gingival health. J. Prosth. Dent., *13*:337, 1963.
29. Schreiber, H. R.: Occlusal equilibration in abnormal occlusions. J. Periodont., *27*:47, 1956.
30. Schuyler, C. H.: Correction of occlusal disharmony of the natural dentition. New York Dent. J., *13*:445, 1947.
31. Schuyler, C. H.: Fundamental principles in the correction of occlusal disharmony, natural and artificial. J. Am. Dent. A., *22*:1193, 1935.
32. Schuyler, C. H.: Freedom in centric. Dent. Clin. N. Am., *13*:681, 1969.
33. Shore, N. A.: Equilibration of the occlusion of natural dentition. J. Am. Dent. A., *44*:414, 1952.
34. Simring, M.: Occlusal equilibration of the dentition. J. Am. Dent. A., *56*:643, 1958.
35. Sorrin, S.: Traumatic occlusion. Its detection and correction. Dent. Digest, *40*:170; 202; 1934.
36. Sorrin, S.: Traumatic occlusion and occlusal equilibration. J. Am. Dent. A., *57*:477, 1958.
37. Stillman, P. R.: Traumatic occlusion. Nat. Dent. A. J., *6*:691, 1919.
38. Thomas, B. O. A., and Gallagher, J. W.: Practical management of occlusal dysfunctions in periodontal therapy. J. Am. Dent. A., *46*:18, 1953.
39. Troest, T.: Diagnosing minute deflective occlusal contacts. J. Prosth. Dent., *14*:71, 1964.
40. Vale, D. F.: Occlusal stability following occlusal adjustment. A stereophotogrammetric study. Typed thesis, University of Michigan, 1970.
41. Weinberg, L. A.: Diagnosis of facets in occlusal equilibration. J. Am. Dent. A., *52*:26, 1956.
42. Westbrook, J. C., Jr.: A pattern of centric occlusion. J. Am. Dent. A., *39*:407, 1949.
43. Wick, A. E.: Treatment of functional occlusal disharmonies. J. Am. Dent. A., *58*:16, 1959.
44. Williams, C. H. M.: Correction of abnormalities of occlusion. J. Am. Dent. A., *44*:748, 1952.
45. Winslow, M. B.: The preventitive role of occlusal balancing of the natural dentition. J. Am. Dent. A., *48*:293, 1954.
46. Zander, H. A., and Hürzeler, B.: Diagnosis of occlusal disharmonies. South. Calif. Dent. A. J., *26*:392, 1958.

Films

1. "Occlusal Adjustment, Part I—Centric"
2. "Occlusal Adjustment, Part II—Lateral and Protrusive Excursions"

May be loaned through:
V. A. Central Office Film Library
810 Vermont Avenue, N.W.
Washington, D.C. 20420

Film Library
American Dental Association
211 East Chicago Avenue
Chicago, Ill. 60611

CHAPTER 14

MINOR ORTHODONTIC THERAPY

Orthodontic procedures may constitute an important and often indispensable part of any correction of occlusal disharmony. Although comprehensive orthodontic therapy requires a very high degree of special training and skill, there are certain simple and predictable procedures that in selected cases may enhance physiologic stress distribution, functional effectiveness, and esthetics. Such procedures may be carried out by well informed practitioners of general dentistry.

What may appear to involve only "minor tooth movements" is often misjudged and proves to be a complex problem. Therefore, some basic principles of orthodontic therapy have to be outlined before appliances and techniques for specific orthodontic purposes are discussed.

FORCE DISTRIBUTION AND IMPACT

The diagnostic acumen that is necessary for selection of patients for minor orthodontic therapy, for referral to specialists, and for palliation or other forms of therapy should rest upon an understanding of the biomechanics of occlusion. Orthodontic forces usually are applied to the crowns of the teeth. The impact of these forces, however, may be directed toward any part of the periodontium through tipping, bodily horizontal movements, vertical movements and rotation of the teeth. In comprehensive orthodontic therapy all these movements are often included in the management of a single patient, while minor orthodontic therapy is chiefly concerned with tipping of teeth and rather simple patterns of force distribution. An unavoidable part of all orthodontic stress distribution is concerned with reciprocal forces or "anchorage," which poses the greatest problem in dentitions disturbed by loss of teeth or periodontal disease.

Teeth may be moved by immediate forces, by intermittent forces, and by continuously acting forces. Regardless of type of force, the impact has to alter the metabolism of the periodontium to the extent that resorption and new formation of bone are induced. The reaction of the periodontal tissues to various types, magnitudes, and frequencies of orthodontic forces has been well described in the orthodontic literature.[4, 5, 9]

Immediate and intermittent forces are tolerated to various degrees without initiating movement of teeth since such forces are normal expressions of masticatory and swallowing function. In patients with bruxism or compensatory hyperplasia of the periodontium as a result of usually heavy function, the periodontal tissues can withstand heavy immediate or intermittent forces without any resultant tooth movement; however, teeth in nonfunction can be moved with much less force. The main part of occlusal stress is transmitted to the alveolar bone as pull or tension when the periodontal membrane consists of heavy collagen fibers; however, compression and resorption inducing pressure on the alveolar bone occur much more readily in the absence of such well developed fibers. Tooth mobility studies have demonstrated a rebound in tooth position from a temporary movement by an intermittent force (probably on a hydrodynamic basis), which explains the normal tolerance to such forces.[7]

Continuously acting forces are not involved in the physiology of mastication and there is no direct compensatory mechanism in the periodontium against such forces. This may explain the common experience that teeth can be moved by continuous forces of much smaller magnitude than is required to move teeth by immediate or intermittent forces. It is also a well known principle of bone physiology that it requires very little continuous pressure to initiate bone resorption.

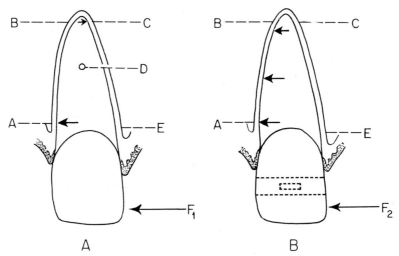

Figure 14–1. *A, Tipping force* (F_1). The impact of the force is concentrated at (A) and (C). Since the center of rotation is at (D), bone resorption at (A) and (C) allows the crown of the tooth to tip rapidly in the desired direction. There is tension (pull) on small areas at (B) and (E). *B, Bodily movement force* (F_2). In this type of movement the impact of force (pressure) involves total alveolar wall from (A) to (B). The restricting pull (tension) involves the area from (C) to (E). Bodily tooth movements require more total force and will be at a slower rate than tipping movements.

The distribution of impact of orthodontic force varies from the concentrated impact of a tipping force (Fig. 14–1, *A*) to the widely dispensed impact of an intrusive force or a force directed toward bodily movement (Fig. 14–1, *B*). It is, therefore, evident that much greater total forces are required to intrude or move teeth bodily in a horizontal direction than are required for tipping teeth. Rotation also has a widespread impact and requires considerable force. The least force is needed for extrusion of teeth, since this type of force corresponds to a natural movement and does not involve any bone resorption unless there is a bend in the root or the tooth has multiple roots. Root length and shape are also important factors for stress distribution, and these factors may be altered by loss of periodontal support associated with periodontal disease or root resorption.

Alteration of the periodontal tissues by inflammation and trauma also may alter the biomechanics of orthodontic movement of teeth. Whether an alteration of polymerization of the ground substance of the periodontal tissues of systemic origin has any practical significance for orthodontic movement of teeth is not known.

HAZARDS OF ORTHODONTIC THERAPY

The impact of the orthodontic forces should be sufficient to induce resorption of alveolar bone, and at the same time remain well below the pressure level that interferes with the normal activity of the cementoblasts on the surface of the root. A considerable range in tolerance to pressure between the bone and the cementum is the necessary basis for orthodontic treatment. Resorption of the cementum is usually the result of a heavy crushing force whereby there is necrosis of the periodontal membrane, including the cementoblasts.[6] The necrotic tissues are removed by the surrounding vital tissues, and as part of this removal process there is resorption both of alveolar bone and cementum. If the resorption involves only a small part of the root surface and represents the result of a transient trauma, the repair usually is complete with no residual gross defect. Microscopic areas of cemental resorption and repair are a common result of incidental traumas.[3] However, if a severe trauma affects a large area of the root and is repeated or continuous, the injuries may result in root resorption of clinical significance. Root resorption of the apical areas of teeth associated with intrusion attempts or movement of the apical areas of teeth is not uncommon when continuous heavy forces are applied. Resorption of the roots may also occur from very heavy immediate or intermittent forces such as extensive bruxism. Roentgenologic evidence of root resorption unquestionably indicates that the physiologic tolerance level for occlusal forces has been exceeded and that the orthodontic forces have to be reduced drastically.

The chances for resorption are very small if removable appliances with controlled restrictions on movement are used. If the patient's own biting force is utilized as an orthodontic force, one will very seldom find that the patient's neuromuscular mechanism will induce periodontal injury of the severity required for root resorption.

Dehiscence of the alveolar process and gingival recession may also develop from moving teeth too far out on the alveolar process. This result should be carefully avoided since it permanently reduces the periodontal support for such teeth and often leads to exposure of the root surfaces. Misguided attempts at correction of extensive crossbites to normal occlusion when the maxilla distinctly is too small in relation to the mandible often will result in dehiscence on the buccal side of the maxilla and the lingual side of the mandible. Expansion of the dental arches may be accompanied by buccal bone formation when several teeth are moved slowly and simultaneously, but movement of a single tooth out of the arch will usually take the tooth through the labial plate of bone. The apical base of the teeth also has to be considered so the teeth are not moved off the basal bone support and left at an unfavorable angle from a functional standpoint.

Formation of periodontal pockets is the third main hazard of orthodontic therapy. A periodontal pocket will not develop from orthodontic therapy if the gingival tissues are healthy. But in the presence of gingival inflammation or periodontal pockets, especially of the intrabony type, there is a definite danger of deepening the pockets and inducing periodontal abscesses. Such changes result from the combined effect of local irritation and disturbance of tissue metabolism induced by orthodontic trauma. Consequently, orthodontic movement of teeth should be delayed till all gingival and periodontal inflammation has subsided following elimination of local irritants. Gingival health should be carefully maintained during the entire period of orthodontic treatment.

ELIMINATION OF CAUSES OF MALOCCLUSION

It may be possible by mechanical means to move teeth into a desired position without a clear understanding of some of the important causes of the malocclusion being treated. However, because of the dynamics of occlusion, relapse will invariably result unless the cause of the malocclusion has been eliminated. All causes of malocclusion should, if possible, be eliminated prior to the orthodontic therapy, otherwise the causative factors will act against the therapeutic devices, induce complications and delay the desired result.

For the purpose of delineating minor orthodontic therapy the causes of malocclusion may be divided into two principal groups: (1) genetic and developmental factors influencing cell development and growth that tend to influence the entire occlusion and which in most instances require comprehensive orthodontics beyond the realm of the nonspecialist; and (2) external or environmental factors. It is from this second group that some types of malocclusion may be corrected effectively by minor orthodontic therapy.

Every tooth maintains its position in the dental arch as a result of balance in the various forces acting on the tooth (occlusal forces, lip, cheek and tongue forces, forces from inflammation or other tissue changes in the periodontium, and the eruptive tendency of all teeth). Since malocclusion resulting from locally disturbed dynamics of occlusion is the type of malocclusion that may lend itself the best to minor orthodontics, some of the common etiologic factors will be discussed.

A disturbed or altered eruption pattern of the teeth and loss of teeth without replacements or position maintaining appliances are very common causes of malocclusion. The sequelae may be grave and complex, but at times, for example, resultant tipping of teeth may be easy to treat.

Faulty dental therapy is another common cause of dysfunctional malpositioning of teeth. This factor has been discussed under the etiology of trauma from occlusion (p. 139).

A number of various occlusal habits may induce malpositions of teeth (bruxism, biting on objects brought into the mouth, tongue, lip and cheek biting, sucking habits, etc.). All these habits will, unless recognized and eliminated, bring a relapse after orthodontic treatment.

Periodontal disease both of the proliferative hyperplastic type and the destructive type will often lead to malpositioning or migration of teeth. Drifting of teeth is very common in patients with advanced periodontal disease.

In general, it is important to find out whether malposed teeth were once in a normal position. If this is the case, it means that the displacement has been the result of disturbed dynamics of occlusion rather than a basic malocclusion. It also means that treatment will be confined to correction of the disturbances of occlusal relationships rather than comprehensive orthodontic therapy.

PROBLEMS IN ORTHODONTIC TREATMENT

There are several problems that have to be considered in minor orthodontic therapy. Included are problems of space, occlusal function, periodontal disease, age of the patient and retention. The effect of these problems should be thoroughly evaluated prior to orthodontic treatment.

Lack of Space

A lack of available space into which a tooth can be moved may often change what first appeared to be a minor tooth movement into major comprehensive orthodontic therapy. A realistic evaluation of space problems is best accomplished on casts and will often require accurate measuring and trial placement of the crowns of the teeth which have been cut away from the casts. The main consideration is always the relationship between tooth size and arch size and whether space can be made for the tooth within the ridges of the jaws, since any alteration of ridge relations is beyond minor orthodontic therapy.

It often has been recommended that the crowns of teeth be stripped interproximally up to 0.25 mm. on each proximal side to gain some space. Even if this removal of tooth substance may be acceptable esthetically and functionally, it may be undesirable from a periodontal standpoint. Interproximal stripping will alter the contact areas and infringe upon the normal space for the inter-proximal papilla, with subsequent interference with self-cleansing of the interproximal gingival crevices. Interference occurs because the buccal and lingual portions of the interproximal papilla will become hyperplastic and the interproximal col deeper than normal because of the more apical position of the contact as a result of the stripping. If there has been a loss of interproximal tissues and the gingival margin is located more apically than normal, it may be fully permissible, and from every standpoint desirable, to bring the teeth closer together by interproximal stripping, providing that sufficient space is left for interproximal oral hygiene.

Anchorage

Any force applied for orthodontic purposes will by necessity evoke an equal reciprocal force. In order to accomplish controlled movement of teeth the reciprocal forces have to be anchored or distributed in such a way that the activated appliances move the teeth into the desired position without disturb-ing the occlusal relationship of the teeth that are used for anchorage. The effects of the activated forces always have to be weighed against the possible reciprocal action upon the anchorage.

Anchorage can be intraoral or extraoral. For minor orthodontic therapy in-traoral anchorage may be intra- or intermaxillary. Both teeth and alveolar proc-

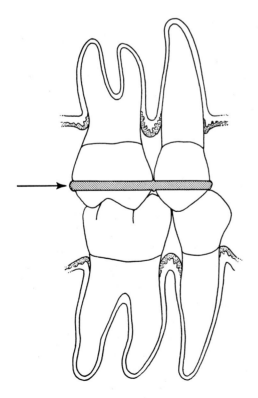

Figure 14–2. Splinting with temporary fixed wire and acrylic assures that forces, for example in the direction of the arrow, will be distributed over all periodontal tissues. Without splinting there would be a long leverage arm and a concentrated impact of tip-ping forces associated with the loss of supporting structures. Note also stability from cuspal interdigita-tion with opposing arch.

esses may serve as anchorage. Since it requires much less force to tip teeth than to move them bodily (the periodontal support being equal), an attempt should always be made to anchor appliances in such a way that the reciprocal forces are supplied as much as possible with a bodily nontipping impact upon the anchor teeth. For teeth that have lost a considerable amount of periodontal support, this may necessitate temporary splinting if removable orthodontic appliances are to be used (Fig. 14–2). Occlusal relationships with the teeth in the opposing arch are also important considerations in relation to anchorage for removable appliances. One may also move one tooth at a time or use a headgear appliance for anchorage.[1]

The alveolar processes are moderately useful for anchorage if the teeth to be moved have minimal bone support and the movement of the teeth will extend over a short period of time.

Occlusal Function

Since occlusal forces determine tooth position to a great extent, it is evident that functional occlusal forces will influence orthodontic tooth movements and maintenance of the desired tooth position after orthodontic therapy. Functional occlusal forces are especially important when removable appliances and intermittent forces are used. It is not advisable to move a tooth against a functional occlusal force with removable appliances unless the action of these forces has been eliminated by a temporary raising of the bite. Therefore, when removable appliances are used for treatment of crossbites or shearing occlusion, provision has to be made for sufficient bite-raising to let the cusps or incisal edges in the crossbite or shearing occlusion pass without being hampered by functional occlusal contacts. The bite-raising device has to be used constantly until the functional occlusal forces start to act in the direction of the desired tooth movement. With fixed orthodontic appliances teeth can be moved against functional occlusal forces, but this may be disturbing to masticatory function and the temporomandibular joint.

Periodontal Disease

Loss of supporting tissues as a result of periodontal disease, especially in young patients, proves that the response to local irritation is not optimal. It is, therefore, extremely important that the orthodontic treatment for such persons be planned and executed in such a way that gingival irritation from appliances will be minimized. In patients with a tendency to periodontal disease, the requirement for good oral hygiene is essential in order to avoid periodontal pocket formation during the orthodontic therapy.

The impact of a given orthodontic force will increase with decrease in support for the teeth. Standard orthodontic appliances may be too vigorous in their action on teeth that have lost considerable support from periodontal disease, and this is especially true for tipping forces caused by increased length of the leverage above the alveolar crest and the concentrated impact of these forces. The loss of periodontal support should be equated with the various dimensions of orthodontic wires and ligatures. Thus, when tissue resistance has been lowered by periodontal disease, orthodontic forces should be reduced and carefully controlled.

Clinical experience has shown that extensive orthodontic movement of teeth can be performed safely in patients with advanced periodontal disease provided precautions are taken with regard to the avoidance of gingival irritation and control of forces.

Extruded teeth or teeth with severe periodontal bone loss may be intruded orthodontically, making suprabony pockets into intrabony pockets and thus facilitate reattachment therapy.

Age of Patients

Age is not by any means as important a factor in movement of teeth as was previously assumed. The periodontal tissues maintain their ability for adaptive changes throughout life. For example, in our autopsy material from a 93 year old patient there is clear histologic evidence of active reorganization of the periodontal structures. Also there is ample histologic evidence of rebuilding of periodontal structures and adjacent supporting bone following change in occlusal function in a patient 69 years old.[8] Clinically, teeth have been moved successfully in patients up to 70 years of age. However, when it comes to comprehensive orthodontics with major changes in occlusal relationships, especially with regard to vertical dimension, youth is a great advantage since one may then guide growth besides moving teeth. The periodontal structures with the collagenous periodontal membrane can also be influenced and altered much easier before the collagenous fibers have matured and a stable functional occlusal pattern has been established.

Retention

The first requirement for retention of teeth after orthodontic movement is elimination of the factors that initially caused the malposition of the teeth. If these factors cannot be recognized and eliminated, relapses will follow the orthodontic therapy unless the teeth are held in position by occlusal splints. Some habits such as tongue, lip and cheek biting are extremely difficult to eliminate, especially in adults in whom the habit pattern may have been established over many years. These habits often have a strong psychic background and act as outlets for emotional tension. In such cases, it may be practically impossible to break the habit, and devices for permanent retention are needed. In many instances, when orthodontic closure of anterior maxillary diastemas associated with habits in itself would be a very simple procedure, it is better for the patient not to initiate any treatment unless the treatment includes fixed splinting of the teeth. Moving the teeth with a Hawley appliance and then allowing the tongue to move the teeth labially establishes a perpetual traumatic occlusion which is a greater hazard for the periodontal tissues than the stable open bite the patient had before the treatment.

It is of essential importance for retention of the teeth in the desired position that orthodontic therapy be followed by occlusal adjustment or other forms of occlusal therapy needed to stabilize the position of the teeth through harmonious well balanced occlusal forces. The less remaining support the teeth have, the greater is their tendency to move from slight changes in occlusal impact; therefore, it becomes increasingly difficult to stabilize teeth with the advancement of periodontal destruction without resorting to splinting.

Movement of teeth may alter the direction of the functional occlusal impacts and thereby jeopardize retention. In a maxillary incisor with a well developed cingulum, a fairly large component of the biting force is directed toward the long axis of the tooth (Fig. 14–3, *A*). When a maxillary incisor has been moved labially in the presence of periodontal disease, the incisor tends to extrude also. If this tooth is moved orthodontically in a palatal direction, the centric stop will be apically to the cingulum (Fig. 14–3, *B*). In such instances, the biting force in centric and lateral excursions will have a very strong labial component and will tend to move the maxillary incisor labially again. This movement should be anticipated and a solution included in the original treatment plan.

Sufficient time for reorganization of the collagenous periodontal membrane after the active treatment is even more important for adults than for children since the collagen fibers of the periodontal membrane in adults are very stable

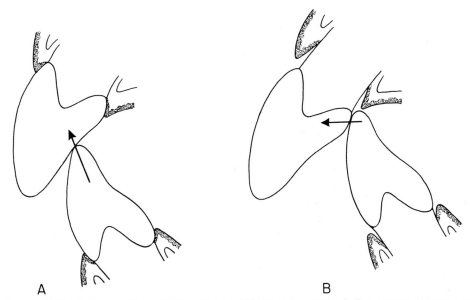

A   B

Figure 14–3. Before periodontal disease and drifting of the teeth, *A*, The impact of forces are directed more axially than shown in *B*, Where the impact of centric closure force has become labially directed.

structures. If orthodontic movement has been accomplished within the physiologic tolerance level of the periodontal membrane, the adaptive changes will have taken place on the surface of the alveolar bone, but it takes a long time to reform mature collagen fibers to correspond in orientation to the functional demand on the tooth in its new position. This problem is greatest following rotation[11] of a single-rooted tooth or when the tooth is maintained in nonfunction. It is important that the tooth be exposed to functional forces during the retention period since such forces provide the stimulus for reorganization of the periodontium of a tooth in its new position. If a tooth is held in a nonfunctioning position with orthodontic bands, reorganization of the periodontium of the tooth will be slow and inadequate. In the young patient with growing teeth, reorganization of the periodontal fibers takes but a short time, but in an adult it is advisable to plan to use a retainer for 1 to 2 years and to maintain close control of the functional relations.

Following correction of crossbite or faulty intercuspidation of teeth, normal occlusal relations are maintained by function, and retention poses no problem.

SELECTION OF PATIENTS FOR MINOR ORTHODONTIC THERAPY

Before any consideration is given to the selection of appliances or methods, it has to be decided whether the malocclusion can be corrected by minor orthodontic procedures, or requires comprehensive orthodontic treatment with referral to a specialist. In many instances of malocclusion in adults, reconstructive procedures are to be preferred to any type of orthodontic treatment. A comprehensive examination, analysis and diagnosis is of basic importance before a decision can be reached with regard to the best treatment for the patient. Knowledge of various types of intricate orthodontic techniques is of much less importance than a thorough understanding of the nature of various types of malocclusion, both with regards to etiology and functional or dysfunctional character. Only a few principles basic to selection of patients for minor orthodontics will be included in this brief discussion.

To attempt to change an adult patient's occlusal vertical dimension or centric by orthodontic therapy is hazardous for the best orthodontist and should be avoided by the nonspecialist. The occlusal vertical dimension of adults is the result of years of adaptation and natural adjustment to the various forces acting upon the teeth. It should be realized that 10 mm. of interocclusal space may be as "normal" for one individual as 1 mm. for another. Attempts to change the relationship between jaws and muscles of an individual to suit an average norm is to invite failure. Intrusion of anterior teeth combined with extrusion of molars and bicuspids is very seldom a satisfactory treatment of a deep overbite in adults since this orthodontic result has to be maintained by appliances that usually perpetuate chronic traumatic occlusion.

Orthodontic therapy that necessitates bodily movement of teeth and controlled movements of the apical base of teeth requires considerable orthodontic experience and technical skill, which are usually found only among specialists trained in orthodontics. Such comprehensive cases are not suitable for minor orthodontic procedures by general practitioners of dentistry.

Rotation, at least of single-rooted teeth, is not necessarily too technically difficult, but retention problems often make the orthodontic treatment impractical since splinting is commonly needed for retention. The problem of malposition may often be solved in a more simple way by a jacket crown on the rotated tooth.

Orthodontic intrusion and extrusion of teeth should be attempted by the nonspecialist only in selected cases of single-rooted teeth.

If one considers the preceding principles, the main field of minor orthodontic therapy for adults is narrowed down to tipping of teeth. If tipping of teeth is done after the gingival inflammation has subsided and precautions are taken for proper control of the forces, this type of treatment can be carried out successfully and without undue risk to the patient by a well informed general practitioner of dentistry. Both the functional and esthetic results of restorative procedures can often be greatly enhanced by simple tipping of teeth.

As a general approach for the selection of patients it is important to know whether the malocclusion has always been present or has been acquired as a result of some reversible dental factors or procedures. The latter type of malocclusion is much easier to treat than the former.

FIXED OR REMOVABLE APPLIANCES

The main advantage of fixed orthodontic appliances is that they provide full control over movement of the entire tooth. They allow good anchorage for reciprocal forces, and teeth can be moved against functional occlusal forces without undue trauma from the occlusion. The disadvantages are related to esthetics, gingival irritation and complexity in technique and management.

Removable appliances are esthetically more acceptable than fixed appliances, especially for adult patients. They are less irritating to the gingival tissues and allow for better oral hygiene than is possible with banded techniques. However, removable appliances do not allow for adequate control of bodily movement of teeth, and their use is restricted mainly to tipping movements of the teeth. Removable appliances may, in selected cases, be used for intrusion, extrusion and rotation of teeth, but they are not so effective as fixed appliances.

Removable appliances may also be used for comprehensive orthodontic treatment, but for the purpose of this book the discussion of their use will be restricted to orthodontic correction of minor occlusal disturbances.

The safe use of most fixed orthodontic appliances requires training and experience beyond what can be included in a brief chapter of this type so no attempts will be made to cover their use in minor orthodontic therapy.

MOVEMENTS OF TEETH

Lingual Movement of Anterior Teeth

The commonly used appliance for tipping of anterior teeth in a lingual direction is the Hawley appliance (Fig. 14–4).[2] Although this appliance is well known, it is often abused, and seldom used to its full advantage.

Anchorage is the first important consideration in the construction of a Hawley appliance. All of the posterior teeth should be used for anchorage and a wire clasp (0.030 inch wire) for retention should be placed distally on the last molar on each side of the arch. The acrylic should fit as snugly as possible into all the lingual interproximal spaces and extend at least to the middle half of the clinical crown. This is done in an attempt to achieve an anchoring effect simulating the bodily anchorage that can be obtained with orthodontic bands. An anchoring effect from a clasp that transmits a tipping force is not by any means so effective as an anchor where the forces are spread over the entire periodontal membrane and require bodily movement forces in order to move the anchor teeth.

If the posterior teeth have poor periodontal support, it may even be advisable to splint these teeth with a wire and acrylic combination splint before the Hawley appliance is inserted in order to secure adequate anchorage for active movement of anterior teeth. If some of the posterior teeth have been lost, it is extremely important that the Hawley appliance fit well into all the spaces of the missing teeth and fill a good part of these spaces to get a stable anchoring effect.

Special care has to be taken when all the posterior teeth are present on one side and only one or two on the other side. Under such conditions there is a tendency to achieve a lopsided result when the Hawley appliance is activated for movement of the front teeth. This may occur especially if there is functional contact between the maxillary and mandibular anterior teeth since such contacts tend to pull the anchorage teeth forward when the Hawley appliance is activated. Because of the absence of teeth on one side (and thus less anchor-

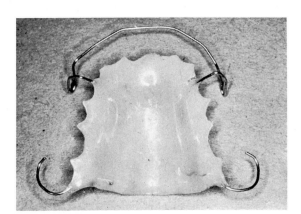

Figure 14–4. Hawley appliance with labial arch wire and clasps for molars.

age) there will be more give on that side. Greatly disturbed total occlusal relationships may occur in such cases.

The labial arch wire should be made of 0.036 inch stainless steel wire if the teeth have normal periodontal support and the wire goes into the acrylic distal to the cuspids; if the teeth have lost some support, 0.030 inch wire should be used. If the wire has to be extended buccally and distally around the last molar because of insufficient embrasure space for the wire on the distal of the cuspid, use 0.036 or 0.040 inch wire. Thus, if the passage of the labial arch wire from the buccal side to the lingual anchorage in the acrylic is to be accomplished without any occlusal interference, it is necessary to extend the wire to the distal aspect of the last maxillary molar. It is extremely important that the labial arch wire be placed incisally to the main contour of the front teeth in order for the resultant force to push the teeth apically as well as lingually when the appliance is activated. The cuspid loops or "rabbit ears" of the labial arch wire can be modified to provide the desired action. Long loops give a more gentle spring action and are used for cases that require considerable tooth movement, while short loops with less spring action are used for retention and stability when these appliances are used as retainers after active movements or for minor movements.

When the Hawley appliance is adjusted in the mouth, heavy palatal occlusal contact between the Hawley and the mandibular incisors should be avoided. To raise the bite on lower anterior teeth by biting against a maxillary Hawley appliance may lead to serious impingement of the palatal gingival tissues, and may also lead to extrusion of posterior teeth if the appliance is used for a long time. It is important to provide ample space for the palatal gingival margin when the Hawley appliance is activated, so that when the teeth move lingually there will be no impingement of the tissue between the teeth and the appliance (Fig. 14–5, *A* and *B*). The relief zone of the palatal acrylic should provide space for about 0.5 mm. movement if the teeth have normal support or for as much as 1 mm. of movement if considerable periodontal support has been lost. The relief zone in the acrylic should be made in such a way that when the teeth are tipped into contact with the acrylic the contact will be made incisally to the main contour of the cingulum of the teeth. After the teeth are in contact with the acrylic, the remaining spring action in the labial arch wire will then move the teeth in an apical direction (Fig. 14–5, *C* and *D*). The labial arch wire should purposely be activated more than is needed to tip the maxillary front teeth into contact with the acrylic to achieve some intrusion. Since this force, after a limited tipping, will result in an apically directed impact, there is no danger of a damaging effect within reasonable limits of forces. In severe maxillary protrusion, it is essential for a good result that the front teeth be intruded as well as tipped lingually, otherwise they will appear much too long and interfere with function when tipped lingually. By combined lingual tipping and intrusion of the maxillary incisors into the alveolar process it is also possible sometimes to convert suprabony palatal pockets to intrabony pockets that are amenable to reattachment therapy (Fig. 14–6).

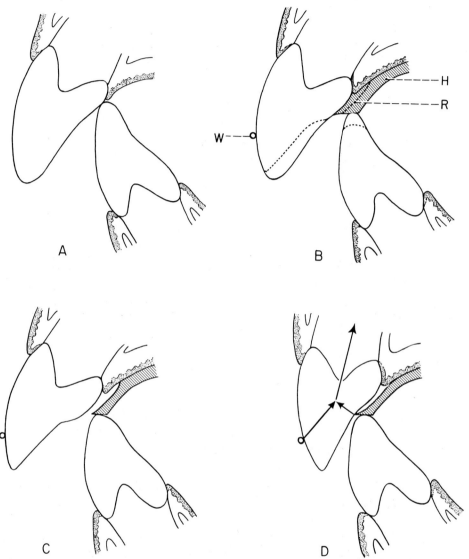

Figure 14-5. *A,* Schematic representation of central incisor in labial version and showing extrusion. *B,* With Hawley appliance (H) in place, relief of appliance is made as indicated by the dotted line (R) to provide space for gingival margin and lingual movement of the tooth. Dotted line on incisor indicates grinding needed to provide functional freedom and space for lingual tipping. The mandibular incisor should be ground according to the dotted line so as to just contact the appliance. The labial wire (W) is placed incisally to the labial contour. *C,* After grinding of appliance and teeth the appliance is activated. *D,* After the tooth has reached contact with the appliance, the resultant forces will move the tooth in an apical direction, and its apex slightly labially, which also helps in uprighting the tooh. A combined intrusion and tipping can be achieved with less force than direct intrusion since less alveolar bone resorption is required at any given time when combined movements are used.

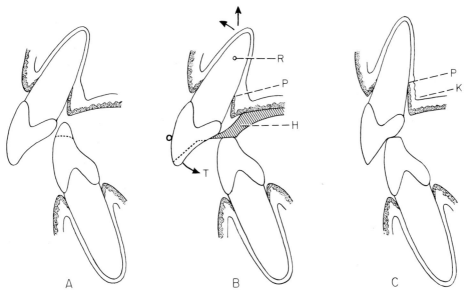

Figure 14-6. *A,* Before orthodontic treatment and insertion of Hawley appliance. Dotted line indicates grinding to be done on mandibular incisor. *B,* With activation of Hawley appliance (H) the tooth will be rotated about center of rotation (R) and intruded. With lingual movement (T), the maxillary incisor must be ground as indicated by the dotted line. Note base of periodontal pocket (P). *C,* After orthodontic treatment new bone has not formed at (K), but the tooth has been intruded into the bone. This does not alter the relationship of the bottom of the pocket (P) to the tooth, which is the same as before the orthodontic treatment. Since the relationship between the pocket and the bone is now altered to an intrabony pocket, the chances for reattachment are greatly enhanced. Also the potential for retention is improved by the more axially directed occlusal forces.

The next step of the activation is to provide space for the teeth to tip lingually if they are in functional contact with the mandibular teeth. Considerable grinding may be needed on the lingual surfaces and incisal edges of the maxillary teeth or the incisal edges of the mandibular incisors. This grinding should not only free the teeth from contact in centric but also provide functional freedom in lateral and protrusive excursions.

If the mandibular incisors are ground so they are not in contact with the maxillary incisors, centric stop contacts should be provided for the mandibular incisors against the palatal surface of the Hawley appliance by adding self-curing acrylic till the teeth just touch the appliance when the patient is biting with posterior contacts.

If there is undesirable spacing between the mandibular incisors, these teeth can also be moved together as well as lingually with the maxillary Hawley appliance. This should be attempted only when there is very good posterior anchorage for the appliance, otherwise the protruded mandibular incisors may, because of reciprocal force, tip the maxillary molars mesially (Fig. 14-7, *A*). In such cases, it is better to use a separate mandibular appliance. When tipping of the lower incisors is attempted by a maxillary Hawley appliance, the adjustment during activation of the appliance is made by reduction of the incisal

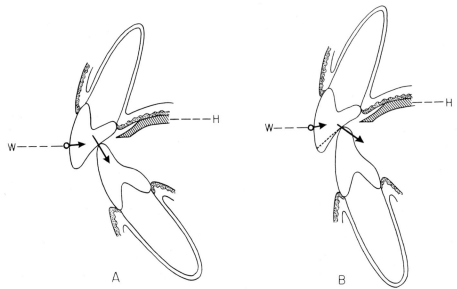

A   B

Figure 14–7. *A,* Incorrect use of Hawley appliance (H) to move both maxillary and mandibular teeth. The impact of the force from the labial arch wire (W) will be transmitted in an axial direction to the mandibular incisor because of the angulation of the incisors. This method is not effective for lingual tipping of either teeth, since the mandibular incisors will resist intrusion and the tendency is for the maxillary posterior anchorage teeth to move anteriorly. *B,* Inclination of mandibular incisor allows for simultaneous lingual movement of maxillary and mandibular incisors. Functional freedom is obtained by grinding according to the dotted line. The labial arch wire (W) is activated incisally to the labial contour.

guidance on the maxillary teeth while the centric stops are left in contact (Fig. 14–7, *B*).

The patient should use the appliance every night and as much as possible in the daytime. An interval of 3 to 4 weeks should be allowed to pass after each activation of the appliance. A typical case is illustrated in Figure 14–8.

In patients with marked protrusion of the front teeth, the labial arch wire may slide up and tend to dislodge the Hawley appliance in the posterior region. Although the appliance can be held up by posterior clasps under such circumstances, it may be better to apply wire ligatures or narrow bands with small labial hooks on the central incisors for the labial arch wire to rest against. The activated wire will then intrude these teeth as well as move them lingually (Fig. 14–9).

The popular use of labial rubber bands attached to side hooks instead of labial arch wire should be discouraged except for selected cases. The rubber bands have a tendency to slip gingivally above the contour of the tooth and produce gingival irritation, besides applying excessive continuous forces.

Figure 14–8. Pictorial history of typical use of a Hawley appliance. *A, B,* and *C* show patient prior to periodontal treatment and insertion of appliance. *D,* After periodontal surgery; testing contact and pressure of activated labial arch wire with dental tape. *E,* Palatal view with appliance activated. *F,* After completion of tooth movement. Note shortening of teeth by grinding and intrusion. *G, H,* Splinting with pin-ledge inlays. Note establishment of centric stops on lingual aspects of the maxillary incisors shown in *H;* also note how contacts have been established in mandibular arch in *I.*

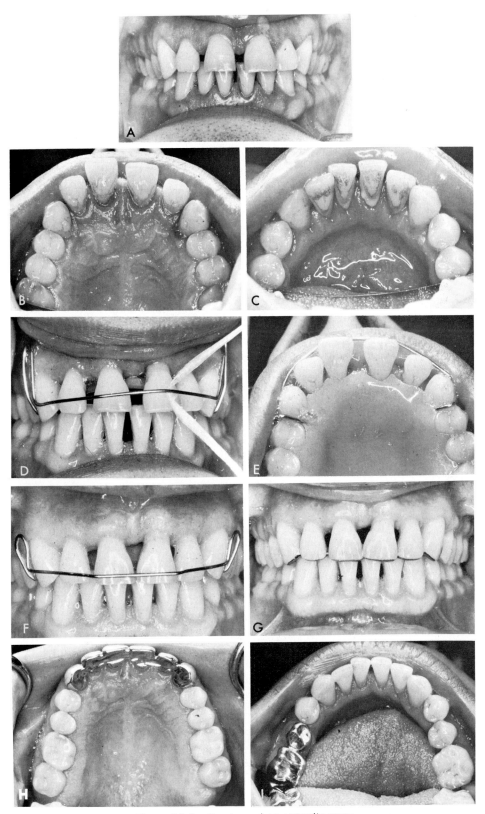

Figure 14-8. See legend on opposite page.

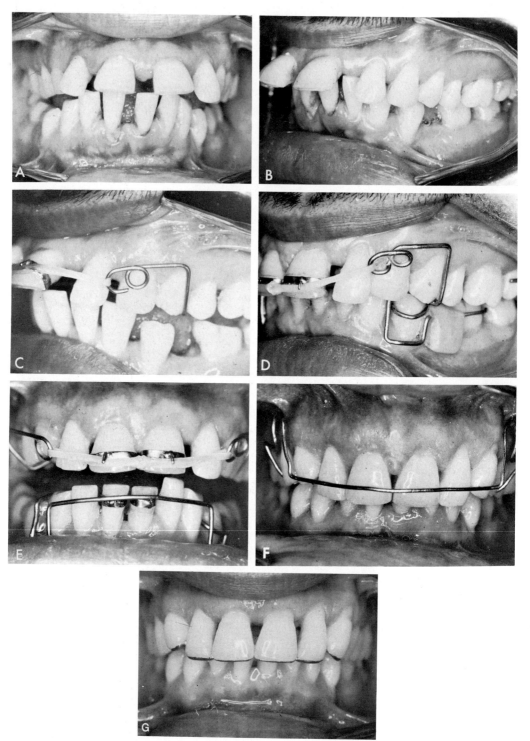

Figure 14–9. Treatment of extreme protrusion of maxillary and mandibular anterior teeth. *A* and *B,* Before treatment. *C,* Modified Hawley appliance in place. *D* and *E,* After use of maxillary and mandibular appliances for 8 months. Note intrusion of mandibular incisors. A band with hook for intrusion of the left lateral mandibular incisor was added. *F,* The movement of the teeth has been completed and the patient is ready for splinting of the maxillary anterior teeth with pin-ledge inlays. *G,* The teeth have been splinted and periodontal surgery has been performed. *H,* Roentgenograms showing banding of teeth. *I,* Roentgenograms one year after treatment completed. (Figure 14–9 continues on pages 331 and 332.)

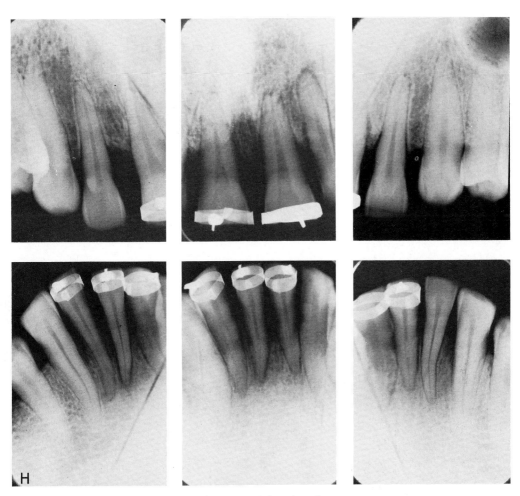

Figure 14–9 (continued).

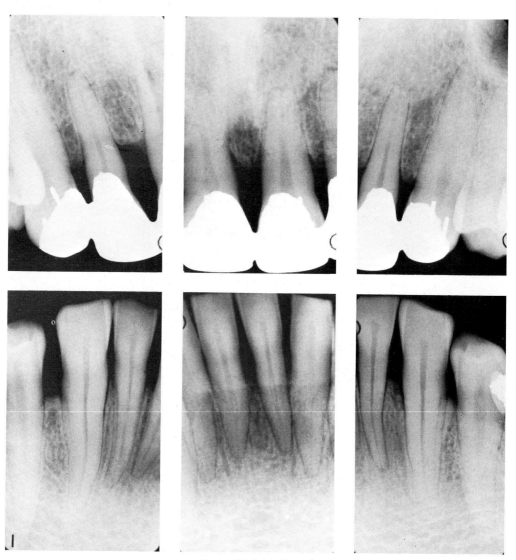

Figure 14–9 (continued).

Also, instead of a desired intrusive component of the active force, as occurs when the wire is properly placed, one may get an extrusive component of force from the rubber band slipping gingivally above the contour of the tooth.

If orthodontic bands or other labial stops are placed on the front teeth, rubber bands can be used. With temporary acrylic crowns present, labial notches can be made either for wire or rubber bands that provide for well controlled action and a favorable distribution of stress. A warning must be given against placing the labial arch wire too high on the crown of the teeth and against having the palatal contact of the Hawley appliance apically to the cingulum (Fig. 14–10). The palatal adjustment of the Hawley may also guide the teeth in a lateral direction and serve as a stop for rotating forces. It is wrong to relieve the Hawley so much on the palatal side that it will not make contact with the maxillary incisors after the teeth have moved the intended distance. The lingual stops on the Hawley behind the maxillary front teeth also prevent traumatic movements of the teeth if the labial arch wire has been activated too much, since with these proper stops the activity of the wire will lead to intrusion of the teeth rather than excessive tipping. This is especially important if the teeth have poor periodontal support.

When the teeth have been moved into the desired position, the Hawley appliance and the occlusion should be adjusted for a period of retention.

In order to use the Hawley appliance effectively as a retainer, self-curing acrylic is added to the margin of the appliance corresponding to the maxillary front feeth. Isolation of the teeth from the soft acrylic may be accomplished with the use of Saran Wrap placed over the teeth and the palate. Then the appliance is inserted and excess acrylic removed. This procedure will then provide a stable and accurate seat for the teeth when the labial arch wire is adjusted with very little pressure on each tooth. The occlusion can then be adjusted with a fairly stable result. The patient is instructed to use the appliance every night for at least 1 year; later every 2 or 3 nights; after 2 or 3 years the appliance may not have to be used. If permanent fixed splinting is used, no period of orthodontic retention is needed.

A Hawley appliance of similar construction may also be used to move mandibular front teeth lingually. It is important, however, to be sure that the new

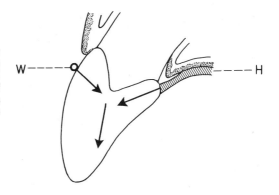

Figure 14–10. Incorrect placement of Hawley appliance. Both the labial arch wire (W) on the labial and the Hawley appliance (H) on the lingual contact the tooth apical to heights of contour of the crown. This placement of wire results in forces (as indicated by arrows) which tend to extrude the teeth.

position of the teeth will not encroach upon the normal tongue space. The best indication of tongue space can be obtained from a history of the position of the teeth prior to their labial version. If the teeth were initially closed together, but moved labially because of lost support resulting from periodontal disease, the prognosis for retention is good. If the mandibular anterior teeth have always been protruded, the prognosis is poor for retention of the teeth in a more lingual position unless permanent splinting is contemplated. Retention is less of a problem if correction of a crossbite is involved since the resultant normal occlusion will provide the retention.

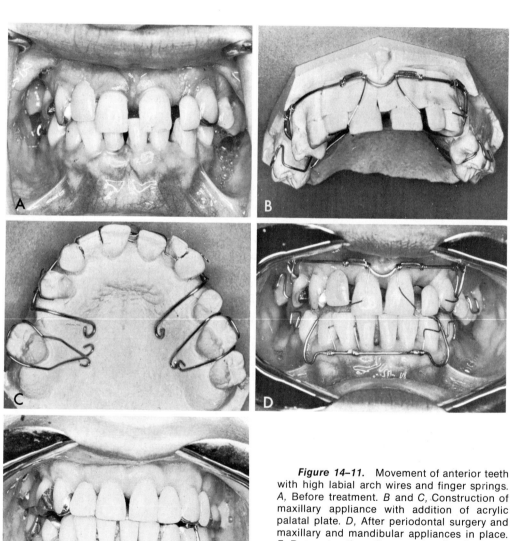

Figure 14–11. Movement of anterior teeth with high labial arch wires and finger springs. *A,* Before treatment. *B* and *C,* Construction of maxillary appliance with addition of acrylic palatal plate. *D,* After periodontal surgery and maxillary and mandibular appliances in place. *E,* Reconstruction after completed orthodontic treatment.

Anterior teeth can also be moved lingually by various types of high labial arch wires and fingersprings (Fig. 14–11). The fingersprings are made of 0.020 to 0.024 inch diameter wire. Although the use of an appliance with fingersprings appears to be a very precise way to pinpoint tooth movements, it has the great disadvantage of being easily distorted. The Hawley appliance is the simplest and most reliable way of tipping anterior teeth in a lingual direction.

Correction of Crossbites

In patients who have anterior crossbites without true mandibular prognathism it is often desirable to move the maxillary teeth labially and the mandibular teeth lingually. This type of movement may be accomplished with removable appliances provided (1) the appliances are used all the time (including eating) and (2) they are used until the maxillary teeth are distinctively in labial version relative to the mandibular teeth in centric closure.

The relationship between the teeth when the jaw is in centric relation is of essential importance for the selection of patients for treatment of anterior crossbite. If the anterior teeth or the cusps of the posterior teeth are in an almost end-to-end position in centric relation and the jaw is deflected into the centric occlusion crossbite, the prognosis for treatment is good since the crossbite is, to a great extent, of a functional nature. If there is a considerable dental discrepancy in favor of the crossbite when the jaw is in centric relation, the prognosis for treatment with removable appliances is poor, and the patient should be referred for comprehensive orthodontic therapy or the crossbite left untreated. Due allowance must be made for the possibility of undesirable dehiscence if teeth are moved outside or inside the alveolar process in correction of crossbite.

The most common type of removable appliance for treatment of anterior crossbite is a biteplane placed in the mandible. Such a biteplane is illustrated in Figure 14–12. The biteplane illustrated should be taken out of the mouth only for oral hygienic procedures. The patient should be instructed not to bite together with the biteplane out of the mouth unless the incisal edges of the maxillary teeth are engaged in a labial position to the incisal edges of the mandibular teeth. This type of treatment will involve some nuisance and discomfort to the patient and should be attempted only in highly motivated patients. Self-curing acrylic can be added to the biteplane as the maxillary teeth move labially. The appliance is more effective with a steep incline and considerable bite opening than if it is made barely extended over the lower incisors. As soon as the teeth grip in the desired relationship, the use of the biteplane should be discontinued. The mandibular teeth can then be moved lingually if there are open contacts and space for them to move. If needed, oral reconstruction should be postponed at least 6 months after orthodontic treatment until the proper occlusal vertical dimension has been established.

Various types of biteplanes with fingersprings can also be used to achieve

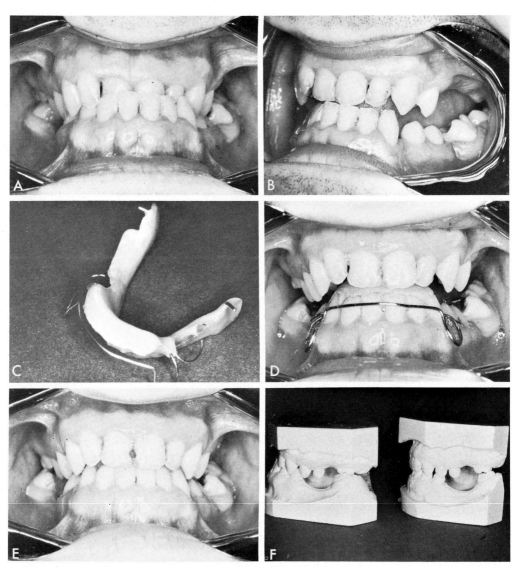

Figure 14-12. Treatment of anterior crossbite with mandibular biteplane. *A,* Functional Class III occlusion. *B,* Relationship of anterior teeth with jaws in centric relation. *C,* Biteplane, showing labial arch and clasps. *D,* Appliance in position, showing contact of maxillary teeth. *E,* Relationship of anterior teeth after movement. *F,* Casts showing relationship of jaws before and after labial movement of the maxillary anterior teeth and repositioning of mandible to centric relation.

the same result. The occlusion is then raised on the biteplane, and the patient has to use it continuously until the crossbite has been directed into a normal relationship. Two such cases are illustrated in Figs. 14–13 and 14–14. These appliances can also be used for posterior crossbite. If patients are carefully selected for treatment of crossbite, appliances should not have to be used more than 1 to 3 months.

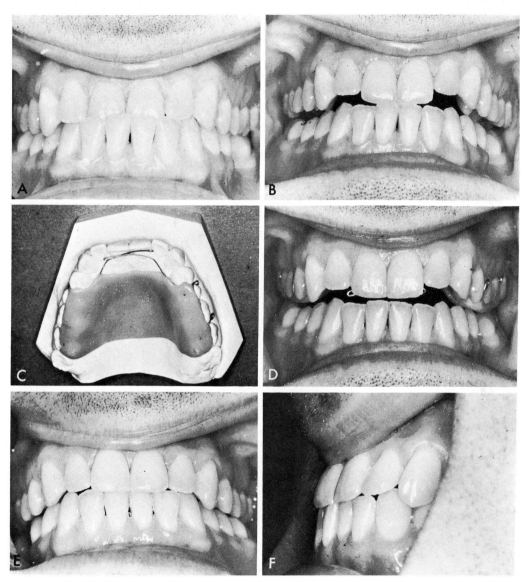

Figure 14–13. Maxillary appliance for correction of anterior crossbite. *A,* Protrusion of mandible to accomplish contact of posterior teeth (functional Class III relationships). *B,* Relationship of teeth with mandible in centric relation. *C,* Acrylic appliance with finger springs contacting maxillary incisors. *D,* Appliance in position with sufficient opening for incisors to be moved labially. *E* and *F,* Position of teeth following labial movement with mandible in centric occlusion.

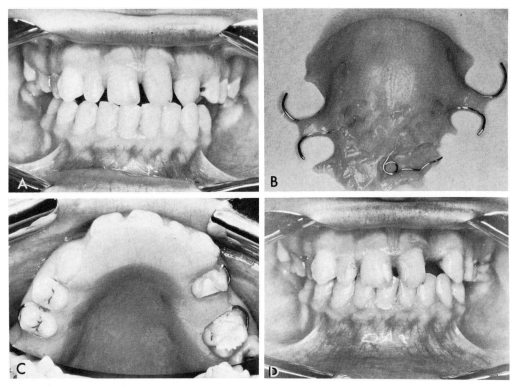

Figure 14–14. Correction of cuspid crossbite. *A*, Relationship of cuspid with mandible in centric relation. *B*, Appliance with small finger spring for movement of cuspid. *C*, Appliance in position and activated and temporary bite raising to allow movement of cuspid. *D*, Mandible in centric occlusion. Note that labial and distal movement of the cuspid has been accomplished.

Mesial and Distal Movements

Mesial or distal tipping of teeth can be accomplished by the use of finger-springs made on either the lingual or buccal aspect of Hawley appliances (Fig. 14–15). High labial arch wires or simple palatal acrylic plates can also be used as anchorage for fingersprings. The thickness of the fingersprings should be from 0.020 to 0.024 inch in diameter, dependent on the periodontal support for the teeth.[10] It is essential for the success of treatment that the teeth be ground to remove the interferences to movement with regards to the occlusion, otherwise the bite has to be raised temporarily to allow for occlusal freedom (Fig. 14–16). Unless the teeth are ground or the bite raised, the teeth will hardly tip against functional occlusal forces when removable appliances are used.

Minor distances between anterior teeth can also be closed by rubber elastics or various types of elastic or silk ligatures. The use of rubber elastics is not recommended since they may easily slip down to the gingival tissues and cause severe injury. The forces exerted by rubber bands are also poorly controlled and often excessive.

Grass lines and other ligatures can be tied on the teeth in such a way that they do not slip to the gingival tissues, and several teeth can be tied together

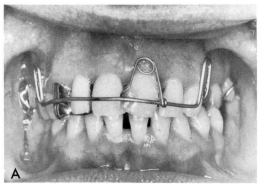
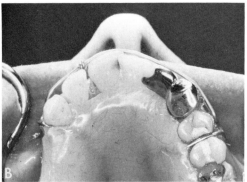

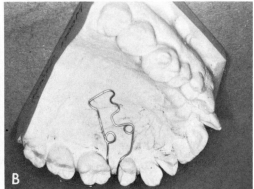

Figure 14-15. Use of Hawley appliance with finger spring to correct overlapping of an anterior incisor. *A* and *B*, Appliance positioned with adequate clearance of acrylic for distal movement of the incisor. *C*, Completion of distal movement of the incisor.

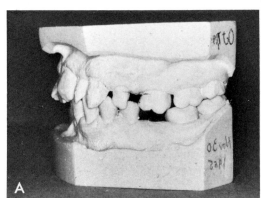
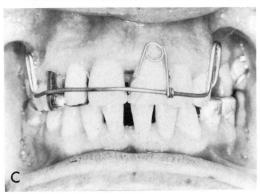

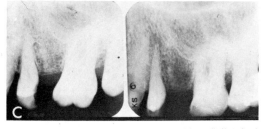

Figure 14-16. Regaining space following drifting of bicuspid and molar. *A*, Casts showing spaces on mesial of biscuspid and distal of molar. *B*, Type of wire arrangement which is imbedded in palatal acrylic for dual action. The spring wire is covered by plaster before placing the acrylic so that the wire is free of acrylic from the loops to the teeth. As the teeth are moved, occlusal adjustments are necessary to allow for movement. *C*, Radiograph showing closure of spaces on mesial of bicuspid and distal of molar (left—before, right—after).

for anchorage. However, it is much more difficult to control the orthodontic forces with ligatures than with fingersprings, and a grass line ligature cannot be left on the teeth for more than 2 or 3 days since it becomes inactive and produces a foul odor. Plastic-coated nylon ligatures can be left on for 4 or 5 days but will then have to be changed by the dentist. Since teeth moved with any type of ligature will move back to the previous position almost immediately when the ligature is removed, this type of tooth movement is most useful for closing of slightly open contacts prior to impressions for bridges or fixed splints. If grass line ligatures are used for teeth that have lost considerable amount of periodontal support, No. 3 single thickness ligature should be used with light pressures since these ligatures may become very traumatic if they are tied on tight and the coronal leverage is long.

Teeth with advanced periodontal disease can also be pulled together by an immediate force using 0.008 inch diameter soft annealed stainless steel ligature wire, but this procedure is not recommended since the force is difficult to control and root resorption or pocket deepening may result if the force is too heavy.

To upright a mesially tipped molar would often be very desirable prior to bridge work or other forms of oral reconstruction. However, this is a much more complex problem than uprightening a tipped anterior tooth. When a molar tips mesially the distal root moves occlusally and this root has to be intruded in order to place the tooth in its previous vertical position. Any tipping orthodontic device will tend to move the mesial root occlusally rather than to intrude the distal root unless a considerable occlusal force is directed toward intruding the tooth at the same time it is being tipped. This type of movement should not be attempted with a removable appliance unless the bite is raised temporarily to free the tooth from occlusal force or the tooth is ground off occlusally as it is tipped. After the tooth has been uprighted and the bite-raising appliance has been removed, the space has to be maintained while the normal vertical dimension is re-established. A more effective way to upright tipped molars is by fixed appliances, but in either case this treatment should be extended over a year's time to allow for proper natural adjustment of the vertical dimension prior to the reconstruction. In most instances, it is more practical to use the tipped tooth for a bridge abutment without uprighting it than to go through these orthodontic procedures. (See also Chapter 15.)

Intrusion

The periodontal structures are very resistant to forces in the direction of the long axis of a tooth, so intrusion requires forces of considerable magnitude over a prolonged period of time. Intrusion of teeth with single roots, especially incisors, is much easier than intrusion of multirooted teeth. In order to get bone resorption started it is often advisable to combine intrusion with some tipping of the tooth. Such a combination of forces will eliminate the functional resistance to pull from a good percentage of the principal periodontal fibers. Otherwise, to intrude vertically a tooth that has been in heavy function over a long period of time will require extremely heavy forces since the collagen fibers of the periodontal membrane transmit vertical or axially directed forces as well tolerated pull or tension forces to the alveolar bone.

Intrusion of maxillary anterior teeth combined with tipping has already been discussed under the use of Hawley appliances. Single teeth can also be intruded by the appliance recommended by Hirschfeld[4] and shown in Figure 14–17. Andersen's[5] biteplanes may also be used as illustrated in Figure 14–18. The bite for making the Andersen biteplane appliance should be taken with the

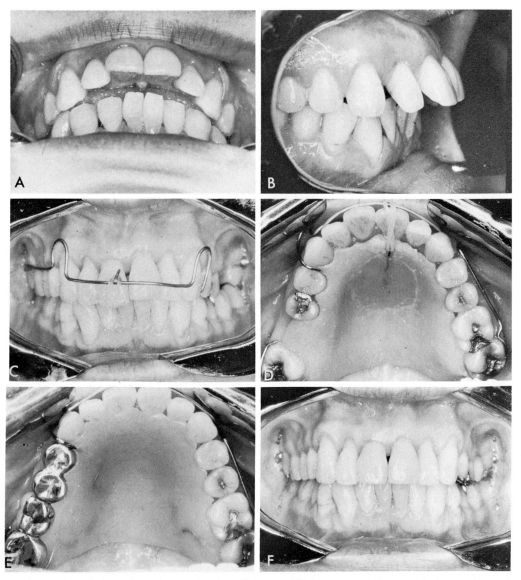

Figure 14–17. Intrusion of single front tooth by modified Hawley appliance and elastics. *A* and *B*, Before orthodontic treatment. *C*, Right maxillary central incisor elongated after faulty use of Hawley appliance. This tooth is now being intruded by rubber elastics hooked on to the labial arch wire. *D*, Palatal view. Hook for rubber band in palatal acrylic. *E* and *F*, Final result. Hawley used as retainer.

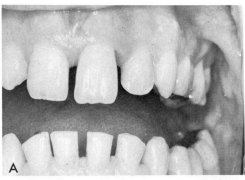
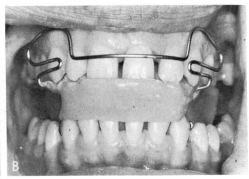
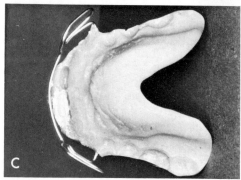

Figure 14–18. Intrusion of a maxillary incisor. *A,* Elongated left maxillary central incisor. *B,* Andersen's appliance for intrusion of front teeth. *C,* Self-curing acrylic added to imprint of central incisor in order to localize the biting pressure to that tooth.

mandible in combined opening and protrusion since this relationship will provide more muscle activity than a bite relationship of simple opening on the path of habitual opening and closure.

None of the methods of intruding teeth mentioned is very effective, and a prolonged period of retention or fixed splinting is required to avoid relapse. Intrusion of multirooted teeth produces severe traumatic injury in the bi- or trifurcation area and is unpredictable with regard to the required force and time. The most difficult part of intruding multirooted teeth is to control the reciprocal force or anchorage so that only the teeth that should be moved are moved. It is not advisable to attempt orthodontic intrusion of molar teeth by removable appliances.

Extrusion

Eruption of impacted or partially impacted cuspids is sometimes aided through orthodontic therapy by moving other teeth to provide space for the tooth or by actual pull on the cuspids. One has to be sure there is no ankylosis before this treatment is started. A hook for rubber band or spring has to be attached to the tooth, and the anchorage should preferably be in the same arch as the impacted tooth since resistance to intrusion is much greater than resistance to extrusion.

Biteplanes with contacts on anterior teeth only are often used to provide opportunity for extrusion of posterior teeth in patients with deep overbites.

This method of treatment is not recommended for adults since the occlusal forces will intrude the posterior teeth again when the biteplanes are removed.

Rotation

Rotation of single-rooted teeth can sometimes be performed with removable appliances by a combination of fingersprings and reciprocal tooth support from a palatal acrylic plate (Fig. 14–19). However, this is difficult and unpredictable to the point of being impractical except when combined with other tooth movements, for example, partial rotation associated with repositioning of front teeth with a Hawley appliance. Rotation of teeth can be accomplished in a much more predictable and efficient manner with fixed than with removable appliances.

Retention

Retention following any orthodontic treatment in adults is always a greater problem and requires a longer period of time than that required in children during their period of growth. Successful retention always requires that the etiologic factors have been eliminated and the teeth established in stable func-

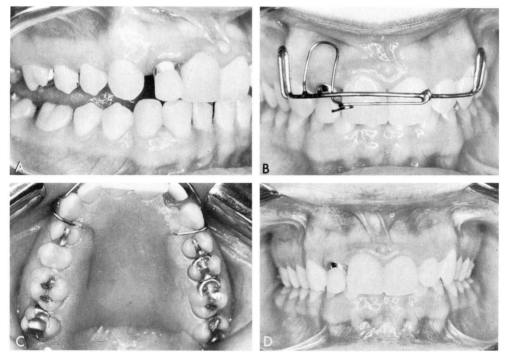

Figure 14–19. Correction of rotated lateral incisor using modified Hawley appliance. *A,* Rotated lateral with some labial version and overlapping of the central incisor. *B,* Appliance in position with tips of finger springs on mesial portion of the lateral incisor. *C,* As distal movement and rotation have started the acrylic is removed on the palatal aspect to make room for lingual movement. *D,* Completion of rotation, and distal and lingual movement.

tional relations. Occlusal adjustment with due regard to stabilization of occlusion should follow all orthodontic therapy. Periodontal surgery following completion of the orthodontic movement also facilitates retention since the regenerating transeptal and gingival fibers will mature with the teeth in their new position if orthodontic retention is maintained for about three months following the surgery.

In the majority of cases of orthodontic therapy in adults, one has to count on more or less permanent mechanical retention of the teeth either by stabilizing permanent splints or removable appliances. Only when the teeth have been moved into normal functional positions (for example, following treatment of crossbite) can one be sure of natural retention. Various types of splints for stabilization of teeth will be discussed in Chapter 16.

It should be understood that many patients with severe malocclusion and periodontal disease can be treated successfully by qualified orthodontists, and patients should be referred for such consultation whenever orthodontic treatment is practical. Whenever one is in doubt about the simple orthodontic problems discussed in this chapter or when encountering unexpected response to the treatment, a specialist in orthodontics should be consulted.

REFERENCES

1. Becher, A.: The retraction of the maxillary anterior segment by simple orthodontic means. Brit. Dent. J., *128*:585, 1970.
2. Hawley, C. A.: A removable retainer. Internat. J. Orthodont., 5:291, 1919.
3. Henry, J. L., and Weinmann, J. P.: The pattern of resorption and repair of human cementum. J. Am. Dent. A., *42*:270, 1951.
4. Hirschfeld, L.: Minor Tooth Movement in General Practice. St. Louis, The C. V. Mosby Co., 1960.
5. Lundström, A.: Introduction to Orthodontics. 2nd ed., New York, McGraw-Hill Book Co., Inc., 1960.
6. Oppenheim, A.: Human tissue response to orthodontic intervention of short and long duration. Am. J. Orthodont. & Oral Surg., *28*:263, 1942.
7. Picton, D. C. A.: Effect of repeated thrusts on normal axial tooth mobility. Arch. Oral Biol., *9*:55, 1964.
8. Ramfjord, S. P., and Kohler, C. A.: Periodontal reaction to functional occlusal stress. J. Periodont., *30*:95, 1959.
9. Reitan, K.: The initial tissue reaction incident to orthodontic tooth movement as related to the influence of function. Acta odont. scandinav., *9*:Suppl. 6., 1951.
10. Reitan, K.: Some factors determining the evaluation of forces in orthodontics. Am. J. Orthodont., *43*:32, 1957.
11. Reitan, K.: Biomechanical principles and reactions. *In* Graber, T. M. (Ed.): Current Orthodontic Concepts and Techniques. Vol. I, pp. 56–159. Philadelphia, W. B. Saunders Co., 1969.

CHAPTER 15

OCCLUSION IN OPERATIVE AND RESTORATIVE DENTISTRY

Optimal functional capacity and stability of occlusal relationships are major considerations in every phase of operative and restorative dentistry. The placement of dental restorations offers an even greater potential for attainment of these goals than mere correction of occlusal disharmony through grinding.

OCCLUSION PRIOR TO RESTORATIVE PROCEDURES

Before operative or restorative procedures are started it should be determined if the patient's occlusal relationships are adequate and merit perpetuation in the restorations or appliances. As indicated in Chapter 6, the very processes that created the need for the operative or restorative procedures (caries, inadequate restorations, periodontal disease, loss of teeth) all predispose and often lead to disturbed occlusal relations. The pathways of masticatory function often become restricted in such conditions. The resulting convenience patterns, through uneven occlusal wear and conditioned occlusal reflexes, limit the function of the dentition. Such restricted movement patterns preclude functional utilization of restorations placed outside the established convenience path unless the obstacles to harmonious smooth gliding occlusal movements are eliminated. The use of the best articulators or functionally recorded occlusal wax patterns are meaningless if unharmonious occlusal relationships in the dentition are being reproduced by the use of these methods. It is therefore of essential importance for the establishment of harmonious multidirectional occlusal function that occlusal interferences be removed prior to the operative or restorative procedures. Only then can the patient obtain the full benefit of the restorations (Fig. 15–1).

In some instances, the functional part of a patient's occlusion may be free

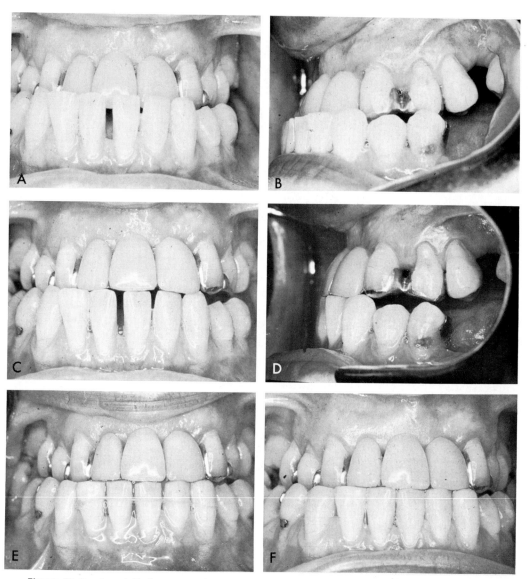

Figure 15–1. *A* and *B*, A seven-unit fixed bridge was made to fit the patient's centric occlusion without adjustment or correction of the malocclusion. The patient developed temporomandibular joint pain and also experienced some difficulty in chewing tough food. *C* and *D*, In centric relation there was an end-to-end relationship on some of the anterior teeth. The occlusion was adjusted until a stable jaw relationship was achieved for centric relation, and the mandibular incisors that had been pushed labially by the bridge were brought into contact by grass line ligatures. *F*, The resultant occlusal relationship has been maintained for several years without the use of a retainer. Because of the discomfort initially experienced with the maxillary bridge, the patient refused to have the missing posterior teeth replaced (female, age 37).

of occlusal interferences, while other teeth not participating in occlusal function may have drifted into malposition because of the loss of antagonists or from other causes. The occlusion with such interferences requires correction before optimal functional relations can be established between the replacement of the lost teeth and the remaining opposing teeth. Occlusal adjustment prior to restorative procedures should, therefore, go beyond elimination of the actual occlusal interferences at the time of the adjustment and include corrections of deviations from an acceptable plane of occlusion. The potential occlusal relationship following the restorative procedures should be considered before the restorations are made, since the functional relations between the restorations and the opposing teeth, to a great extent, can be determined by grinding and/or by orthodontic movement of the remaining teeth.

Standardized occlusal *templates* are, in most instances, unacceptable as indicators of the plane of occlusion, since there is an individual optimal occlusal pattern for each patient. A thorough analysis of the occlusion and considerable clinical judgment are required in order to determine the optimal occlusal relationship of those patients with grossly-deranged occlusions. It is often advisable to mount casts in an individually adjustable articulator as indicated in Chapter 10. A trial adjustment of the occlusion, with subsequent trial waxing of restorations and tooth replacements, will provide an opportunity to establish the best occlusal patterns and relations for the patient.[1,3]

A standardized template approach is justified when an insufficient number of teeth are available for reproduction of the previous pattern of occlusion. Templates are, therefore, used mainly in extensive oral rehabilitation when the patient has relatively few remaining teeth. Even so, a standard template cannot be used without due consideration for the optimal occlusal pattern for each patient.

In patients with severe bruxism and/or temporomandibular joint pain it is often impossible to determine the proper centric relation at the time of the initial examination. These patients often change the terminal stationary hinge position of the jaw after elimination of the occlusal interferences and pain. Occlusal reconstruction should always be oriented to a normally functioning temporomandibular joint. This orientation may require use of occlusal bite-planes or splints for a couple of weeks or more and some occlusal adjustment before the patient's stable or true centric relation can be recorded and used as the basis for the reconstruction.

SINGLE RESTORATIONS AND OCCLUSION

Stable tooth position is predicated upon an axially directed resultant of biting forces in centric occlusion for bicuspids and molars. In the anterior region there has to be balance between the impact of the functional forces and the lip and tongue pressure. In dentitions with evidence of minimal occlusal wear the contacts in centric relation are often on opposing inclines and embrasures (Fig. 15-2). Such a contact relationship is difficult to reproduce in occlusal restorations, especially if they are carved directly in the mouth. If the centric stops or contacts are on inclines which do not balance the occlusal forces, the teeth are apt to move and new occlusal interferences may result (Fig. 15-3). It is, therefore, most practical to place the centric stop for the opposing cusp on

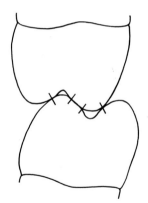

Figure 15-2. Normal stability of unworn teeth with centric stops on opposing inclines.

a flat surface in the bottom of the fossa (Fig. 15-4), so that biting forces in centric occlusion are dissipated in the direction of the long axis of the teeth. The most common mistake is to overcarve occlusal restorations to the point that centric stops are removed (Fig. 15-5), leading to interferences in lateral excursions. Such an effect may be exaggerated when restorations are placed in opposing teeth and centric stops are removed by overcarving both restorations.

Another common mistake in operative dentistry is to forget to test the retrusive closure both between centric relation and centric occlusion. This path will not be registered by having the patient simulate masticatory movements or by doing command swallowing without a bolus. There is also a tendency to reproduce balancing side contacts in restorations following the generated wax technique. These balancing side contacts should be removed later if balanced occlusion is not wanted as an end result.

Occlusal restorations should have approximately the same hardness and potential for wear as the teeth; otherwise, the restorations will wear away at a faster rate than the surrounding enamel and create occlusal interferences in lateral excursions. Marked cuspal interferences in lateral excursions are often

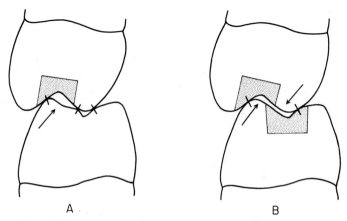

A   B

Figure 15-3. Although there are centric stops for the buccal mandibular and lingual maxillary cusps, there would be a tendency for occlusal instability.

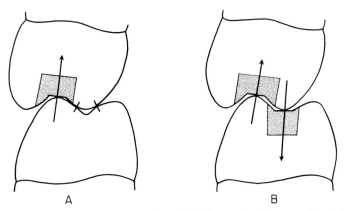

Figure 15–4. The biting forces in centric against the restorations are directed axially.

seen in dentitions with a large number of soft, poorly condensed amalgam restorations.

Faulty interproximal contacts (too loose or too tight) may disturb the occlusal relationships for a number of adjacent teeth. The use of soft restorative materials for interproximal contacts may allow for accelerated wear and unharmonious mesial drift and may predispose to occlusal interferences. If the restorative material is very hard (such as glazed porcelain), such hardness may not allow for the normal amount of wear and will result in occlusal interferences.

Occlusal restorations made of a material harder than the teeth usually do not result in occlusal interferences in the posterior part of the mouth. However, anterior crowns of porcelain or other very hard materials that do not wear in harmony with the rest of the teeth often result in an anterior displacement of the maxillary teeth. As a result, the lip will exert more force on the labially

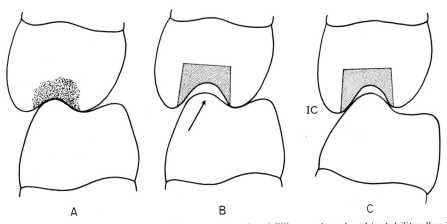

Figure 15–5. *A,* Occlusal caries. *B,* Overcarved occlusal filling and occlusal instability allowing tipping of lower tooth and resulting in occlusal interferences in lateral excursions. *C,* Indicates one of the interfering cusps (IC) after the tipping.

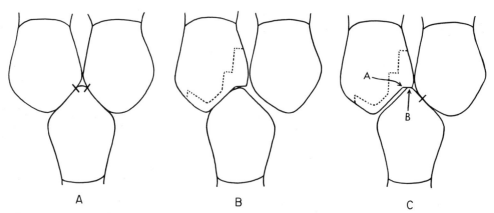

Figure 15–6. *A,* Centric occlusion before occlusal adjustment. *B,* Centric relation after occlusal adjustment. If a restoration is placed as indicated by the dotted line, the restoration should be carved to the same surface pattern as established by the grinding at the time of the previous occlusal adjustment. *C,* Centric occlusion after placement of restoration. Note "long centric" between A and B in the drawing.

displaced teeth than the other teeth, and a "jiggling" traumatic occlusion may be the result.

Following occlusal adjustment to centric relation, the established freedom in centric or *long centric* should be reproduced in any new restoration involving occlusal relations.[5] If the patient is told to close or tap his teeth together from rest position and the new restoration is carved or ground to fit this pattern of closure without any specific attempt to bring the jaw back to centric relation, the restoration will often interfere with closure in centric relation. The failure to consider this source of interference when one or more new occlusal restorations are placed in patient with a previous history of bruxism and temporomandibular joint pain is a common source of recurrence of such disturbances. The "long centric" between a patients centric relation and his previous centric occlusion should be reproduced in the restorations, and definite occlusal contacts should be established and maintained without occlusal prematurity in any jaw relation between these two positions (Fig. 15–6).

ORAL RECONSTRUCTION OR REHABILITATION

Following the establishment of a normal jaw-to-jaw relationship, either by occlusal adjustment or biteplanes, it is of essential importance that these relationships be transferred into the restorations (Fig. 15–7). A large number of articulators and techniques have been devised to secure such transfers. Several of these methods will provide acceptable results when used within the limitations of the instruments and the techniques. (See Chapter 10.) Relatively simple procedures using a Hanau or Dentatus articulator may be used for any kind of dental reconstruction. These instruments are not satisfactory if the purpose is to restore bilateral balanced occlusion with equal occlusal stress on the working and balancing side; however, this type of restoration is not essential or may not

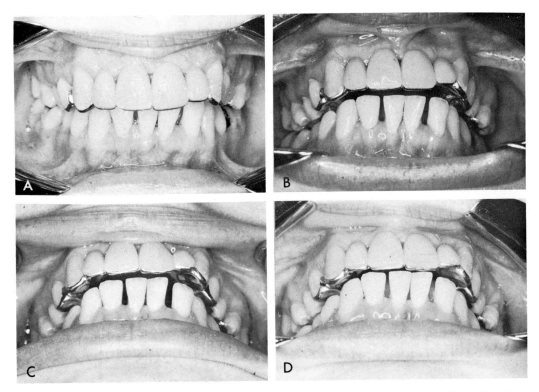

Figure 15–7. *A,* Eight-unit anterior fixed bridge which esthetically looks fairly good. The patient had had temporomandibular joint pain which had been relieved by occlusal adjustment prior to the construction of the bridge. The pain recurred immediately after cementation of the bridge which, in centric occlusion, fitted perfectly. *B,* In centric relation the patient contacted the bridge on steep forward and, in part, laterally directed inclines. *C,* When these inclines were ground back to centric relation, the pain and discomfort subsided but recurred again within intervals of 3 to 6 months. *D,* By repeated adjustments and gradual movement of the teeth, a stable occlusion in centric relation was achieved. The patient has been without recurrence of symptoms for 4 or 5 years. The recurrence of pain and discomfort after insertion of the bridge could have been avoided if the occlusal relation had been made to fit centric relation as well as centric occlusion (female, age 36).

even be desirable for good function of the natural dentition. In this respect, Schuyler's[6,7] concept is subscribed to, in which the working side contacts lift the teeth slightly apart on the balancing side in lateral excursion when the excursion is more than 1 to 2 mm. from centric.

Initially, a provisional inlay or crown is made for a mandibular bicuspid or molar that has opposing teeth and is going to be included in the reconstruction. If the reconstruction is going to involve both the left and right sides of the mandible, similar provisional crowns are made for both sides. These crowns should be fitted as accurately as possible to the previously established occlusal pattern of the patient. Then reference marks are made for the relationship between these crowns and the opposing maxillary teeth with the mandible in centric relation. Later, all the other abutments in the same jaw may be prepared and impressions secured. Before the bite is taken, the previously fitted temporary crown should be inserted. This is done in order to secure a controlled positioning of the jaw in the previously determined centric relation and with the same occlusal vertical dimension as before the preparations were made.

The casts should be mounted in an individually adjustable articulator and the provisional temporary crowns placed on the dies for guidance during the carving of the other crowns or inlays. This use of the provisional crowns will allow for duplication of both vertical dimension and functional pathways within the adaptive range of almost all patients.

If the oral rehabilitation involves both the maxilla and the mandible, provisional crowns or inlays may be fitted in opposing areas in both jaws before the rest of the preparations are made and the subsequent bite is obtained. Both the mandibular and maxillary restorations can then be carved at the same time, as described, for example, by Lucia[4] or Granger.[2] While indisputably the ideal procedure is to complete restorations in both jaws at the same time, this procedure is considerably more difficult technically than completing those in the mandible first and then those in the maxilla. If the patient has considerable overbite and a well defined cuspid guidance, temporary crowns or inlays on these teeth should be fitted to the occlusal pattern before the rest of the maxilla is prepared. The desired cuspid guidance can then be transferred to the articulator with these crowns. Even if one wants to use functionally generated wax patterns or "chew-in" methods, it is important to have temporary crowns to provide proper guidance in lateral and protrusive excursions.

It is not permissible to open or close the occlusal vertical dimension in an articulator unless the stationary hinge axis has been recorded by a kinematic face bow and instruments allowing for an accurate transfer have been used. However, if for some reason it is necessary to increase the vertical dimension and a conventional Hanau or Dentatus articulator with a nonkinematic face bow is to be used, the vertical dimension should be raised to the desired height on provisional crowns before the bite is taken.

Oral rehabilitation started in the maxilla and followed by mandibular restorations may result in poor functional relations or sometimes embarrassing and time-consuming problems, especially in previous edentulous areas (Fig. 15–8).

To start an oral rehabilitation with preparation of all the remaining teeth in the mandible and/or the maxilla without leaving centric stops or having made provisional crowns is a haphazard procedure which easily may lead to unacceptable results. Even the use of a kinematic face bow and stationary hinge axis location may give misleading results.

Temporary bridges or appliances used during the oral rehabilitation have to be fitted well; otherwise, displacement of teeth, faulty occlusal pathways, and disturbed temporomandibular joint function during this critical period may jeopardize the final result.

Whether oral rehabilitation should be based on gnathological principles[2,4] of centric relation or made to allow for "freedom in centric" ("long centric") is still a controversial issue (Fig. 15–9, *A* and *B*). No scientifically proved advantage has been established for either approach.

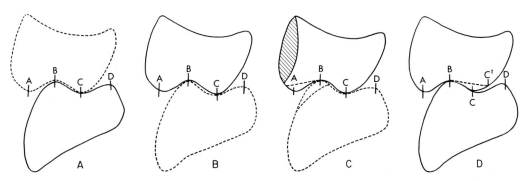

Figure 15–8. *A,* As acceptable, the mandible was reconstructed first and maxilla (dotted lines) afterward. This procedure provides for control of occlusal relations involved in working function from A to C. The buccal incline of the mandibular lingual cusp (C–D) has already been established, but that area is of minimal significance for masticatory function compared with the A–C area. Balancing side contacts are only to some extent controlled by this procedure, and it may involve sacrifice of centric stops at C if the mandibular central fossa is carved too deep at the time of the mandibular reconstruction. *B,* Unacceptable is the reconstruction of the maxilla first, followed by the mandible (dotted lines). With the maxillary pontic already made, one has control over working side functional relations only in the unimportant area from C to D. There is no control over working functional relations from A to C and poor control over balancing side occlusal relations. *C,* If the maxillary pontic has been made first and one attempts to establish good functional occlusion, the lingual incline of the buccal maxillary cusps at A may have to be ground. This grinding may jeopardize occlusal protection of a porcelain facing. If an attempt is made to clear a working side interference by reduction of the buccal aspect of the mandibular buccal cusp, there is a tendency to lose functional contact for this cusp, which has its most important functional field close to centric occlusion. *D,* If there are opposing teeth present in the area of occlusal reconstruction, treating the mandible first, and then the maxilla, provides control over the entire field of occlusion. If the mandible is done first, one has working side occlusal control for the area C to D and balancing side control from B to C. When the maxilla is reconstructed next, one has working side control from A to C and balancing side control from B to C. This provides an opportunity to restore ideal functional relations in areas in which it was necessary to sacrifice centric stops during the occlusal adjustment. (See, for example, dotted line from B to C¹ which might have been the result of correction of a balancing side occlusal interference.) If the occlusal relations of the teeth to be restored are good, it does not make any difference whether the maxillary or the mandibular arch is reconstructed first.

If the maxillary teeth remain and some of the mandibular teeth are missing, one may have problems similar to the ones described under C. It is advisable to mount casts of such a case, adjust the occlusion on the casts, do trial waxing of the missing mandibular teeth, and adjust the maxillary teeth in the edentulous area until there are good occlusal relations. Then do an adjustment in the mouth resembling the adjustment of the casts as closely as possible prior to construction of the replacements of the missing mandibular teeth.

If the mandibular teeth remain against missing maxillary teeth, the situation is similar to *A.* A functionally acceptable result can usually be obtained by simply grinding the malposition of the occlusal surfaces of the mandibular teeth relative to the plane of occlusion after completing the elimination of occlusal interferences.

From the standpoint of clinical dentistry, it is much easier to do oral rehabilitation with a slight range of 0.3 to 0.8 mm. between centric relation and centric occlusion (Fig. 15–9, *A*) than using gnathologic principles (Fig. 15–9, *B*). As long as there is no scientific evidence to indicate that such a "long centric" (Fig. 15–9, *C, D,* and *E*) places the patient under any disadvantage compared with a gnathologic reconstruction, it appears that the "long centric" and the principles described in this chapter are, for reasons of convenience, to be preferred in the general practice of dentistry. Reconstruction to point centric relation (gnathology) requires exact instruments for recording of the Bennett movement, as well as for the hinge axis; therefore, attempts to carry out such

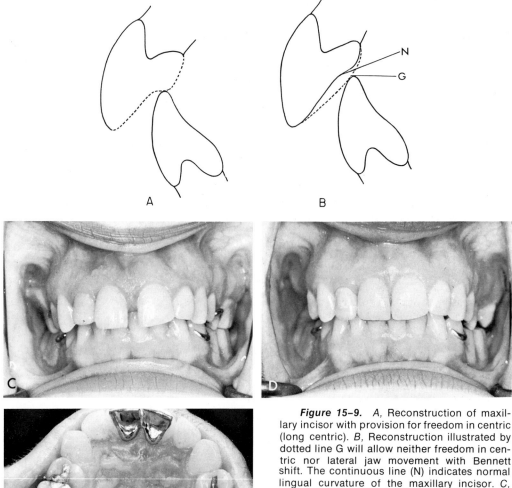

Figure 15–9. *A*, Reconstruction of maxillary incisor with provision for freedom in centric (long centric). *B*, Reconstruction illustrated by dotted line G will allow neither freedom in centric nor lateral jaw movement with Bennett shift. The continuous line (N) indicates normal lingual curvature of the maxillary incisor. *C*, Impinging overbite and separation of anterior teeth following loss of molars. The mandibular incisors were reduced in length and the maxillary incisors brought back into contact. *D*, Two pin-ledge inlays were constructed and soldered together to splint these teeth. *E*, Note "long centric" in the inlays providing axially directed forces both in centric relation and centric occlusion. This reconstruction prevents the teeth from tipping labially again and provides additional stability.

procedures on the conventional Hanau or Dentatus articulator are not fair tests of the validity of gnathologic principles.[4]

It appears from limited electromyographic studies that immediately following the insertion of a maxillary appliance which guides all occlusal movements to centric relation, there is tension in the posterior part of the temporal muscles and some slight discomfort. However, this reaction seems to disappear rapidly, and the muscle adaptation to such an occlusion is good (Fig. 15–10). Similarly,

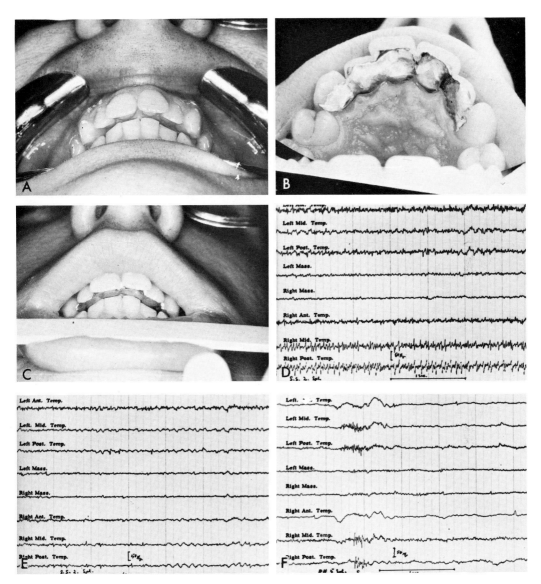

Figure 15–10. Experimental repositioning of the mandible to centric relation. Male with severe bruxism, age 26. *A,* After occlusal adjustment, considerable opening appeared between the maxillary and mandibular front teeth when the patient closed in centric relation. A long centric had been ground into the posterior teeth, and lateral excursions were cleared from centric relation. B, A splint was constructed, following hinge axis mounting of the casts, for cementation to the maxillary front teeth. *C,* The splint was constructed so that when it was in place the patient could only close to centric relation, and all his lateral excursions were guided to centric relation by the splint. The splint was inserted after electrodes were in position for electromyography. *D,* The initial reaction to the splint was one of added contraction of the posterior and middle fibers of the temporal muscle, even when the patient was sitting with the mandible in rest position (D). Initially the patient complained about the splint being uncomfortable. *E,* After 15 minutes with the splint in place, the muscles had adapted to it and relaxed in rest position. *F,* Following occlusal contacts in swallowing, the muscles also relaxed with the splint in place. Then masticatory function was normal clinically and electromyographically. (The synchronized temporary increase in amplitudes is associated with tooth contacts in swallowing.)

good muscle balance is also found with "long centric," and much more research under well controlled conditions is needed before this old controversy regarding "long centric" and "point (gnathologic) centric" can be solved.

REFERENCES

1. Beyron, H.: Det. adulta bettet och bettanalys. Nordisk Klinisk Odontologi. Vol. II. Kapitel 8. Copenhagen, 1959.
2. Granger, E. R.: Practical Procedures in Oral Rehabilitation. Philadelphia, J. B. Lippincott Co., 1962.
3. Lindblom, G.: Balanced occlusion with partial reconstructions. Internat. Dent. J., *1*:84, 1951.
4. Lucia, V. O.: Modern Gnathological Concepts. St. Louis, The C. V. Mosby Co., 1961.
5. Mann, A. W., and Pankey, L.: Oral rehabilitation. Part I: Use of the P-M instrument in treatment planning and in restoring the lower posterior teeth. J. Prosth. Dent., *10*:135, 1960.
6. Schuyler, C. H.: An evaluation of incisal guidance and its influence in restorative dentistry. J. Prosth. Dent., *9*:374, 1959.
7. Schuyler, C. H.: Freedom in centric. Dent. Clin. N. Am., *13*:681, 1969.

CHAPTER 16

SPLINTS IN OCCLUSAL THERAPY

A splint is a rigid or flexible appliance used to keep in place and protect an injured part. The term splint is also used to indicate the act of fastening or confining with a splint a displaced or movable part, or the support or bracing of such a part. In dentistry, splinting designates tying together or uniting two or more teeth in order to gain occlusal stability.

CLASSIFICATION AND PURPOSE OF SPLINTS

Splints may be classified as (1) temporary, (2) diagnostic or provisional, and (3) permanent. In each of these groups either fixed or removable splints may be used. External splints may be placed outside the crown of the teeth, internal splints are fitted or attached inside the circumference of the teeth.[9]

The purpose of a temporary splint is to reduce occlusal forces for a limited period of time. Temporary stabilization is important: (1) following accidental loosening of teeth by trauma; (2) as a supportive measure in the treatment of advanced periodontal disease; (3) for stabilization of teeth during extensive occlusal reconstruction; (4) until restorative procedures are completed in other areas of the mouth, allowing for redistribution of functional occlusal forces; and (5) for anchorage in orthodontic therapy.

The diagnostic or provisional splint is used in borderline cases in which the final result of the periodontal treatment cannot be predicted with certainty at the time of the initial treatment planning.

Permanent splints are constructed to provide stability for teeth that have lost so much of their periodontal support that they cannot carry out normal function if they are left as single units. Permanent splints are also used for retention of teeth following orthodontic procedures and to prevent eruption of teeth without antagonists. Various types of fixed or removable splints are used as abutments for replacement of lost teeth. All splints should enhance stability and function of the dentition.

BIOMECHANICS OF SPLINTS

Reduction of Mobility

The clinical effect of splinting is the reduction of mobility of teeth. Considering that tooth mobility = force/resistance, it is apparent that tooth mobility can be reduced either by decreasing the occlusal force or increasing the periodontal resistance. The origin of the force, where the force contacts a tooth, and the direction, magnitude and frequency of the forces have to be considered in the analysis of forces. The extent of the periodontal area receiving the impact relative to the total support of the tooth and the integrity of the supporting tissues have to be considered in an analysis of periodontal resistance.

An analysis of all these factors as they apply to a single tooth has been presented in Chapter 4 under Periodontal Reaction to Physiologic Forces (p. 98). Splinting of teeth will radically change the periodontal distribution of impacts from occlusal forces. The impact area will always increase to various degrees following splinting, and this means a reduction of stress upon each given unit of the pressure-receiving parts of the supporting tissues.

Lateral or tipping forces are most apt to induce trauma and abnormal mobility of teeth. The degree of benefit from splinting with regard to tipping forces depends to a great extent upon the direction of the forces relative to the alignment of the splinted teeth. When two single-rooted teeth are splinted together, the impact of a tipping force in a facial or lingual direction is distributed to the periodontal support of both teeth. Although there is some gain in stability by the joint periodontal resistance of two teeth, the force still acts as a tipping force with concentrated impacts in the alveolar crest and lateral apical areas. Thus, little is gained by splinting two single-rooted teeth, since the traumatic forces commonly are directed facially or lingually. Such a splint, however, provides a very marked increase in stability to forces directed mesially or distally (Fig. 16–1).

Center of Rotation

The impact of the horizontal component of a mesially or distally directed force is evenly distributed over the periodontal structures, inducing a bodily movement of the teeth, rather than tipping. The center of rotation for the splint and the teeth is between the teeth, and mesially or distally directed tipping forces will act chiefly as intruding vertical forces upon the tooth toward which the forces are directed.

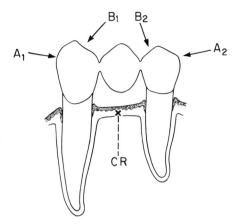

Figure 16–1. Schematic drawing of splinting of two single-rooted teeth to illustrate maximum stability afforded in a mesiodistal direction. Forces in mesiodistal direction (A_1 or A_2) will not have a tipping impact but will engage the entire remaining periodontal membrane (mesially and distally) with a bodily moving force. Buccolingual forces will still have a tipping impact with a concentration of forces at the alveolar crest and apical areas. Combined vertical-occlusal and mesiodistal forces (B_1 or B_2) will have some tipping impact with the axis approximately at CR. However, there will never be the concentration of tipping forces in a small part of the periodontal structures that is seen when, for example, single-rooted teeth are used as abutments for free-ending saddle partial dentures.

Intrusive Forces

Intrusive forces are very well tolerated, since their impact is spread over a maximal number of principal periodontal fibers. If a tipping force on a splint is directed mesially, the distal abutment tooth could conceivably become extruded and the whole splint tipped mesially like a two-rooted mandibular molar. However, if the distal abutment tooth has an antagonist in the opposing jaw, the antagonist has to be intruded in order to allow extrusion of the splinted tooth. The chance for a mesial or distal tipping of the splint will therefore be very small, since this would involve intrusion of both maxillary and mandibular teeth. Bodily movement of a group of splinted teeth may occur if the horizontal components of the occlusal forces are very strong.

In order to achieve an equally favorable stabilization in the faciolingual as in the mesiodistal direction, a splint has to connect posterior and anterior segments or to engage teeth in the opposite side of the arch for support. Such a distribution of abutments produces the so-called "tripod effect," which means that a tipping force will act as a well tolerated intrusive force upon one or more of the abutments. The functional stability of the splinted teeth is enhanced, also, by the stabilizing effect of contact with the teeth in the opposing jaw.

Functional Contacts

It is also important to have functional occlusal contacts, as much as possible, in a straight line between the abutments of the splint in order to avoid tipping forces when biting forcefully together. A reduction of lateral forces on splinted teeth with poor periodontal support may be achieved, also, by avoiding, when possible, construction of functional contacts in lateral excursions. For example, use "cuspid rise" if the cuspid has good support and the posterior teeth, poor support.

The total impact of functional forces may be minimized by sharp occlusal anatomic surfaces, by directing function to the areas that have the best periodontal support, and by making the occlusal anatomic features functionally more attractive in these areas than in areas with poor support. As the result of conditioned reflex activity, masticatory function is directed toward the area that is most convenient and efficient for the function.

Mechanical Stability

The greatest mechanical stability obviously is achieved from a rigid, fixed splint. Some concern has been expressed about the fixed, rigid splint leading to partial degeneration and atrophy of the periodontal structures from lack of functional stimuli. However, no clinical or histologic evidence has been submitted to indicate that any such detrimental changes of periodontal significance occur. The only unfavorable biomechanical phenomenon associated with rigid splints is an increase in tolerance to total occlusal forces. This means that a patient can increase the pressure from habitual clenching and biting (with or without objects between his teeth) beyond the tolerance level prior to the splinting and might thereby compromise the temporomandibular joint(s) and jaw muscles. The slight compression of the mandible of about 0.5 mm. in wide opening of the jaw does not seem to affect splints on the teeth.[1]

Since fixed splints provide much greater stability than removable appliances, fixed splints are preferable for teeth with a minimum amount of residual support. However, other considerations such as avoidance of gingival irritation, esthetics and economics may favor the construction of removable splints if adequate functional support is available.

Periodontal Resistance

An increase in periodontal resistance to occlusal forces may follow successful periodontal therapy. Occasionally, some functional support may be regained by reattachment therapy. More common is an increased functional capacity of the remaining periodontal tissues following elimination of irritation, inflammation and traumatic occlusion. A moderate increase in mobility beyond the normal limits is well tolerated periodontally if the teeth are kept clean. Splinting should be done only when mobility interferes with normal masticatory function.

TEMPORARY SPLINTS

Fixed, External Types

Temporary splints may be utilized for a period of 2 to 6 months, or even longer, during periodontal or other dental therapy. The most frequently used temporary splint is an external wire-acrylic combination illustrated in Figure 16–2. Annealed stainless steel ligature wire (0.010 or 0.012 inch), single or

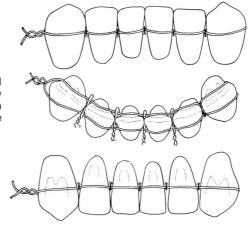

Figure 16-2. Temporary combination wire and acrylic splint. The horizontal wires should be loosely connected until all interproximal loops have been tightened and bent into the interproximal spaces; the horizontal wires should then be tightened lightly.

double, is adapted to the teeth facially, lingually and slightly gingivally to the contact areas (incisally to the cingulum of anterior teeth). The ends of the wire are tied together very loosely. Then ligature wires (0.010 or 0.008 inch) are placed interproximally and tightened, starting at the interproximal area closest to the loop of the horizontal supporting wires. It is important to tuck the end of the interproximal wire loops under the horizontal wire interproximally, in order to avoid gingival irritation. Tighten the horizontal supporting wire after all the interproximal wires have been placed. Then a moderately thick layer of self-curing acrylic of the proper shade is brushed over all the wires, making sure the acrylic is adapted well interproximally. Avoid contact of the acrylic with the gingival tissues and interference with the occlusion. A heavy layer of vaseline or silicate lubricant may be applied to the gingival tissues before the acrylic is brushed on the teeth. The teeth must be dry before applying the acrylic, since poor adaptation with leakage predisposes to decay.

A wire ligature splint without acrylic is a very poor splint; but wire combined with acrylic constitutes an effective splint for mandibular anterior teeth and a fairly useful temporary splint for maxillary anterior teeth. When bicuspids are loose, but firm molars and cuspids are present, this type of splint may also be used. Teeth included in such a splint may be ground out of occlusion temporarily without erupting while orthodontic procedures are performed in the opposing dental arch. Grinding the teeth will shorten the leverage arm of occlusal forces, and moving the opposing teeth may change the direction of the functional forces into a more axial direction and thereby enhance future stability of the teeth (Fig. 16–3).

Ligatures (wire, grass line, nylon) should not be used alone for splinting of teeth, since they are ineffective as stabilizing splints and are potentially traumatic.

Orthodontic bands welded together were popular as temporary splints a few years ago, but these splints do not have much advantage over properly applied wire and acrylic combination splints. Orthodontic band splints are more

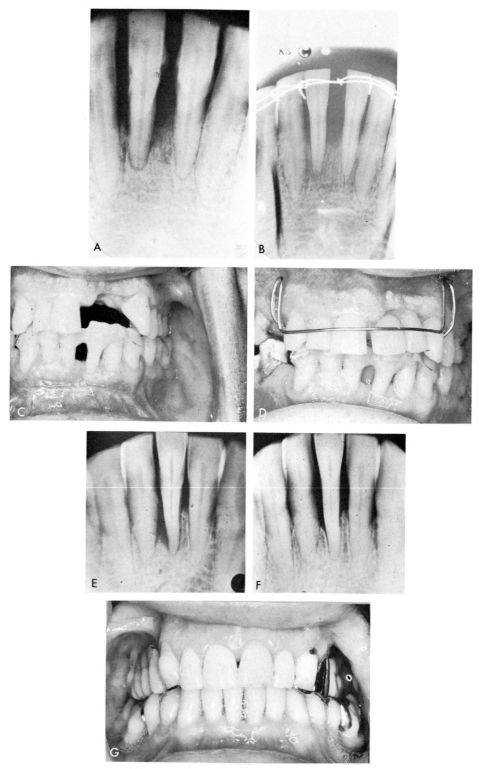

Figure 16–3. See legend on opposite page.

cumbersome to make and less esthetic than the wire and acrylic splints. They also require some space interproximally, so the stabilization of the teeth in the exact desired position is not possible with the orthodontic band splint in place.

Various cast splints of gold or chrome-nickel alloys can be cemented to the teeth temporarily and the facial and lingual parts tied together with ligature wires. Usually these splints have one open end and fit just over both sides of the line of contour of the teeth. Acrylic wire combinations have also replaced these cast metal splints, at least for temporary splinting of teeth.

Fixed, Internal Type

Temporary splints with internal fixation to the teeth can be worn for up to 2 to 3 years if so desired. Since all these splints require preparations of the teeth, they should be used only when permanent splinting is scheduled at a later date. The most popular internal temporary splints are various types of full coverage acrylic crowns united as bridges. In order to enhance stability and fixation, some of them have metal cores or bands to fit the prepared teeth. In other instances, the splint may consist of interproximal box preparations with marked retention grooves and the teeth held together by amalgam or acrylic reinforced by metal wires (Fig. 16–4).

Removable Temporary Splints

Removable temporary splints do not provide as much stability as fixed splints; but in cases in which stability is not critical, removable splints may be used because of convenience of construction and the opportunity for good oral hygiene. Practically all removable temporary splints are of the external type. Hawley's orthodontic appliance and various types of occlusal splints (also called "bite guards" or "night guards") have been used for stabilizing splints. These appliances have been described in Chapters 11 and 14. None of these splints is recommended when there is severe periodontal involvement or when maximal stabilization is desired.

Cast metal splints of the Elbrecht[3] type can be used both as temporary and permanent removable splints (Fig. 16–5). These splints are esthetically un-

---

Figure 16–3. *A,* Roentgenograms before periodontal therapy (male, age 42). *B,* Splint has been in place for 4 months. Periodontal treatment has been performed and the crowns of the teeth reduced considerably in length. *C,* Splint in place with acrylic supports around the splinted teeth. The acrylic should not touch the gingiva. *D,* Maxillary front teeth being moved lingually as mandibular teeth are shortened. More axially-directed forces, less leverage, and improved esthetics resulted from this treatment. Later, a mandibular partial denture and a maxillary fixed bridge were made for this patient. Temporary splinting and subsequent periodontal and other dental care may eliminate the need for permanent splinting. *E,* Before temporary splinting in 1949 (male, age 37). *F,* Twelve years (1961) following therapy. Note filling-in of bone and functional stability after 12 years without permanent splinting. G. Clinical picture, 1961. Excellent oral hygiene and restorative dentistry in other areas of the mouth contribute to the success of the treatment.

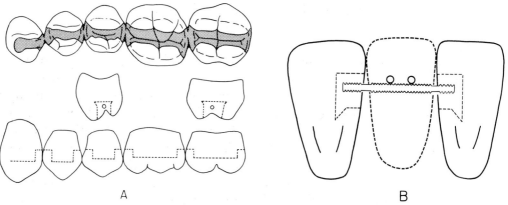

A   B

Figure 16–4. *A,* Amalgam or acrylic and wire combination splint. A well-fitted, heavy wire with a rough surface is placed in the middle of the box preparations. Undercuts in the preparations will enhance the stability of this splint after placement of amalgam or acrylic. *B,* Splint where a missing tooth is replaced temporarily by an acrylic denture tooth. First boxes are made with undercut retention on the lingual aspect of adjacent teeth. Then heavy steel wire with roughened surfaces connecting the preparations is placed. After insertion of the wire, acrylic is used to fill the preparation and the lingual aspect of the artificial tooth.

satisfactory and allow for considerable individual movement of the teeth within the splint. For temporary splinting they do not have any advantage over a wire-acrylic combination splint.

In order to obtain optimal benefit from the use of temporary splints, the patients should receive the best of periodontal and occlusal therapy while wearing the splints. The occlusal therapy should include both occlusal adjustment and reconstruction for equal distribution of stresses and maximal stability. The success or failure of temporary splinting cannot be fully assessed until after the splint has been removed for some weeks. If the teeth are still loose after removal of the splint, or become loose, permanent splinting is needed.

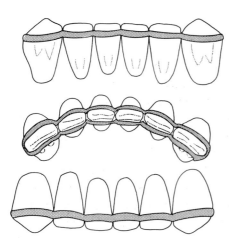

Figure 16–5. Removable cast Elbrecht splint. Such a splint can be extended around the entire dental arch. This splint has been used extensively in many countries for 30 to 40 years.

DIAGNOSTIC OR PROVISIONAL SPLINTS

Diagnostic splints are used in borderline cases when the result of the periodontal and occlusal therapy is unpredictable. The use of diagnostic temporary splints for 3 to 6 months in order to ascertain whether the teeth can withstand normal functional demands after periodontal and occlusal therapy is a recommended procedure. However, the rather common inclusion of teeth with a hopeless periodontal prognosis in diagnostic splints in "heroic" attempts to keep teeth in the mouth as long as possible is a highly questionable form of therapy. There are fairly well established guidelines in periodontics with regard to when periodontal disease can be cured or is incurable. With advanced bi- or trifurcation involvement, a temporarily cemented splint may prolong the course of the periodontal disease and lessen the chances for occurrence of periodontal abscesses, since there is less possibility for trauma from occlusion to initiate such abscesses. However, this is an uncertain truce which should not be misconstrued to mean that the periodontal disease has been cured. In the overwhelming majority of cases, both the dentist and the patient are better off without hopeless teeth being included in a splint.

It is recommended that the use of diagnostic splints be limited to temporary external splints for teeth that can be treated successfully from the standpoint of pocket elimination and future cleanliness of the exposed tooth surfaces.

PERMANENT SPLINTS

Permanent splints may be fixed, semirigid or removable, and may be anchored internally or externally to the teeth. A number of different techniques are available for making permanent splints of these various types; it is beyond the scope of this book to discuss their construction in detail. A permanent splint is indicated when the teeth cannot maintain their functional stability following dental and periodontal therapy, including temporary or provisional splinting.

Fixed Permanent Splints

As with temporary splints, optimal stability is achieved with rigid fixed splints, and this type of splint is usually the first choice for permanent splinting. There are certain main principles to be considered when fixed splints are made: (1) Avoid all sources of gingival irritation from the splint. (2) Allow good access for oral hygiene. (3) Provide excellent retention in all abutment preparations (this is of increasing importance with increased mobility of teeth). (4) Provide adequate thickness or bulk of the splint and good solder joints. The pressure on splints is often uneven, especially in individuals with bruxism who have both maxillary and mandibular splints. For example, after a few years there is a tendency for the labial cervical margins of three-quarter crowns to open as a re-

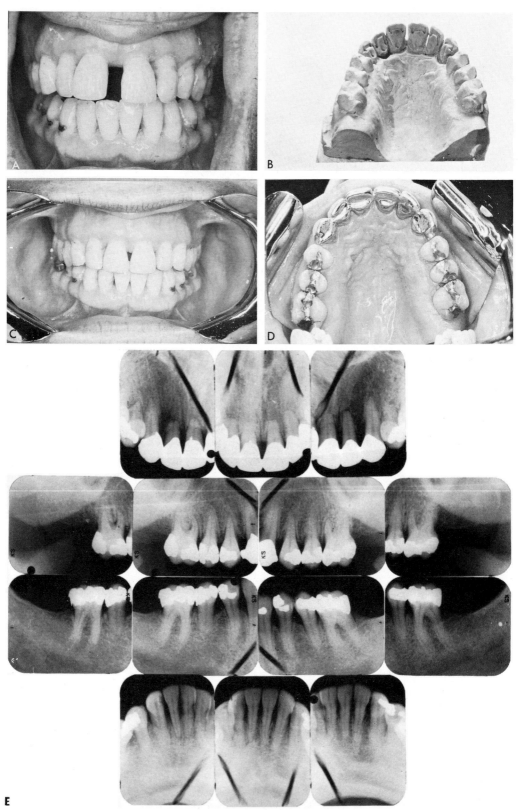

Figure 16-6. See legend on opposite page.

sult of repeated slight deformation of the splint associated with heavy occlusal forces.

Technical, esthetic and economical considerations all favor including the minimal number of teeth to provide the support needed for the splint. Often this decision is based upon poorly defined and intangible clinical judgment, but a thorough understanding of occlusion and the principles of splinting is invaluable. Sometimes the decision can be reached by the use of diagnostic or provisional splints, starting out with the fewest possible abutments and increasing the number of abutments until stability and comfort are secured.

Whenever it is feasible from technical, functional and esthetic standpoints, the pin-ledge type of abutment retainer should be used for fixed splints (Fig. 16–6). Recently, there has also been a revival of the use of horizontal pins for attachments of splints[7] of the type initially used by Köhler[5] and others.

The full coverage type of preparation is the last choice from the standpoint of periodontal acceptance, retention and long-term esthetics. Full coverage crowns should be used only when unavoidable, i.e., on the basis of esthetics or when caries activity is high.

Next to fixed rigid splints in stability and controlled stress distribution come semirigid or precision attachment connections between the various parts of the splint. These connections should always be made deep, parallel and as rigid as possible, and used only when it is not practical from a technical standpoint to make rigid fixed splints.

Removable Permanent Splints

The best splinting effect from removable splints is obtained by telescoping crowns and precision attachments. In some instances, these splints may be even more stable than fixed bridges. They may derive part of their support from alveolar ridges in edentulous areas. By use of cross-palatal bars,[6] lingual bars and telescoping crowns or precision attachments, lateral support can be obtained for posterior teeth without including the anterior teeth in the splint.

Cast metal splints with continuous labial and lingual clasps of the Elbrecht[3] type have been used extensively for removable permanent splinting of teeth, with or without inclusion of lost teeth. These splints give only fair support for the teeth and are esthetically unsatisfactory in the anterior regions of the mouth.

Various types of clasp-supported partial dentures with continuous lingual bars, embrasure hooks and other supporting arrangements are not very effective as splints (Fig. 16–7). Often abutment teeth for partial dentures are splinted with fixed appliances before they are used as abutments. Fixed splinting of two

Figure 16–6. *A,* Hypermobile anterior teeth with large crowns and short roots. *B,* The front teeth were moved into contact and prepared for pin-ledge restoration. *C,* Pin-ledge splint in place. *D,* Lingual view of splint. Note "long centric" with flat impact area for mandibular incisors, so that the main forces in centric are directed axially on the anterior teeth with the inadequate root support. *E,* Roentgenograms with splint in place (female, age 38).

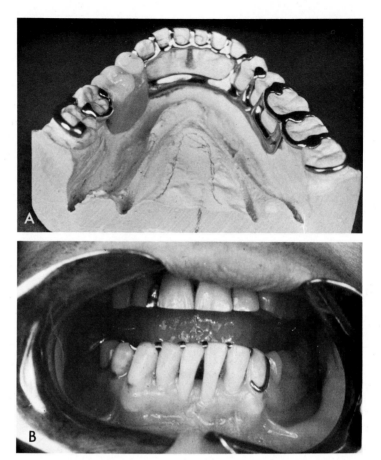

Figure 16–7. *A* and *B,* Combined partial denture and removable splint with embrasure hooks on loose mandibular anterior teeth. Extensive preparation was needed to provide space for occlusal stops, parallel surfaces for reciprocal clasp arms, and for insertion of the appliance.

abutment teeth on each side of the arch for free-ending saddle partial dentures increases the stability of the abutments greatly in mesiodistal directions. Stability is increased in the faciallingual direction by the proper arrangement of well fitting bilateral reciprocal arms of the partial denture clasps.

Other permanent removable splints include various arrangements of bars or connectors fitted into occlusal and lingual inlays or crowns. These splints are not so effective as fixed or removable precision-attachment type splints and can hardly be recommended.

Elbrecht splints[3] and clasp arrangements are satisfactory as splints only when there is a minimal need for splinting. When there is need for maximal effectiveness of splints in patients with advanced loss of periodontal support, rigid fixed or semirigid constructions are always preferred.

Regard should also be given to the oral occlusal forces exerted by the patient. In persons with bruxism, dysfunctional forces usually far exceed functional forces; therefore, these patients need better abutments and heavier, more rigid splints than patients without the tendency for bruxism.

COMMON DYSFUNCTIONAL PROBLEMS IN SPLINTING AND ORAL REHABILITATION

Tipped Abutment Teeth

Tipped Molars. Mandibular second and third molars are often tipped mesially following the loss of the first molars. After tipping of the molar begins, the occlusal stresses resulting from biting are no longer axially directed, but have a marked tipping impact on the tooth. Because of the lack of a mesial interproximal contact, the tooth tends to tip more, and the tipping component of the occlusal force will gradually become greater. The unfavorable sequelae to the entire dentition associated with this phenomenon have been described in a classical manner by Hirschfeld.[4] Because of the hazards to the health of the dentition with such tipped molars, treatment should be instituted unless stabilization has occurred and existed over a number of years without any evidence of unfavorable sequelae.

Uprighting of Teeth. One obviously ideal solution to the problem of tipped molars appears to be uprighting of the tooth to its normal position, and then use of it as an abutment for a fixed or removable appliance which replaces the lost tooth or teeth. As indicated in Chapter 14, this is a somewhat cumbersome procedure since, besides uprighting the tooth, the distal root has to be intruded in order to regain the normal vertical dimension. Fortunately, there are in most instances other acceptable alternatives to uprighting tipped molars. Orthodontic treatment is advocated only when there is extensive combined mesial and lingual tipping of the second or third molars after loss of first molars.

Overcontouring. If there is a relatively narrow (1 to 2 mm.) open contact between a mandibular tipped molar and a bicuspid, restorations that are overcontoured to provide interproximal contact are sometimes inserted in an attempt to stabilize the tipped tooth (Fig. 16–8). In most instances, this is not an acceptable procedure, since the tipped molar acts as a single unit. An extension of the restorations increases the tipping momentum by moving part of the occlusal force even farther away from the axis of rotation of the tooth than before extension of the restorations. The impact of this tipping force upon the bicuspid is in an unfavorable horizontal direction. Although the bicuspid may

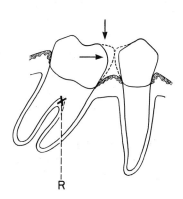

Figure 16–8. Illustration of the undesirable effects resulting from overcontouring of interproximal restorations between tipped teeth. Impact of tipping force from vertical function will be horizontal against the bicuspid after the interproximal contacts have been established. Rotation center for the tipped molar is at R.

be well supported mesially by good contacts, there is often enough movement induced to disturb interarch occlusal relations. Since there is also a tendency for lower molars to tip lingually, the use of overcontouring to provide contacts and to stop tipping will often allow for further lingual tipping.

Overcontoured restorations always have undesirable periodontal effects because of the associated deep gingival crevices and poor self-cleansing. The only time an overcontoured restoration may be used to stabilize a tipped molar is in those cases in which tipping is slight, no lingual tipping is present, the open contact is narrow, the periodontal support is good, and there are good occlusal relations with the maxillary teeth. Ideal stress distribution can never be achieved by this procedure.

Fixed Bridges.   The most effective and desirable splinting procedure is to include the tipped tooth in a fixed bridge extended to one or two mesially positioned teeth (Fig. 16–9). A fixed bridge will radically change the impact of vertical forces upon the periodontal structures of the tipped tooth. Without splinting, forces from biting on a tipped molar are transmitted horizontally; with splinting, such forces are to a great extent transmitted by the splint to the mesial abutment tooth as a vertical or intrusive force. Vertical force is well tolerated, both from stability and potential trauma standpoints. Furthermore, because of the splinting there will be even pressure on the periodontal structures of the tipped tooth; and the previously concentrated impact of vertical stresses with traumatogenic potentials at the alveolar crest and apex of the tipped tooth will have been eliminated.

The entire mesial periodontal membrane on both roots of such a tipped tooth will be exposed to an even compression, and all the principal periodontal fibers on the distal aspects of the roots will be engaged in a well tolerated pull action. As far as ability to withstand vertical occlusal forces is concerned, a tipped lower molar is a much better abutment for a fixed bridge than usually realized. However, this type of splint does not provide very good buccolingual stability. Since the abutments are on a straight line, buccolingual forces will act as tipping forces. If a long span bridge is involved or the teeth have weak support, it is recommended that the buccolingual forces be reduced by grinding (Fig. 16–10) for elimination of posterior contacts in lateral excursions (lingual incline of buccal cusps of the maxillary teeth and buccal incline of lingual cusp of mandibular teeth for working side, and relief for balancing contacts). This relief of functional lateral contacts may decrease capacity for ideal masticatory function, but the over-all effect of stability of occlusion for both arches is far superior to that obtained from removable appliances in the same area.

If the periodontal conditions are good, long-spanned mandibular fixed bridges can be constructed with better prognosis than generally realized. A long span might be considered as one extending from a tipped second or third molar to a first bicuspid or cuspid. This is one case in which the "cuspid rise" in lateral function is recommended in order to minimize lateral forces.

Abutment Crowns.   Technically, severely tipped lower molars provide limited possibilities for retention of abutment crowns or inlays. Preparations of

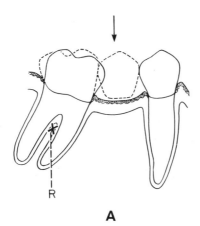

A

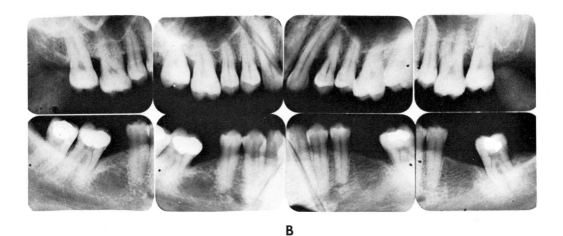

B

C

Figure 16-9. *A,* Dotted lines indicate a fixed bridge. Vertical pressure at the arrow is transmitted to the total periodontal structures of the teeth, and the rotation axis at R of the tipped molar no longer acts as a rotation center when vertical occlusal forces are applied to the molar in the bridge. B. Tipping of teeth following loss of first mandibular molar. *C,* After treatment with fixed bridges.

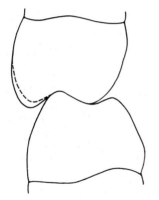

Figure 16–10. To reduce lateral force on a long-span mandibular bridge, make buccal incline of lingual mandibular cusps short and relatively flat. Grind off buccal cusps of maxillary posterior teeth as indicated by dotted line.

deep buccal and lingual slots and use of pins should always supplement conventional preparations. Occasionally, the use of telescoping crowns is indicated in order to utilize severely tipped teeth as abutments for fixed bridge constructions.

Semirigid Connections. If the distance between a tipped molar and mesially positioned teeth is short (less than the width of a molar tooth), a satisfactory splinting effect may be achieved from a semirigid joint or connection placed in the mesially positioned tooth (Fig. 16–11). The semirigid connection eliminates the requirement for parallel preparations in cases of severe tipping, and coverage of the cusps in the anterior abutment is not essential. However, the semirigid bridge will never be as effective a splint as a fixed bridge, and semirigid constructions should never be used for teeth with poor or questionable periodontal support. When such bridges are made, the joints should be as deep and parallel-walled as possible — preferably, flat precision attachment type joints.

Removable Splints. Removable splints may also utilize tipped teeth for abutments. The precision attachment appliances may provide a splinting effect almost equal to a fixed bridge. Such appliances will also transmit some of the occlusal forces to the alveolar ridge. A removable precision attachment appliance is sometimes preferable to a fixed bridge when the abutment teeth have minimal periodontal support or when long edentulous spans are involved (see Fig. 16–12).

Partial Dentures. Partial dentures with conventional clasp arrangements are much less suitable for splinting of a tipped lower molar than any of the previously listed appliances. Since the tipped tooth is not firmly splinted to other teeth, it will act as a single unit when submitted to occlusal forces. With the use of well fitting and rigid reciprocal clasps and connectors, this tipping momentum can be transmitted to several teeth and will thus minimize the potential harmful effect. The occlusal rests may also be placed on the distal marginal ridge to minimize the tipping effect from biting on the partial dentures. However, the maximum benefit of splinting, with transmission of vertical occlusal tipping forces into axial forces on the bicuspids, cannot be achieved with a partial denture of this type. Furthermore, since there is a tendency to

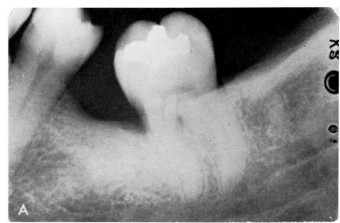

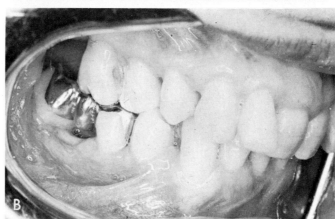

Figure 16–11. A and B, Semirigid joint on distal aspect of second bicuspid to splint tipped second molar. There should be good access for oral hygiene.

develop some play and give between the partial denture and the teeth over a long period of time, the splinting effectiveness of the partial denture is reduced.

When the tipped molar is tipped considerably in a lingual as well as a mesial direction, the splint has to be extended over to the other side of the arch for stability. This tripod effect is essential for stabilization against buccolingual forces and can be achieved either by extending a fixed bridge over to the other side of the arch or by removable appliances with bilateral support. If the anterior teeth do not require extensive dental restorations or splinting, it is often more practical to use precision attachment removable appliances to achieve bilateral stability of posterior teeth than fixed bridges. Occasionally, fixed posterior bridges may be connected with the other side of the arch by precision attachment bars, which are usually cemented temporarily.

Properly utilized, the periodontal structures of a tipped tooth will provide a much more effective and stable response to occlusal forces than is obtainable from alveolar ridges under free-ending saddles of partial dentures. Every effort should be made, therefore, to utilize the periodontal structures of these tipped teeth, rather than extracting them for "convenience" reasons.

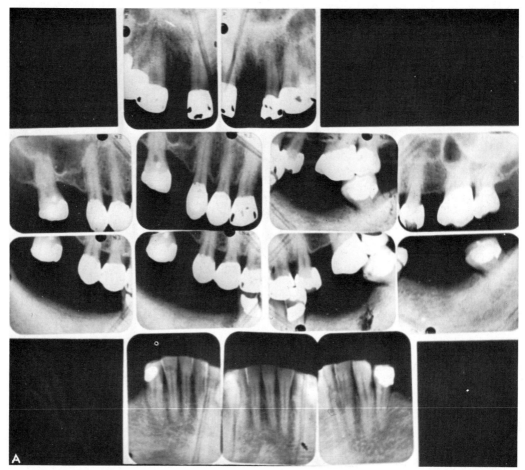

Figure 16–12. *A,* Roentgenograms after periodontal therapy in 1951. The remaining mandibular third molar was extensively tipped, clinically loose, and tender to touch. Patient had bruxism. Reconstruction was done in 1951 with a mandibular precision attachment partial denture and a maxillary fixed bridge. *B,* Roentgenograms in 1964, 13 years after the restorative dentistry was completed. Note that there is no loss of bone and the alveolar crests are well defined. *C, D* and *E,* Clinical pictures of mandibular removable appliance and maxillary fixed bridge. The gold restorations were extended under gingival margin because of a high caries rate. A long centric was present on the maxillary anterior teeth. *E* and *F,* There were no functional contacts posterior to cuspids for more than 1 mm. of lateral excursions. Since the posterior teeth had poor periodontal support sharp carvings of occlusal anatomy (*D*) were made to minimize masticatory pressure on posterior teeth. Later, gold occlusals were made for the mandibular partial denture instead of the plastic, which was too soft and wore out of normal function in a short time (male, age 37).

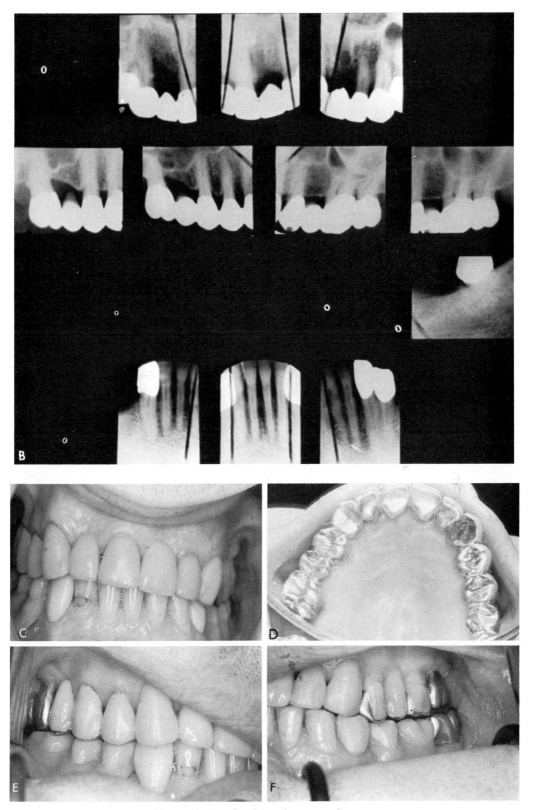

Figure 16--12. See legend on opposite page.

Deep Overbite (Vertical Overlap)

Deep overbite (vertical overlap) is an occlusal anomaly that is often incorrectly treated. Many adult patients with deep overbite have ended up with more problems, as a result of attempted bite-raising procedures, than they ever would have had if the deep overbite had been left untreated. The common mistake is to raise the bite in the molar and bicuspid region and to grind off the mandibular and maxillary anterior teeth in order to create "ideal" occlusal relations—often more important to the dentist than to the patient.

Many patients with deep overbite have excellent occlusal function in centric and lateral excursions; and there may be no pathologic changes in their periodontium, temporomandibular joints or jaw muscles. If the function is good and no harmful effect is evident from the overbite, the adult patient should be discouraged from having the deep overbite treated for the reasons that it may represent a potential periodontal hazard or an esthetic handicap.

Injury to Gingivae. Certain types of deep overbite definitely require

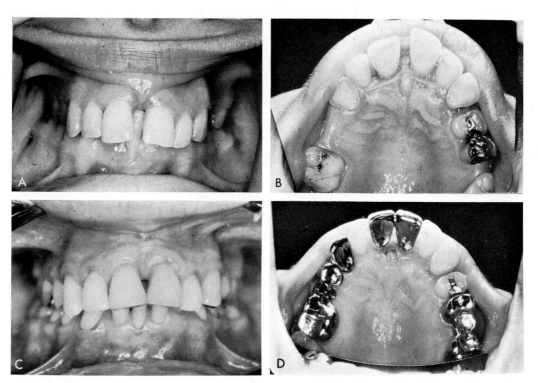

Figure 16–13. *A* and *B,* Impinging overbite. Mandibular incisors had been shortened numerous times by patient's dentist, but this had provided only temporary relief from impingement on the palate. Also note Stillman's cleft on mandibular incisor. *C* and *D,* Clinical pictures 8 years after periodontal treatment which included minor orthodontic movement and restorative dentistry. Flat steps were made on the lingual aspect of the maxillary incisors to prevent impingement by the mandibular incisors. The mandibular front teeth also were moved lingually (note the healing of the Stillman's cleft). *E,* Roentgenograms prior to treatment. *F,* Roentgenograms 8 years after treatment. Note regeneration of bone following periodontal and orthodontic treatment of the maxillary anterior region (female, age 40). Figure 16–13 continues on pages 377 and 378.)

treatment. For example, when the lower incisors bite into the gingival crevice of the maxillary incisors (Fig. 16–13) or the incisal edges of the maxillary incisors bite into the marginal labial gingiva of mandibular incisors, periodontal injury is unavoidable and treatment is required. The possibility of orthodontic treatment should always be explored for such patients. If for various reasons orthodontic treatment is not practical or acceptable to the patient, occlusal adjustment and/or restorative procedures should be considered. However, the vertical dimension and the freeway space should, as much as possible, be left unchanged even if the patient has a freeway space much wider than commonly quoted "normal values" of 2 to 3 mm. A deep overbite (vertical overlap) becomes a great liability when posterior teeth are lost. This loss may lead to closure of occlusal vertical dimension with forced forward positioning of the mandible and pressure on anterior teeth and/or gingival impingement.

Grinding on the incisal guidance and incisal edge of the maxillary incisors will provide relief for impingement on the mandibular gingiva and often free restricted lateral function. Grinding off the incisal edge of the mandibular

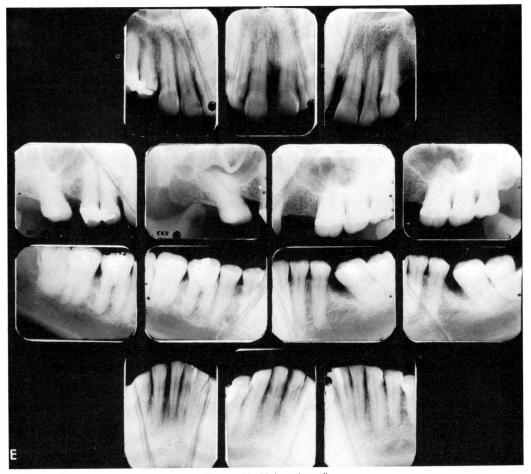

Figure 16–13 (continued).

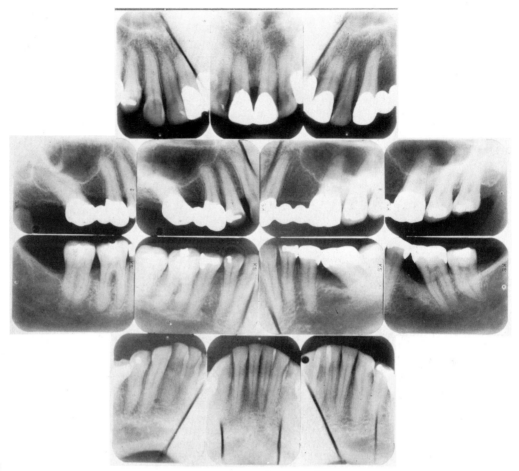

F

Figure 16–13 (continued).

incisors, however, will provide only temporary relief from palatal impingement unless some type of centric stop can be placed on the lingual aspect of the maxillary incisors. This is sometimes accomplished by placement of pin-ledge gold inlay with flat occlusal centric stops on the palatal aspect of the maxillary incisors after the mandibular incisors have been shortened as much as possible. If there are open contacts between the maxillary incisors, they may be moved together orthodontically and splinted (Fig. 16–14). Pin-ledge types of splints are often needed for permanent stability of the maxillary anterior teeth following orthodontic repositioning.

If freedom of lateral function and stability of occlusion in centric can be established without impingement into the gingival crevice, the prognosis for the dentition may be excellent, both in terms of function and periodontal health, in spite of the persisting deep overbite.

Splinting.   In oral reconstruction and splinting of maxillary anterior teeth, it is important that the splint be properly articulated in lateral excursions, allowing lateral movements without undue pressure being placed on the splint.

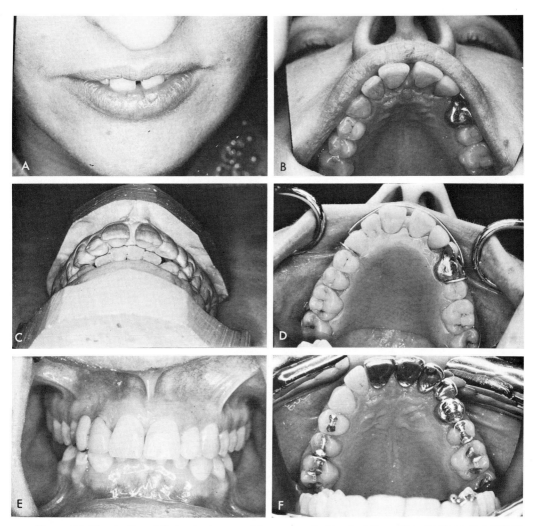

Figure 16–14. *A, B* and *C,* Impinging overbite aggravated by lip biting. The diastema and palatal impingement occurred following the loss of mandibular molars. The mandibular incisors were shortened as much as possible without risk of pulpal involvement. *D,* A Hawley appliance was inserted with palatal contact for the mandibular incisors, but without raising the bite on the appliance. *E* and *F,* After the teeth had been moved into contact, a pin-ledge anterior splint was made with palatal stops and a long centric. Also a mandibular partial denture was made without any increase in vertical dimension. There has been no relapse after treatment during 5 years of observation (female, age 33).

If the cuspid teeth have good periodontal support, it is advisable to have these teeth carry the main burden of the occlusal contacts in lateral excursions. However, if the posterior teeth have good support and the anterior teeth have lost a main part of their support, it is often preferable to construct steep cusps on the posterior teeth so they carry the main functional load and any unavoidable load existing from possible bruxism in lateral excursions. There is no demonstrated neuromuscular benefit from "cuspid raise" in any type of occlusion; the only consideration is with regard to optimal stress distribution. This opinion is not universally accepted.[2]

Provision for Overjet.   It is always important to provide sufficient overjet with a deep overbite so the patient can do unrestricted lateral excursions. Otherwise, a patient with a tendency for bruxism can break the splint, break facings, move the whole splint anteriorly, and develop temporomandibular joint and muscle pain.

Maintenance of Incisors.   In patients with deep overbite and a markedly curved arch in the anterior region it is very important for the stability of the splint that maxillary incisors be maintained for abutments, even if these teeth have extensive loss of support and appear very loose (Fig. 16–15). The loss of

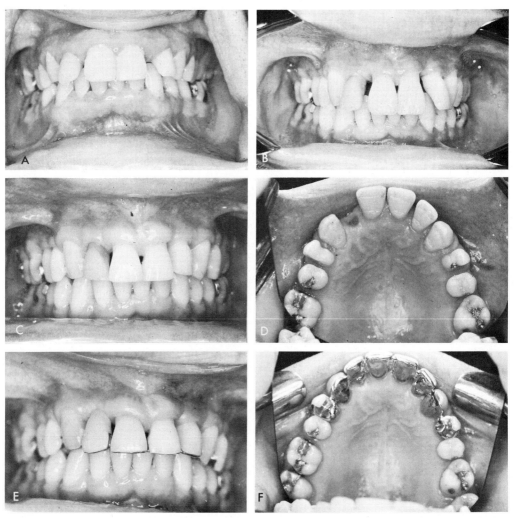

Figure 16–15.   *A,* Advanced periodontal disease. *B,* After pocket elimination the esthetic result was very poor. *C,* The anterior teeth were reduced in length and brought lingually by a Hawley appliance. *D,* The discolored lateral incisor was extracted and preparations were made for a pin-ledge splint. *E* and *F,* The splint in place shows a result which is both esthetically and functionally satisfactory. If the maxillary incisors had been extracted and replaced by a fixed bridge, there would have remained an undesirable tipping force to the abutments because of the position of the incisors in front of a straight line between the cuspids. Extraction would probably also have led to more resorption of the protruded maxillary process. The functional and restorative phase of treatment of teeth with advanced periodontal disease should always be planned and discussed with the patient prior to the periodontal treatment (male, age 33).

the incisor teeth will lead to torque on the splint and its posterior abutments. On the other hand, if the maxillary incisors are not in a protruded position relative to the cuspids, excellent functional and esthetic results may be obtained following loss of the maxillary incisors by placement of a fixed bridge from cuspid to cuspid, with possible inclusion of the first bicuspids in the bridge.

DISADVANTAGES OF SPLINTING TEETH

All splints have a tendency to interfere with oral hygiene and self-cleansing of the teeth and the gingival tissues.[10] Whenever splints make contact with the gingival tissues, it is almost impossible to avoid completely gingival irritation and inflammation. It is especially crucial for patients with a tendency for destructive periodontal disease who, unfortunately, are the patients who most often need splints. It is also difficult to achieve proper contour of a splint at the gingival margin, especially in the interproximal areas. If the roots of the teeth that are to be splinted are very close together, it may be impossible to achieve periodontal health in the interproximal areas after the splinting. Splints, especially of the full coverage type, may allow the development of extensive caries without symptoms under loose abutments. It is very important that splints be inspected regularly and the patient examined for development of caries. There is a tendency for teeth that are very loose to move slightly from the pressure of the cement at the time of seating of the splint; thus, cement-filled open margins may later lead to separation between the tooth and the gold casting. The tooth then becomes loose in the splint after a few years.

Splints require a great degree of accuracy with regard to occlusal relations at the time they are made, since after the insertion of the splint there is no adaptive movement of the teeth to accommodate various occlusal discrepancies. A splint will also interfere with normal interproximal wear and mesial drift. If there is a large fixed splint in one arch and no splint in the opposite arch, a lack of harmonious interproximal wear may conceivably lead to some occlusal interference, and periodic check of occlusal relations is indicated. It has been claimed that single teeth with poor periodontal support opposing an extensive fixed splint will suffer more from trauma from occlusion than before the insertion of the splint; however, this claim apparently is not true.[8]

Splints may occasionally pose problems of speech in that patients have a feeling of weight or fullness in their mouth. For some patients such sensations may persist for some time.

Since splints have many disadvantages accompanying their obvious stabilizing advantages, splinting of teeth should be restricted to the minimum needed to achieve occlusal stability and adequate masticatory function. Splints should never be used as a "shot gun" substitute for accuracy and exactness in occlusal therapy of the individual teeth.

REFERENCES

1. Burch, J. G., and Barcheres, G.: Method for study of mandibular arch width change. J. Dent. Res., *49*:463, 1970.
2. D'Amico, A.: The canine teeth — Normal functional relation of the natural teeth of man. South. Calif. Dent. A. J., *26*:6; 49; 127; 175; 194; 239; 1958.
3. Elbrecht, A.: Systematik der abnehmbaren partiellen Prothese. Leipzig. Meusser, 1937.
4. Hirschfeld, I.: The individual missing tooth: A factor in dental and periodontal disease. J. Am. Dent. A., *24*:67, 1937.
5. Köhler, G.: Om frontalfixering vid paradentosbehandling. Odont. Rev., *2*:275, 1951.
6. Nilson, E.: Avlastningsbarens användning vid fasta och avtagbara broar. Sv. Tand. Tidskr., *49*:129, 1956.
7. Overby, G. E.: Esthetic splinting of mobile periodontally involved teeth by vertical pinning. J. Prosth. Dent., *11*:112, 1961.
8. Ramfjord, S. P., Nissle, R. R., Shick, R. A., and Cooper, H.: Subgingival curettage versus surgical elimination of periodontal pockets. J. Periodont., *39*:167, 1968.
9. Romine, E. R.: Relation of operative and prosthetic dentistry to periodontal disease. J. Am. Dent. A., *44*:742, June 1952.
10. Simring, M., and Posteraro, F. F.: Hazards and shortcomings of splinting. New York Dent. J., *30*:19, 1964.

DIAGNOSIS AND TREATMENT OF FUNCTIONAL DISTURBANCES OF TEMPOROMANDIBULAR JOINTS AND MUSCLES

In order to arrive at a proper diagnosis it is essential that all information regarding the patient and his condition be collected and recorded in a well organized and useful manner.[49, 75] This can be done without collecting pages of irrelevant information.

HISTORY AND EXAMINATION PROCEDURES

History

Local History

It is logical to start with the chief complaint and a history of the present illness since the patient is most interested in talking about his chief complaint. In order to save time and obtain pertinent information it is best to ask questions related to the local symptoms first, and in the following order: (1) onset of symptoms, (2) type and distribution of pain, (3) pain associated with type of movements, mastication, time of day, bruxism, etc., (4) any restriction or locking of jaw movements, (5) clicking or snapping noise in the temporomandibular joints, and (6) any symptoms peripheral to the temporomandibular joints.

Systemic History

It is also essential for the diagnosis to obtain information with regard to arthritis or rheumatism elsewhere in the body, occupational and postural myalgias, psychic or emotional stress, physical stress and fatigue, and systemic diseases or disorders.

Previous Treatment

Experience with previous treatment may provide helpful information. However, the fact that a patient has had occlusal adjustment, splints, or any other occlusal therapy, does not by any means rule out occlusion as an important factor in the etiology of the patient's problem. Therapy of functional disturbances may be extremely difficult and often is inadequately performed. For a considerable number of patients, it may also be found that faulty therapy has compounded their disease.

Physical Examination

The physical examination includes a systematic examination of local areas (temporomandibular joint, head and neck), certain observations of the whole body, and radiographic examination and therapeutic tests when indicated.

Local Areas (temporomandibular joint, head and neck)

Examine for asymmetry of the face and head as well as for any irregularities that might indicate hypertrophy or atrophy of muscle(s), swelling, and evidence of traumatic injury. Scars and related traumatic injury or surgery are occasionally of importance in arriving at a diagnosis.

Observe the patterns of mandibular movements. Deviations of the mandible from smooth gliding movements may be related to occlusal interferences, fractures, muscle paralysis and temporomandibular joint disturbances.

Palpate the temporomandibular joints with the teeth in occlusion, at rest, with the jaws open wide, and during movements of the mandible. Snapping and jerky movements within the joint may be sensed even when audible sounds are not produced. Deviations of the mandible can be related to joint or occlusal interferences.

Listen for noise in the joints. Clicking and snapping of the joint(s) may be audible when severe, but may be slight and only sensed on palpation unless a stethoscope is used.

Palpate the entire side of the head and neck for soreness. A light tap on the surface may locate areas of tenderness not discerned by regular palpation. Palpate also the muscles that can be reached intraorally. Tenderness in muscles as well as in the immediate area of the joint(s) is important in the diagnosis of functional disturbances of the joints or muscles.

Do a clinical functional analysis of the masticatory system. The analysis should include an attempt to locate centric relation and occlusal interferences in centric relation as well as in lateral and protrusive excursions of the mandible. Note wear facets on the teeth, mobility of the teeth, and any indication of traumatic, unstable or unbalanced occlusion.

Look for signs of bruxism and muscle hyperactivity. The signs of bruxism have been discussed in Chapter 11. Muscle hyperactivity may be evidenced by twitching or flexing of involved muscles.

A functional analysis of the masticatory system is extremely difficult and never completely reliable in patients with traumatic temporomandibular joint arthritis and muscular hyperactivity. It has been observed at numerous times in patients with temporomandibular joint arthritis that what was initially thought to be centric relation gradually changes position during treatment until relief of pain and muscle tension is provided.[18] In some instances, a patient cannot even open his mouth enough to allow for any inspection of occlusal relationships.

Total Body Examination

The physical examination should include those observations likely to be of value in relating generalized disease to disturbances of the temporomandibular joints and muscles.

The patient's gait and posture should be observed for indications of bone and joint diseases, muscular disorders and diseases of the nervous system.

Observe the joints of fingers and other areas for signs of generalized forms of arthritis. Although not common, other forms of arthritis such as rheumatoid arthritis may also involve the temporomandibular joints.

Laboratory studies are indicated on the basis of an evaluation of signs observed in the physical examination that may relate to systemic disease, or when related to symptoms brought out in the history. Laboratory studies may occasionally be desirable for purposes of differential diagnosis.

Roentgenographic Examination

Although roentgenograms are of no direct value in the diagnosis of traumatic temporomandibular joint arthritis, they are extremely important in a differential diagnosis of other conditions that may give the same clinical signs and symptoms as traumatic temporomandibular joint arthritis.

It is of essential importance to secure roentgenograms that provide an acceptable view of the joint region (Fig. 17–1). Several roentgenographic techniques are available for this purpose. However, because of individual anatomic variation,[24] it is difficult to obtain consistently good roentgenograms of the temporomandibular joints. At least one exposure in the closed and another in wide open jaw position should be available for each joint.

The roentgenograms should be studied with regards to contour and outline of the articular surface of the condyle, the glenoid fossa and the articular tuberculum. The position of the condyle in closed and open view should be

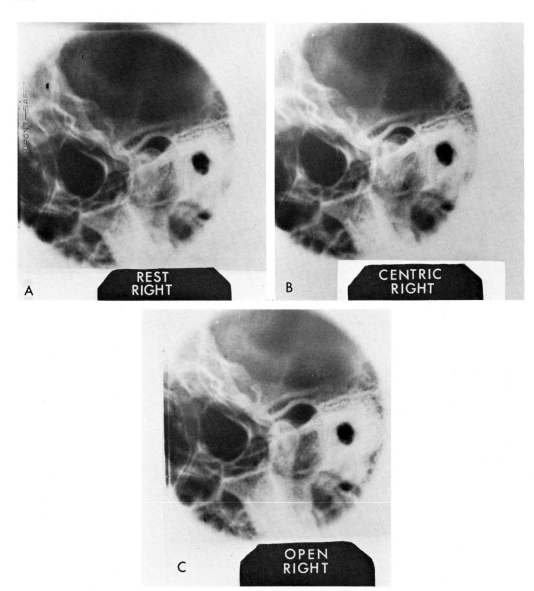

Figure 17–1. *A,* Normal temporomandibular joint with mandible in rest position and showing well-defined outline of joint structures. *B,* Normal closure in centric occlusion. The condyle is curved deeper into the glenoid fossa than in rest position. *C,* Normal opening. The degree of anterior movement of the condyle varies from person to person in normally functioning temporomandibular joints.

observed and all adjacent structures carefully studied for any evidence of pathologic changes. Too much significance has often been given to the position of the condyle in centric occlusion as an expression of distal displacement and mandibular overclosure (Fig. 17–2). Roentgenograms of the temporomandibular joints, regardless of angulation and position of exposure, are totally unreliable for the purpose of assessment of optimal condyle position in centric occlusion.[6]

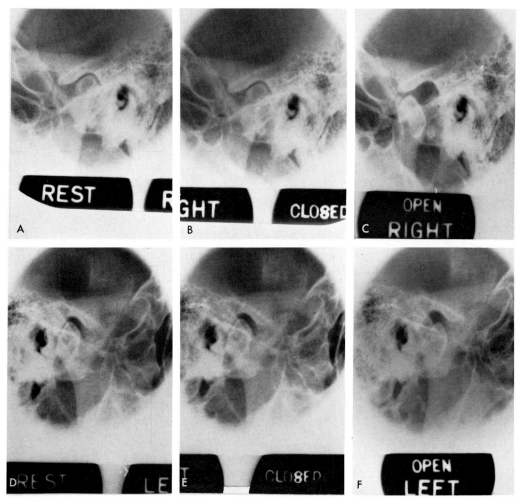

Figure 17-2. *A,* Asymptomatic right temporomandibular joint, rest position. *B,* Centric occlusion closure (note distal position of condyle). *C,* Jaw open with normal anterior condylar movement. The left temporomandibular joint of the same patient had severe symptoms of functional disturbances, viz., pain, limited and jerky jaw movements, and clicking of the joint. *D,* Rest position with the distally placed condyle the same as on the symptom-free right side. *E,* Centric occlusion with the condyle in distal position as in the symptom-free right joint. Note that the condyle moved forward from rest position to centric occlusion. Jaw muscles tend to hold condyle distally if there is pain in the joint, since this takes pressure off the painful area. *F,* Attempted full opening, but condyle is held back by splinting muscle action (female, age 53).

So-called hypermotility or subluxation of the mandible has often been diagnosed on the basis of the condyle moving anteriorly to the articulate tuberculum in maximal openings of the jaw. However, this position of the condyle is often observed as part of an entirely normal maximal opening and, if unaccompanied by any undesirable signs and symptoms, is of no clinical significance. A restriction of condylar movements in opening can be observed roentgenographically but can also be observed easily by clinical inspection (Fig. 17-2, *F*).

Roentgenograms are essential in order to rule out fractures or abnormally healed fractures; for the diagnosis of osteoarthritis, ear, sinus and paranasal disease; for diseases of the teeth and periodontal disease; for unilateral hyperplasia of the condyle;[81] and for neoplastic disease.

Therapeutic Tests

In some borderline cases (in which it may be very difficult to establish the differential diagnosis between traumatic temporomandibular joint arthritis and dysfunctional muscle symptoms and other conditions with similar manifestations), a functional occlusal therapeutic trial may be instituted, usually in the form of occlusal splints or biteplanes. However, the result of such a test is significant only if the patient can be kept free of symptoms over a long period of time. Because of the strong psychic component and the tendency for remissions and exacerbations of several of the conditions of differential diagnostic importance, it is difficult to assess the true significance of relief of symptoms in a therapeutic test. Therapeutic tests using occlusal splints or biteplanes should not be used for patients in whom headache is the main symptom and no dysfunctional joint or muscle symptoms are present, since symptomatic relief of psychic tension and headache is often obtained from any treatment that provides attention and sympathy. Whenever such patients are exposed to stressing situations, their headaches return and the dentist is often faced with a difficult problem, since the patient may conclude that since occlusal therapy once gave relief, something must still be wrong with the occlusion; he will not consider the headache to be related to his psychic tension.

SIGNS AND SYMPTOMS OF ACUTE TRAUMATIC TEMPOROMANDIBULAR JOINT ARTHRITIS AND MUSCLE SPASMS

The manifestations of acute temporomandibular joint arthritis may occur as a response to injury of extrinsic or intrinsic origin. There are no epidemiologic data available that specify the prevalence or incidence of the acute type of traumatic temporomandibular joint arthritis, since all of the published surveys include both acute and chronic conditions. The clinical manifestations of acute temporomandibular joint arthritis may include unusually sharp pain when movement of the jaw is attempted, painful restriction of mandibular movements, unusual deviation of the mandible to the involved side, varying degrees of trismus or muscle spasms, tenderness to palpation, an inability to make contact between the posterior teeth on the involved side, sometimes radiographic evidence of increased joint space, and visible swelling, although this is rare.

Manifestations of traumatic temporomandibular joint arthritis or muscle spasms in the jaw muscles may be in response to a known external traumatic injury, such as accidents or removal of impacted teeth.[44] Manifestations may come on suddenly during yawning or biting on a hard object, or the patient may awake during the night or morning with a sore jaw without any apparent reason. The onset may be related to a change in occlusal relations associated with insertion of dental restorations and appliances. It may follow change in the masticatory pattern from pericoronitis around mandibular third molar gumflaps, periodontal surgery, loss of teeth, open cavities, ill-fitting restorations, etc. Anything that changes the habitual path of mastication may throw the patient into a new path in which there are marked interferences that precipitate acute joint and muscle discomfort. It may also occur in relation to an emotional crisis without any change in occlusal relations.

Restriction of Jaw Movements

The dominating symptom of acute traumatic temporomandibular joint arthritis and acute muscle spasms is a painful restriction of mandibular movements with various degrees of trismus. There is often a sharp stabbing pain in acute cases when jaw movements are attempted. This sharp pain is followed by a dull ache, and there is often tenderness to palpation of the involved temporomandibular joint. However, there is rarely any visible swelling and no redness in the joint area. The involvement is usually unilateral, with a deviation of the mandible toward the involved side when attempts are made to open the jaw.

Inability to Make Contact

During the acute stage the patient is often unable to make contact between the posterior teeth on the involved side. There is also often roentgenologic evidence of increased temporomandibular joint space on this side. Whether this results from edematous effusion within the joint (hydroarthrosis) or is entirely the result of abnormal muscle activity and spasms is not known.

Tenderness to Palpation

In some instances of acute muscle spasms and associated pain there are no signs or symptoms directly referable to the temporomandibular joint(s). Careful palpation will usually reveal areas of soreness in the jaw muscles. Without doubt, muscle spasms and pain may originate within the muscles following sustained muscle tension which has built up during attempts to accommodate occlusal interferences. The muscle spasms and the pain resemble postural or occupational myalgias.[76] A combination of joint and muscle signs and symptoms is the usual occurrence, and the muscle spasms may have been precipitated by impulses from the injured and painful joint in an attempt to splint or restrict the jaw movement and avoid painful contact between the traumatized joint surfaces.

SIGNS AND SYMPTOMS OF CHRONIC TRAUMATIC TEMPOROMANDIBULAR JOINT ARTHRITIS AND RECURRENT MUSCLE PAIN

Most cases of chronic temporomandibular joint arthritis and recurrent dysfunctional muscle pain have a gradual onset; however, a number of acute cases of traumatic temporomandibular joint arthritis or muscle spasms, if untreated, or inadequately treated, go into a chronic stage with characteristic remission and exacerbations that are often related to the patient's emotional status or psychic tension.

Practically all reports agree that traumatic temporomandibular joint arthritis and muscle pain in the adjacent area are about four times as common in women as in men.[21, 33, 72, 76, 103] It may appear in any age group but seems to be most common between 20 and 50 years of age. Since the severity of occlusal disturbances appears to be the same for men and women, it is obvious that besides occlusion there must be other factors responsible for the development of this disorder. The symptoms include ache or dull pain, which is usually unilateral, painful restrictions of mandibular movements, unusual deviation of the jaw toward the involved side during opening of the mouth, crepitation or clicking noise in the joint(s), occasional tenderness to palpation of jaw muscles, and swelling or visible deformity, which is rare.

Pain

Pain is the most disturbing symptom, according to Campbell's survey of 1109 patients with temporomandibular joint disorders.[14] He found the most common sites of pain to be in the following descending order: (1) the temporomandibular joint area, (2) the gonial angle, (3) the ear, (4) the zygomatic arch, (5) the anterior part of the temporomandibular region, (6) the submandibular space, and (7) the suboccipital space. Pain was also found in other adjacent areas but with lesser frequency than elsewhere. The pain is usually a dull ache but may also be sharp and stabbing in character. Occasionally, the patient characterizes it as a "drawing" pain. The pain is usually unilateral, but occasionally may be bilateral when involvement of both joints occurs.

Restriction of Mandibular Movements

The second most common complaint is a painful restriction of mandibular movements and/or an inability to open the mouth to a normal extent.[33] Sometimes patients indicate that they have a "locking of the jaw" and it is necessary to massage the jaw muscles or to grasp the jaw in order to initiate further jaw movements. Hypertonus and poor muscle control are expressed by an awkward coordination of mandibular movements and a tendency to bite the tongue and cheek accidentally. A jerky movement pattern[12] can also be observed by inspection and palpation of the condyles during movements of the jaw.

Deviation of Jaw

There is usually deviation toward the involved side during opening of the mouth,[44] and that side is preferred also for mastication since these joint positions provide for minimal stress on the injured joint. For the same reason, there is usually more pain associated with jaw movements away from the involved side than toward this side, even with the teeth apart.

Tenderness to Palpation

There may be mild pain or tenderness to palpation of the posterior aspect of the condyle, but there is rarely any swelling or visible deformity. Palpation of the jaw muscles may reveal painful areas, especially along the anterior border of the masseter and the internal pterygoid muscles or at the mandibular insertion of these muscles.[86]

Crepitation

Crepitation or a clicking noise in the temporomandibular joint is another common complaint.[2,3,11,20,33,43,98,103] This condition may be accompanied by pain,[44] although crepitation or a clicking noise is more often annoying than painful. The clicking may be caused by (1) roughness or cracks on the meniscus and the articulating joint surfaces; (2) anterior or lateral subluxation of the condyle over the edge of the meniscus in wide opening or extreme lateral movement; (3) disturbed neuromuscular coordination (as seen sometimes in patients with bruxism when their mandibular teeth in contact with the maxillary teeth pass over incisal or cuspal ledges); and (4) stickiness of joint surfaces when there is inadequate lubrication with synovial fluid. This last condition is completely without pain and of no pathologic significance.

Phonograms or phonoarthrograms have been made of the noise of temporomandibular joints in persons with and without temporomandibular joint disturbances; however, there does not seem to be any characteristic sound pattern for various temporomandibular joint disturbances.[28,32]

Hypertonicity of the external pterygoid muscle[74,107] probably plays an important role in the so-called "subluxation of the temporomandibular joint," which may involve disturbed relationships between the meniscus and the condyle, with the condyle moving on the border rather than over the central aspect of the meniscus.[2,3,27,43,50,78,95] This condition was described more than 100 years ago,[20] and it is notoriously accompanied by a clicking or snapping noise. It was observed by Boman[11] that the click can also be associated with the passage of the condyle over roughness on the articulating joint surfaces.

It has been observed that most clicking or snapping noise in the temporomandibular joint will disappear following functional occlusal therapy except in cases of marked osteoarthritic deformity of the joint structures. The clicking noise associated with hypertonicity and asynchronous action of the jaw muscles will subside rapidly after occlusal therapy. However, the gritty or grinding noise associated with roughness of the joint structures (often with the jaw close to centric occlusion) may gradually decrease over a period of 4 to 6 months after the therapy as the joint structures gradually regain their normal anatomy. Since these tissues are, in part, avascular, the healing potential is poor and some cases will not regain their normal anatomic characteristics. Even so, the clicking will be much less audible after good occlusal therapy than before because of less pressure on the joint structures and smoother, better coordinated movements. A decrease in tonicity of the jaw muscles is of essential importance for all alleviation of clicking noise in the temporomandibular joint(s).

COSTEN'S SYNDROME

In 1934 Costen[23] listed a number of symptoms that he felt were caused by overclosure of the mandible following loss of teeth. The symptoms associated with the syndrome were impaired hearing (continuous or intermittent), stuffy or stopping sensations in the ears (marked about mealtimes), tinnitus, vertigo, and pain of a dull type within and about the ears. Associated with obstruction of the eustachian tube was a headache localized to the vortex occiput. Impingement of the auriculotemporal nerve and chorda tympani was also considered to cause pain and burning sensations in the throat, tongue, side of the nose and sinuses. Most of these symptoms had been described before Costen's famous article. About 1920 several investigators claimed that loss of posterior teeth without replacement could cause damage to the temporomandibular joint,[73, 100] and Monson's[60] distal displacement theory, in 1921, also included potential deafness from pressure on the ear structures by the distally displaced condyle. A similar report was published in 1920 by Wright.[112] Also published prior to Costen's were Goodfriend's[41, 42] and Decker's[25] articles listing symptoms similar to those of Costen.

Costen's syndrome (and specially his explanations for the listed symptoms) has been under severe criticism ever since its inception. It has been convincingly demonstrated by Sicher[96] and other anatomists[113] that the anatomic basis for Costen's syndrome is not acceptable. Impingement of the main branch of the auriculotemporal nerve between the condyle and the postglenoid spine cannot take place, as suggested by Costen. Neither are the impingement of chorda tympani from direct pressure on the ear structures and the closure of the eustachian tube likely to be caused by loss of posterior teeth. Schwartz[86] stated, after clinical study of 2500 patients with temporomandibular joint and muscle disturbances: "The symptoms we found were not those emphasized by Costen, nor did the symptoms comprise the complex described by him. Where individual symptoms of Costen's syndrome were met, we were unable to relate them to bite closure."

The majority of the pain symptoms listed by Costen have been shown to be "myofacial" pain,[36] with a dull ache aggravated by function or pain from traumatized joint structures. The ear symptoms listed by Costen are still controversial. There has never appeared scientific evidence which definitely has established that impairment of hearing has any relationship to mandibular overclosure or other temporomandibular joint disturbances.[19] Many attempts have been made to link temporomandibular joint and ear disturbances on an anatomic basis: Pinto,[71] by a ligament; Thonner,[104] by vascular supply from the internal maxillary artery to the inner ear passing through the fissure system of the glenoid fossa; and Carlson[15] and Myrhaug,[64, 65] by increased tonus in the tensor tympani muscle increasing the intralabyrinthine pressure through action on the ossicular chain and footplate of the stapes. It is possible that one or more of these mechanisms may explain an improvement in vertigo and tinnitus reported following occlusal therapy.[52, 53] It has also been reported that blocking a myofacial trigger mechanism in the mandibular muscles has eliminated loss of hearing, stuffiness and tinnitus in some patients.[34, 106] However, no good explanation has been offered for these observations.

Vertigo has also been produced by a myofacial trigger area in the sternocleidomastoid muscle,[108] so there may be some relationship between vertigo and dysfunctional muscle spasms in the masticatory system.

It appears that Costen's theories have almost all been disproved, and other explanations are now available for most of the symptoms that were included in his suggested "syndrome."

SIGNS AND SYMPTOMS OF OSTEOARTHRITIS OF THE TEMPOROMANDIBULAR JOINT

The local etiology and most of the signs and symptoms are the same for osteoarthritis as for traumatic arthritis of the temporomandibular joint. The systemic potential for response to repeated traumatic injury is probably the factor which determines whether a traumatic temporomandibular joint will eventually develop into osteoarthritis. This systemic factor is in some way related to age and sex, since osteoarthritis is seldom seen in patients less than 40 to 50 years of age and is seen less frequently in men than in women. The importance of local trauma in the pathogenesis of this disease is well demonstrated by the observation that a patient may have a severely deformed temporomandibular joint on one side associated with occlusal disharmony and a normal joint on the other side associated with corresponding normal occlusal relations (Fig. 17–3).

The clinical manifestations of osteoarthritis of the temporomandibular joint are essentially the same as described for chronic traumatic temporomandibular joint arthritis, with the exception of the osseous changes which may be visible and palpable as deformities of the joint. There is no direct re-

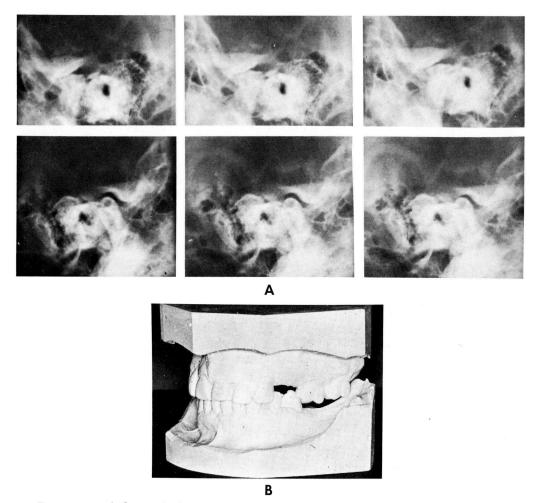

Figure 17–3. *A,* Osteoarthritis in left temporomandibular joint (upper three pictures). From left to right are rest position, centric occlusion, and centric relation. Note severe deformity of the left condyle. Lower pictures are from the right, asymptomatic and normal-appearing temporomandibular joint in the same patient and the same positions. *B,* Casts showing occlusal instability on the left side corresponding to the deformed joint. Occlusion on the other side was normal. The patient became asymptomatic after functional occlusal therapy (female, age 55).

lationship between the magnitude of the bony changes of osteoarthritis and the severity of the symptoms.[7] There may also be bony changes of osteoarthritis present without any temporomandibular joint symptoms.[30] It seems that the symptoms are to a great extent dependent upon the presence or absence of trauma at the time of observation. This is also indicated by the observation that these patients often can be made symptom-free, or at least free of pain, by functional therapy without any improvement of the pathologic changes in the joint.

It should be emphasized that osteoarthritis represents a continuation of a traumatic arthritis, and the difference in the two is more in degree than in kind. The difference is similar to that existing between simple gingivitis and periodontitis where differentiation is made on the basis of the bone involvement rather than cause, since both have the same pathogenesis. However, the differential diagnosis of osteoarthritis and traumatic arthritis is of importance since their significance, management and prognosis do differ.

The muscle symptoms accompanying osteoarthritis are similar to those of traumatic temporomandibular joint arthritis. This means that psychic tension and occlusal interferences are also of essential importance for the development and clinical manifestations of osteoarthritis of the temporomandibular joint.

ROENTGENOGRAPHIC SIGNS OF FUNCTIONAL TEMPOROMANDIBULAR JOINT DISTURBANCES

There are no characteristic or diagnostic roentgenographic signs of traumatic temporomandibular joint arthritis[35] since there are no bony changes. It has been claimed that distal displacement of the condyles could be assessed from roentgenograms (Fig. 17–2);[79] however, such interpretations are valueless because of the normal anatomic variations of the joint structures.[6] A similar statement can be made with regard to wide opening of the jaws and the placement of the condyle(s) in relation to the articular tuberculum. An anterior placement of the condyle relative to the articular tuberculum in wide opening is often seen in roentgenograms of the normal temporomandibular joint and does not necessarily indicate a subluxation of pathologic nature.[57] Some authors claim a relationship between the anatomic factors of size and shape of the condyle and fossa to temporomandibular joint disorders.[46, 55] This has not been substantiated by recent reports.[57] Restriction of movements can, of course, be seen on roentgenograms, but this can be studied better clinically. The most revealing technique for roentgenography of the joint(s) is arthrography,[67] but the method is difficult and painful. Roentgenograms are of value for differential diagnosis in that other pathologic conditions having signs and symptoms similar to traumatic temporomandibular joint arthritis may be distinguished by roentgenographic changes. Lindblom[57] has recently completed a comprehensive account of the radiography of the temporomandibular joint, and in another article Boering[10] discusses in detail various approaches to temporomandibular joint roentgenography.

Roentgenographic changes associated with osteoarthritis of the temporomandibular joint are (1) lack of definition of the anterior aspect of the condyle, (2) peripheral lipping of the bone of the condyle with flattening of the articular surface, (3) resorption of bone on the posterior aspect of the articular tuberculum toward the glenoid fossa, (4) fragmentation of the meniscus (seen only with special roentgenographic technique utilizing contrast media),[37, 67] and (5) dystrophic calcification of the meniscus (difficult to see on roentgenograms) (Fig. 17–4).

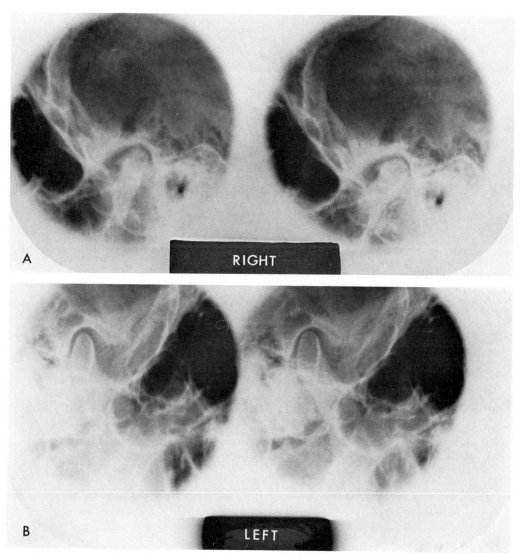

Figure 17–4. *A,* Osteoarthritis of right temporomandibular joint. There is marked deformity of condyle seen in the closed and rest jaw positions. *B,* The same patient's left, perfectly normal, temporomandibular joint. The patient obtained relief from pain and functional discomfort following prolonged use of an occlusal splint and repeated occlusal adjustments, in spite of the persistent anatomic changes in the right joint (female, age 35).

PRINCIPLES FOR DIAGNOSIS OF TRAUMATIC TEMPOROMANDIBULAR JOINT ARTHRITIS AND RELATED CONDITIONS

The logical basis for treatment of temporomandibular joint arthritis, as well as for other diseases, is to make a comprehensive diagnosis with the emphasis on differentiation and recognition of the etiologic factors for each individual case. Besides elimination of the causative factors, the problem of residual arthrodial defects has to be considered. Unfortunately, a common approach has been to treat this disease experimentally and empirically in an attempt to eliminate the symptoms without recognizing and understanding the cause and without elimination of the etiologic factors.

Any of the etiologic factors previously described in Chapter 8 may be responsible for the development of temporomandibular joint arthritis, but it is of fundamental importance that the basic role of increased muscle tonus in the pathogenesis of traumatic arthritis be understood. Except for a few patients with a history of external trauma, traumatic temporomandibular joint arthritis and associated muscle disturbances are the result of abnormal activity of the jaw muscles related to psychic tension, pain and occlusal interferences. When the functional disturbances have reached the stage that painful injury occurs, the pain will increase the muscle activity, and the increased muscle activity will increase the potential for injury, while increased injury will result in more pain, etc. As pointed out by Travell,[106] Schwartz[86] and Freese,[36] it is extremely important that this feedback mechanism be broken up by elimination of the pain, but the diagnosis and treatment should not result in only symptomatic, temporary elimination of the pain.

The diagnosis of functional disturbances of the temporomandibular joint and jaw muscles should be based on the signs and symptoms revealed during the examination and a thorough understanding of the etiology (p. 176), and the signs and symptoms previously outlined in this chapter.

Differential Diagnosis

The diagnosis of functional disturbances of the temporomandibular joints and muscles may require the diagnostic differential elimination of other disturbances which may produce confusing signs and symptoms similar to those associated with acute or chronic traumatic temporomandibular arthritis. The following disturbances should be considered in the differential diagnosis.

Rheumatoid Arthritis

Rhematoid arthritis is a systemic disease of unknown etiology. About 8 to 12 per cent of patients with systemic rheumatoid arthritis will experience an involvement of the temporomandibular joint(s) by this disease.[4, 21, 58, 68] The pathology, signs and symptoms are basically the same as found in other joints involved by the disease. Very seldom is the temporomandibular joint the only joint involved by rheumatoid arthritis. Eighty per cent of all cases occur in the age group of 25 to 50 years, with the peak at 35 to 40, and the sex ratio is 3 women to 1 man.

The management of rheumatoid arthritis is not within the realm of dentistry, but in many instances traumatic temporomandibular joint arthritis may have preceded, occurred simultaneously with, or been superimposed upon an existing rheumatoid arthritis. The signs and symptoms may then be those of traumatic temporomandibular joint arthritis.

Patients with rheumatoid arthritis elsewhere may also develop traumatic temporomandibular joint arthritis of strictly local origin which may have nothing to do with their systemic disease and will, consequently, respond very well to local functional therapy. Even patients with rheumatoid temporomandibular joint arthritis may experience some improvement from local functional therapy, since this will lessen the tension of their jaw muscles and the demand upon the involved joint. It has been observed in a few patients that rheumatoid arthritis had deformed the temporomandibular joints to the extent that the patients had extensive open bite or marked mandibular deviation.

Infective Arthritis

These arthritides are produced by infection with the various pyogenic cocci[102,110] (gonococcus, meningococcus, pneumococcus, staphylococcus and streptococcus). The infection can be either by direct extension or by the hemotogenous route. Involvement of the joint(s) results in an acute, suppurative inflammation. The synovial tissue is hyperemic, swollen, thickened, and infiltrated mainly with polymorphonuclear leukocytes. The articular cartilage may be destroyed and ankylosis may be the end result. Abscesses may form in the marrow of the subchondrial bone, and the soft periarticular structures are often acutely inflamed.

This type of arthritis may occasionally involve the temporomandibular joint following a direct extension of infection from the pterygomandibular space, mandibular osteomyelitis, and otitis media, or it may develop from a blood-borne infection, mainly gonococcal. There are violent signs and symptoms unrelated to injury. The systemic symptoms and the laboratory findings enable the differential diagnosis to be made. Be especially aware of an increase in body temperature that is commonly found associated with any kind of infection.

Tuberculous arthritis is seen mainly in children under 14 years of age and occurs chiefly as tuberculous spondylitis in patients with pulmonary tuberculosis. Syphilitic arthritis may occur at any age as a complication of either congenital or acquired disease.[49] The chances for these diseases to involve the temporomandibular joint are extremely small.

Odontalgia, Sinusitis, Myalgias

The complex system of distribution and intercommunications of the trigeminal and facial nerves accounts for the often bizarre pain patterns in the neck and head region. The actual source of irritation may often be obscured by so-called "referred" pain, which may occur at distant and seemingly unrelated sites. This phenomenon is best known among dentists from cases of pulpal involvement and pain referred from the temporomandibular joint to neck, ear, temporal region, etc., in traumatic temporomandibular joint arthritis; but this type of pain may also be referred to the joint and surrounding areas from the teeth, sinuses, ears, muscles, etc. The differential diagnosis can only be made following a thorough search for the primary site of irritation.[14, 92, 97] An excellent symposium on facial pain has been presented with the papers edited by Alling.[1] This review is recommended for further study of a complex subject.

Neuralgias

Trigeminal neuralgia or tic douloureux affecting one or more of the branches of the trigeminal nerve may also pose differential diagnostic problems.[17, 29, 45] However, the paroxysmal pain in this disease is usually quite different and more severe than the dull ache and even the occasional stabbing pain in traumatic temporomandibular joint arthritis. The sudden pain provoked by trigger zones in trigeminal neuralgia usually lasts for only a short time, rarely over 5 minutes, and this is followed by a period of freedom from pain which is in contrast to the lasting dull ache in traumatic temporomandibular joint arthritis or dysfunctional muscle pain.

Meniere's Disease

This is a disease of the semicircular canals of the ear resulting in vertigo, nausea, pallor, tinnitus, deafness and, sometimes, nystagmus.[109] In early stages of Meniere's disease tinnitus may be the only symptom present, and it may then be confused with the tinnitus which supposedly can occur in association with traumatic temporomandibular joint arthritis.[65] Sometimes the dizzy spells of Meniere's disease are attributed to temporomandibular joint disturbances.

Headache

Various types of headaches pose very difficult problems in differential diagnosis,[38] since some patients notoriously experience headaches associated with muscle tension in the masticatory system.[5] This muscle tension is a result of combined central nervous system tension and the influence of occlusal interferences.[69] The patient may also have tension headaches, vascular headaches, including migraine, hypertension headaches, posttraumatic headaches, headaches from sinus, nasal, paranasal, ear and eye diseases, fever, brain tumor, etc. Since there are so many types of headaches[111] and practically every patient also has occlusal interferences in which the psychogenic factor has great influence, it is very difficult even with therapeutic tests to assay the role of occlusion in the etiology of headaches.

Temporal Arteritis and Other Collagen Diseases

Temporal arteritis may pose a differential diagnostic problem because its symptoms may closely resemble those of traumatic temporomandibular joint arthritis.[91] A hard distended temporal artery felt by palpation may suggest this condition, but a final diagnosis ·can only be made following biopsy and microscopic examination.

Neoplasms

Neoplastic diseases may involve the temporomandibular joint and adjacent structures and produce symptoms similar to the ones described for traumatic temporomandibular joint arthritis.[8, 102] Roentgenograms may be of help for establishment of a diagnosis in such instances.

Rheumatic Fever

Rheumatic fever is an acute or chronic inflammatory disease initiated by a preceding infection by Group A hemolytic streptococci. It involves the connective tissues of various joints and many other organs. There are chances for this systemic disease, which occurs mainly in childhood, to be a differential diagnostic problem; it may be confused with arthritis of the temporomandibular joint.

Rheumatism

Nonarticular Rheumatism.   Two types are generally included; (1) fibrositis and myositis, and (2) bursitis, tendonitis and tenosynovitis. The cause of fibrositis and myositis is unknown. They may appear either as localized lesions or may, in some cases, be widely disseminated. The disease is thought by some to be caused by a metabolic physiochemical disturbance producing inflammation. It is usually seen in young or middle-aged adults and may have an insidious or sudden onset. Gout is another metabolic disturbance which may involve the temporomandibular joint.[54]

Bursitis, tendonitis and tenosynovitis are localized forms of fibrositis and may involve any area in which bursae and tendons are located. Thus, these disturbances may be a part of traumatic temporomandibular joint arthritis. In some cases, the etiology may be unknown.

The prevalence and role of nonarticular rheumatism in temporomandibular joint disease is impossible to ascertain from available literature and observations.

Psychologic Rheumatism.   This disturbance is seen in psychoneurotic persons with emotional conflicts and may be manifested as an interference with joint motion.[101] There are no joint changes present and no systemic laboratory findings. Patients receive no real benefit from analgesics, heat or physical therapy.

Angina Pectoris

The pain associated with coronary occlusion and angina pectoris radiate to the left neck and ear region and even appear to be located in the left jaw and temporomandibular joint.[35] The pain from traumatic temporomandibular joint arthritis and associated muscle spasms may also radiate to the neck and left arm and thus be confused with the pain from angina pectoris. Administration of nitroglycerin or oxygen will provide relief for angina pectoris but not for muscle or joint pain. The lack of definite temporomandibular joint symptoms and of painful areas during palpation of the masticatory system in patients with angina pectoris is also of help in the differential diagnosis.

Otitis

Pain from pathologic processes in the ear may also provide problems in differential diagnosis. In doubtful instances patients should always be referred to an otologist for diagnosis of possible ear involvement.

PRINCIPLES OF TREATMENT

In spite of the voluminous literature and almost fashionable interest in temporomandibular joint arthritis and related problems, there is no field in dentistry in which the confusion is so great as that which is concerned with the treatment of patients with these disorders. Often the treatment that a patient receives does more harm than good. Fortunately, patients with temporomandibular joint arthritis and muscle disorders often experience remissions, with relief of symptoms, with or without treatment.[56] Even irrational treatment may occasionally give apparently good results because of a concomitant natural remission of the disease coincidental with the treatment. A large number of patients also resign themselves to live with their discomfort. However, based on current knowledge of the physiology of occlusion, a rational approach has been developed for understanding and successfully treating functional disorders of the masticatory system.

The recognition and elimination of etiologic factors is the first step in the rational treatment of any disease and, obviously, this is also the first requirement for a cure of temporomandibular joint arthritis and muscle disorders. However, this is not always sufficient to achieve complete cure, since residual arthritic defects and gravely disturbed muscle function may be self-sustaining conditions even after removal of the original cause. Restitution of normal joint function or elimination of defects is not always possible.

Treatment of Acute Traumatic Temporomandibular Joint Arthritis and Muscle Spasms

Treatment of acute traumatic temporomandibular joint arthritis and muscle spasms is dependent to some extent on whether the injury causing the disturbances is of extrinsic or intrinsic origin. The treatment usually includes elimination of gross occlusal interferences by biteplanes or occlusal splints, application of moist heat, the prescription of drugs for relief of pain and muscle and psychic tension, the use of local anesthetics for severe pain and trismus to facilitate occlusal grinding, and the prescription of a soft diet.

Treatment for Injury of Extrinsic Origin

Although occlusion may not be directly related to the trauma that caused the acute traumatic temporomandibular joint arthritis, occlusion is very important for the healing and relief of symptoms. The pain following the trauma will increase the muscle activity or tonus. With the increase in basic muscle activity, occlusal interferences that previously were within the adaptive range and well tolerated may become annoying and act as triggers for further increase of muscle activity or spasms. The injury may also have changed the relations within the masticatory system and have brought on more occlusal interferences than before. A feedback from tense jaw muscles may, in such cases, prevent complete resolution of the acute injury. If not properly treated, the acute injury may develop into chronic traumatic temporomandibular joint arthritis.

Immobilization of the mandible is not needed if there is no fracture. The patient should live on a soft diet for a few days. In the case of unilateral involvement, it is less traumatic to chew on the involved side than on the other side.

For relief of pain, applications of moist heat and pain-relieving systemic drugs should be prescribed. Barbiturates should be prescribed for use at night for a period of a week. Meprobamate or Librium in small doses should be prescribed for use during the daytime in order to keep the muscle tension as low as possible during the healing of the injury. Barbiturates and meprobamates are administered in order to keep the central nervous system effect upon muscle tension at a minimum. Furthermore, it is important to remove gross occlusal interferences if the patient can open the mouth sufficiently, since such interferences will contribute to muscle tension.

If the patient has severe pain and trismus, it may be advisable to inject a local anesthetic such as Xylocaine into the painful area.[88] The anesthetic breaks up, at least temporarily, the feedback involving the pain and the muscle spasms and enables the patient to open the mouth so the operator can eliminate the major occlusal discrepancies. No attempt should be made to do a comprehensive occlusal adjustment at this stage of treatment because the joint and its function have been altered by the trauma, and the muscles are not functioning normally.

The outlined management will usually give almost complete relief of symptoms in a few days. The need for further occlusal therapy depends on whether the symptoms disappear after a couple of weeks. If there are residual symptoms of discomfort or pain at that time, the patient should be given the same treatment as patients with chronic traumatic temporomandibular joint arthritis (with or without muscle symptoms).

Treatment for Injury of Spontaneous or Intrinsic Origin

Acute intrinsic traumatic temporomandibular joint arthritis and painful muscle spasms may occur suddenly without any change in occlusion or they may be precipitated by occlusal changes. The patient may indicate that the pain came suddenly when yawning, biting on an apple or under other circumstances of opening the mouth widely. The pain may have started as a sprain associated with subluxation or even luxation. In other instances, the patient may complain of awaking from sleep with a sore jaw. Sometimes the symptoms are initiated by faultily constructed dental restorations and appliances or misguided attempts at occlusal adjustment.

Since an acutely traumatized joint and spastic muscles are involved, it is important to provide an environment that is conducive to healing and relief of muscle spasms and pain. The same management, therefore, should be followed for these patients as that outlined for patients with externally caused disorders.

Patients with intrinsic trauma or spontaneous muscle spasms almost always had an abnormally increased muscle activity prior to the injury. Subluxation and luxation of this type are the result of a snapping action of hypertonic or spastic jaw muscles. A careful history will usually reveal that patients have had clicking of the temporomandibular joint before the pain started and also, practically always, have signs and symptoms of bruxism.[76]

Although the pain symptoms may subside completely following the initial palliative treatment, or even without treatment, these patients are apt to have recurrences of their symptoms unless they receive a complete occlusal therapy. As soon as the acute symptoms have subsided following the initial treatment, these patients should routinely have a complete occlusal adjustment or any other dental therapy that may be needed in order to give them a stable, well balanced occlusion.

Treatment of Chronic Temporomandibular Joint Arthritis and Functional Muscle Disturbances

Various types of therapeutic procedures have been used for treatment of chronic temporomandibular joint arthritis and related conditions. Some of these procedures are indicated while others are contraindicated and even harmful. The most commonly advocated procedures are use of occlusal biteplanes and splints, occlusal adjustment, occlusal reconstruction, immobilization, muscle relaxing exercises, periodontal and dental therapy, barbiturates, muscle relaxants and other drugs, heat or diathermy, sclerosing solutions, psychotherapy, and surgical therapy.

The treatment should start with an explanation to the patient about the nature of his disorder and the close relationship between the local and psychic factors that are causing the symptoms.

Principles for Successful Treatment

There are three principles involved in successful treatment of traumatic temporomandibular joint arthritis and muscle pain: elimination of occlusal and temporomandibular joint disharmony, lowering of psychic tension, which is the main cause of the abnormally high muscle tonus, and elimination of pain and discomfort from other causes in the oral region.

For an optimal result, all these approaches should be considered, but by far the most practical and successful avenue of treatment is elimination of the functional disharmony between the occlusion and the temporomandibular joint. However, elimination of pain or discomfort and psychic tension will also, to a great extent, enhance the favorable prognosis.

The occlusion is the part of the etiologic complex that the dentist should be best qualified to treat. If it is possible to eliminate the occlusal interferences acting as trigger factors to the functional disturbances, this treatment will usually cure the disease. Also, in some instances, when the result of the occlusal therapy is less than perfect, the occlusal relationship may be brought within the adaptive tolerance level of the patient and will, thereby, eliminate the dysfunctional manifestations.

Occlusal Biteplanes and Splints

Biteplanes or occlusal splints, as described in Chapter 11, are of great value in the functional treatment of temporomandibular joint and muscle disorders. A simple Sved biteplane may give relief of symptoms after a few days and nights of constant use.[72] The major and obvious occlusal interferences should be removed at the time of insertion of the biteplane. However, a much better appliance is the occlusal splint (p. 248).

A biteplane may eliminate the disturbing input upon the neuromuscular mechanism from occlusal interferences in centric and balancing excursion.[70] This facilitates muscle relaxation and decreases the dysfunctional muscle forces.[51] It also eliminates the misguiding influence upon jaw movements from occlusal interferences so the condyles are no longer forced into a traumatic position during closure or lateral excursions. This decrease in muscle tonus and magnitude of the forces, combined with elimination of faulty guidance both from occlusion and traumatized structures in the temporomandibular joints, allows the mandible to seek a normal position, with proper balance between muscles and temporomandibular joint. The occlusion can then be adjusted to the pain-free, normally functioning temporomandibular joint in less time and fewer appointments than would be needed without the biteplane.

Biteplanes of the Sved type should not be used continuously for several weeks since they may initiate tooth movements which may complicate the occlusal therapy greatly. Properly made, and used only during transient periods of tension such as premenstrual tension, these appliances do no harm; but the need for prolonged use should be eliminated by proper occlusal therapy.

For patients who do not obtain relief of their symptoms from the Sved biteplane and for patients with few remaining teeth, flat occlusal splints should be made (Chapter 11). These appliances eliminate all occlusal interferences, including the working and protrusive excursions not included in the Sved biteplane. The main advantage of the occlusal splint is that it does not act as an orthodontic appliance. After such a splint has been used continuously for 2 or 3 weeks, the patient's occlusion should be adjusted and the splint used only if the pain recurs, or if the teeth are extremely worn down. In cases of severe traumatic temporomandibular joint arthritis the patients may have to use such occlusal splints for as long as 2 to 3 months before full relief of pain is achieved.

The flat occlusal splint principles are also used for patients with complete dentures and functional disorders of the masticatory system, if the patients are not willing to go without the dentures till their symptoms have subsided. A very few will have symptoms even without teeth or dentures. For denture patients, or edentulous patients in general, the flat occlusal biteplane is used in the mandible against the maxillary denture and adjusted until it allows for free movements in every direction. Relations for new dentures or reconstruction should not be recorded until the patient has been free of symptoms for 3 to 4 weeks.

Faulty Occlusal Splints and Onlays. The common practice of constructing bite-raising onlays in the molar and bicuspid regions for patients with temporomandibular joint arthritis and associated disorders should definitely be abandoned. These appliances usually lead to intrusion of the posterior teeth and extrusion of front teeth, subsequent occlusal interferences with the onlays in the mouth, and a mutilated occlusion when the onlays are removed. Without doubt, temporomandibular joint pain can be eliminated by any biteplane or splint that eliminates the previous occlusal interferences; posterior onlays may also temporarily serve that purpose. However, the common rationale for the use of posterior onlays or "pivots"[89] is founded upon a mechanistic concept of distribution of stresses upon the jaw and the temporomandibular joint based on the following observations: When a patient bites on a cotton roll in the molar region on the side of a painful temporomandibular joint, the pain will subside because pressure is taken off the joint of the working side. It is also evident that the muscle pattern of the masticatory system is arranged in such a way that great pull can be applied on the mandible by the muscles without much pressure on the temporomandibular joint if the occlusal impact is in the molar regions. Therefore, arranging the occlusion in such a way that the impact will be in the molar region would protect the temporomandibular joint from heavy forces.

Unfortunately, the occlusal pivot therapy lacks appreciation for the physiology of the occlusion and the jaw muscles. In the first place, it is futile, at least in the natural dentition, to raise the bite on a pivot since the normal tendency for the masticatory system is to re-establish occlusal or incisal contact for all the teeth, and to re-establish the vertical dimension that is optimal for the individual with his particular muscle tonus, etc. That a patient can temporarily adapt to an increase of vertical dimension in the molar region does not by any means indicate that this new vertical dimension is ideal. Teeth can notoriously be intruded in a slow painless way and a normal balance re-established between the tonus of the jaw muscles and the patient's interocclusal space. But in the meantime the anterior teeth have erupted and, as the intrusion of the posterior teeth catches up with and goes beyond eruption of the anterior teeth, occlusal interferences will always develop. Thus, the short term relief of pain is turned into a loss because a much greater occlusal disharmony exists than before the treatment.

That such treatment as occlusal onlays is not needed in order to obtain relief from pain is evident, since pain can also be relieved by anterior biteplanes (which mechanically should result in greater stress on the temporomandibular joints) with a flat occlusal splint with even stress on all the teeth, or with occlusal adjustment providing even stress on all the teeth. Relief of pain is obtained by all these methods because the malpositioning of the mandible by the occlusal interferences is eliminated and the traumatized area within the joint is thereby relieved from the undue pressure. However, even more important is that fact that the elimination of the interferences stops the input to the neuromuscular mechanism from the faulty occlusal relations and thereby decreases the abnormal muscle tension and the tendency for muscle spasms. In this respect, much less occlusal force is applied in empty jaw closure, and the tendency for bruxism with the most undesirable forces is greatly reduced.

In order to re-emphasize some of the warnings about faulty occlusal splints and to explain a method to overcome the undesirable effects from such splints, the following case report is presented in an abbreviated form.

Case History.   *Past history.*   A 43 year old female, Mrs. X, came for diagnosis and treatment of pain in the temporomandibular joints. Her chief complaint consisted of pain in both joints, particularly on the left side. She had suffered from intermittent pain of the temporomandibular joints for 10 or 11 years, and had had several bite-raising appliances placed on the posterior teeth during that time. Following each bite-raising procedure she had been fairly free of joint symptoms for 3 to 6 months. When the symptoms recurred, new onlays or appliances were made and Mrs. X again had a period of freedom from symptoms. During the years of treatment, several of the posterior teeth became loose and sore under the appliances, and these teeth were extracted after root canal therapy failed to relieve the soreness.

Mrs. X had been told to continue to wear the appliances and not to concern herself with the loss of the teeth. At the time she came for diagnosis and treatment she could not recall how many times these appliances had been remade. About one and one-half years prior to her first visit she was told that the only treatment that could be advised would be extraction of all maxillary teeth and construction of a complete maxillary denture against a lower partial denture. She was also advised that it would be even better for her occlusion if a complete lower denture were made. When Mrs. X refused that treatment plan, she was told that it was the only treatment that could be done short of surgery to the joint. However, she would not accept dentures or surgery and suffered from almost constant pain for the one and one-half years prior to coming to us for diagnosis and treatment.

Clinical Examination. Mrs. X was wearing both maxillary and mandibular onlay types of bite-raising appliances (Fig. 17–5, *A, B, C*). When she closed her jaws with the appliances removed there was an opening of 4 or 5 mm. in the bicuspid region (Fig. 17–5, *D*). The bicuspids had a high degree of mobility and were moderately sore to percussion. The gingival crevices were deepened as a result of the intrusion of the teeth, but the epithelial attachment was at the cemento-enamel junction.

The left temporomandibular joint was slightly tender to palpation. The opening movement of the mandible was jerky and irregular, with clicking noises in both joints, and there was a deviation to the left when a wide opening of the jaws was attempted. The opening movements were very painful. Roentgenograms of both joints appeared normal.

Diagnosis. Chronic traumatic temporomandibular joint arthritis.

Treatment. The patient's appliances were discarded and an acrylic occlusal splint was made (Fig. 17–5, *E*). She was instructed to wear the splint as much as possible. Alternating areas of relief were made in the acrylic which would provide space for the bicuspids to erupt back to their normal position. The appliance was designed so that occlusal pressure would be maintained on the front teeth. The bicuspids became firm in about 3 to 4 weeks, and erupted into contact in 3 to 4 months (Fig. 17–5, *F*). The maxillary teeth erupted at a much faster rate than the mandibular teeth, but the end result was controlled by the space provided in the acrylic splint.

The pain subsided immediately after the splint was inserted, and the opening movements of the jaw gradually became normal over a period of 3 months. When the bicuspids reached occlusal contact, the occlusion was finally adjusted and crowns were made for all her remaining posterior teeth (Fig. 17–5, *G, H, I*). These crowns were made to fit her centric relation and to conform to her cuspid guidance in lateral excursions. There were no balancing side contacts. There was no need for either esthetic or functional reasons to replace the teeth distally to the remaining second bicuspids; thus, no removable or distal extension appliances were made. The reconstruction was completed one-half year after treatment was started. After treatment Mrs. X was observed for 5 years and did not have a single recurrence of temporomandibular joint pain, and the function of her masticatory system remained excellent.

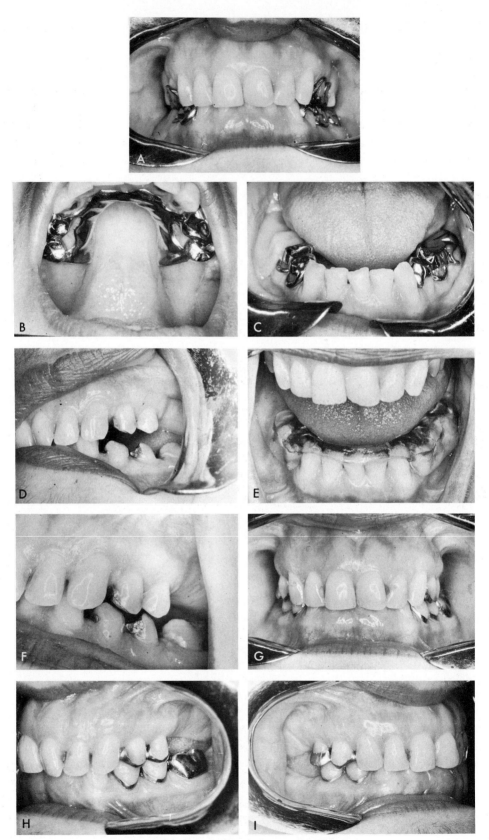

Figure 17–5. See legend on opposite page.

Occlusal Adjustment

The functional occlusal therapy may start with an occlusal adjustment, but is most often postponed until the patient has used an occlusal splint and had relief of symptoms. The occlusal adjustment emphasizes removal of premature occlusal contacts with the mandible in centric relation and elimination of balancing side interferences.[55, 94] The adjustment is carried out according to the principles discussed in Chapter 13. This therapy can be ultimately successful only if there are sufficient teeth present for the establishment of a stable occlusion with even stress distribution after completion of the adjustment. The adjustment should be done in several short appointments, with 2 or 3 days between the first two or three appointments and a couple of weeks between subsequent appointments. Both centric relation and the paths of jaw movements change as the pain and muscle tension subside, and the normal centric relation for the patient cannot be established or recorded until all the disturbing symptoms and abnormal muscle activities have been eliminated.[18] Only then will the condyles assume the ideal seat against the meniscus in the glenoid fossa. Undue pressure on the mandible or extensive manipulation by the operator should be avoided if there is considerable joint pain present.

A common mistake in treatment is to terminate the occlusal adjustment too quickly following disappearance of the initial symptoms. When such patients do come back with recurring symptoms, one will often find that the last molars are in premature contact in centric relation or interfere in balance in lateral excursions. It appears that the condyles settle higher up and probably slightly forward in the glenoid fossa after the initial symptoms have been relieved and, thus, the molar interferences develop. This phenomenon is probably the result of changes in proprioceptive guidance from the temporomandibular joint ligaments following elimination of pain. The occlusal adjustment therapy should not be terminated until the centric relation is reproducible and the occlusion stable, with 4 weeks between the last two appointments. If the occlusion cannot be stabilized by adjustment and new interferences keep appearing, there is an obvious need for restorative procedures or new dental appliances.

Occlusal Reconstruction

In many patients with functional disorders of the masticatory system, dental restorations and replacement of lost teeth are needed in order to establish and maintain a well balanced stable occlusion. However, the common practice of "raising the bite" to compensate for alleged loss of vertical dimension

---

Figure 17–5. Traumatic temporomandibular joint arthritis. *A, B* and *C,* Onlay type of bite-raising appliances, which had been remade several times during the last 8 years, provided only transient relief of pain. *D,* With the appliances out and the patient biting together there was an opening of 4 to 5 mm. in the bicuspid region. *E,* An occlusal splint was made over the mandibular teeth and provision was made for the teeth to move back to their normal position. *F,* After 3 to 4 months the bicuspids were making contact. *G, H* and *I,* Final reconstruction by gold crowns soldered together (female, age 43).

is usually contraindicated since the symptoms can be brought under control by proper occlusal therapy.[59,85] Furthermore, raising the bite will often lead to intrusion of the posterior teeth, with compounded occlusal problems, unless it is done on all the teeth; even then, the neuromuscular acceptance of a decrease in interocclusal space is unpredictable and becomes more critical the more the bite is raised.

Permanent restorative, reconstructive or prosthetic appliances should not be inserted until a month after all pain and discomfort have subsided in order to be assured that the recorded jaw relations represent normal functional relationships. The vertical dimension should, as much as possible, be restored to the patient's previous interocclusal space, unless an increase in vertical dimension is needed to provide space for restorations and a satisfactory esthetic and functional result.

Immobilization

Immobilization of the mandible is never indicated in the treatment of chronic functional disorders. The only time this procedure should be considered is at the initial stage of the treatment of habitual luxation of the temporomandibular joint. Although immobilization may give temporary relief of symptoms, the pain usually will reoccur after the ligatures are removed. Also, this treatment has an unnecessary factor of discomfort that can easily be avoided by functional therapy.

Muscle Relaxing Exercises

Various forms of muscle relaxing exercises have been recommended for treatment of temporomandibular joint and muscle dysfunction.[13,83,86,90] Since this therapy will not eliminate any occlusal trigger factors, and will have only a moderate influence upon psychic tension, the main beneficial effect is upon the local muscle spasms and their associated symptoms. As supportive therapy, in addition to functional occlusal therapy, muscle exercises may occasionally have some value, but when used as the only form of therapy they fail to eliminate the cause of the disorders and will, therefore, in most instances lead to a recurrence of symptoms.

Periodontal Therapy

Any dental and periodontal therapy that eliminates pain and discomfort in the mouth will have a tendency to lower the muscle tonus and thereby support functional occlusal therapy. However, such therapy is rarely sufficient in itself to be of primary importance in the treatment of temporomandibular joint disorders.

Drug Therapy

Barbiturates, muscle relaxants and tranquilizers have all been recommended for the treatment of functional disorders.[9,82] All these drugs may give temporary relief of symptoms as a result of lowering of muscle tonus, either by influence on the fusimotor system or through effect on the peripheral neuro-muscular mechanism. Again, these drugs should only be used as supportive measures to functional occlusal therapy. In most cases of chronic disorders it is undesirable to prescribe tranquilizers, since these patients often have long-standing psychic tension problems which may easily make them seek more drugs and may eventually pose the problem of addiction.

Another form of symptomatic muscle or joint therapy is injection or surface application of anesthetics.[40,87,105] Such therapy may facilitate functional therapy by breaking up muscle spasms and relieving trismus, thus allowing the occlusal disharmony to be corrected. Although an anesthetic may break up an acute attack of muscle spasm or eliminate the "splinting" of an injured temporomandibular joint, it will fail to eliminate the cause of the spams or splinting of muscles. Thus, a new combination of psychic tension and the still-present occlusal interferences will precipitate another painful attack.

Injections of hydrocortisone or hyaluronidase into and around the joints are other forms of symptomatic treatments for relief of pain and restricted mandibular movement.[26,39,47,48] Since this treatment also fails to eliminate the cause of the pain, the recurrence will commonly follow a period of temporary relief of 1 to 3 weeks. The only justification for such therapy is the temporary relief of temporomandibular joint pain and trismus so functional therapy may more easily be instituted.[22] However, these injections have an unpredictable and sometimes very painful effect on the joints; psychologically they may have an undesirable effect upon some patients, who come to believe that they only need further injections instead of complicated occlusal therapy. Whenever the patient can open his mouth enough to allow occlusal adjustment or construction of a biteplane, this is preferable to any injection therapy, and if he cannot open it at all, Xylocaine injections into the painful areas are used so access can be gained for the functional therapy.

Heat

The application of heat or use of diathermy will result in hyperemia with increased circulation in the temporomandibular joint and adjacent areas with muscle spasms. Some relief from severe pain may thus be obtained by enhanced removal of noxious products from injured tissues. However, such relief of symptoms without elimination of cause will not provide a cure, and the pain will recur subsequent to new injuries. Heat should, therefore, be used only as a palliative adjunct until functional therapy can be instituted.

X-ray therapy for pain in the temporomandibular joint is contraindicated because of its accumulative harmful effect, although such therapy may also provide temporary relief of pain resulting from hyperemia.

Sclerosing Solutions

Sclerosing solutions should never be used for the treatment of traumatic temporomandibular joint arthritis or muscle spasms.[66, 84] The unpredictable damage to the joints by such agents makes future functional therapy very difficult, and the end result commonly is a deformed joint with restricted jaw movements. There is no sensible rationale for the use of these agents except perhaps in the most persistent cases of habitual luxation after all other forms of treatment have failed. No case in which a sclerosing solution was needed has ever been seen by us, so this form of therapy is not recommended.

Psychotherapy

Psychotherapy has to be considered a rational treatment since it will lower the muscle tonus and increase the patient's adaptive capacity to occlusal interferences.[61] However, it is often very difficult for a dentist to assess the psychic or psychoneurotic state of a patient with complaints referable to the head and neck region. Thus, the dentist should be very careful about involving himself in psychotherapy beyond the stage of simple counseling.[80]

If the initial interview reveals a potentially dangerous psychoneurosis, the patient should be referred for psychiatric care as soon as possible and before any local therapy is attempted. However, in many instances in which patients obviously could benefit from psychotherapy, they are not ready to seek psychiatric help or to accept referral to a psychiatrist. In such cases, counseling combined with some local therapy may be indicated in order to convince the patient that there is a close connection between his symptoms and his psychic or emotional problems, and that complete elimination of his symptoms will require psychotherapy. It should be emphasized that of all patients with functional disturbances of the masticatory system, less than 5 per cent actually are in need of psychotherapy. Although the psychic factors are of extreme importance in the etiology of these disorders, almost all the patients can be successfully treated by elimination of the local dysfunctional trigger factors, which is much easier and quicker than psychotherapy.

Surgical Therapy

Surgical therapy should not be used for the treatment of traumatic temporomandibular joint arthritis and related disorders. There is no acceptable rationale for such therapy, and controlled observations over a prolonged period of time have revealed that most patients are worse after meniscectomy than before.[63] Attempts to provide surgically a condylar guidance which is acceptable to the occlusion (rather than adjusting the occlusion to fit the temporomandibular joint) have been made by various forms of condylectomies or plastic surgery of the articular tuberculum.[62] This treatment is an unnecessarily crude and unpredictable procedure, especially since the majority of these patients can be cured easily by adequate occlusal therapy. Recommended muscle surgery[31] also seems contraindicated for treatment of functional disorders. Only in patients with extreme deformity and severe limitation of functional movements,[77] or with consistent habitual luxation, should surgical therapy be considered; even then, only after all attempts at functional therapy have failed.

Treatment of Osteoarthritis of the Temporomandibular Joints

The treatment of osteoarthritis of the temporomandibular joint(s) is essentially the same as the treatment of chronic traumatic temporomandibular joint arthritis. Although functional therapy will not cure the deformities of the joint(s), it will often provide relief of symptoms and restore normal masticatory activity. Many persons actually have osteoarthritis of the temporomandibular joint(s) without having symptoms.[30] The prognosis of functional therapy is not necessarily dependent upon the degree of joint changes; viz., patients with severe joint changes may respond very favorably to treatment, while those patients with minimal changes may respond less favorably.

Although patients with osteoarthritis may become free of pain and discomfort following treatment, there often will be persistence of signs of the disease such as clicking joint(s), and jerky movements of the joint(s) and mandible. Some of these patients may require the use of occlusal splints for an indefinite period of time. Surgical therapy to correct the deformity of the condyles or condylectomy is very seldom, if ever, indicated as a treatment of osteoarthritis.

REFERENCES

1. Alling, C. C. (Ed.): Facial Pain. Philadelphia, Lea and Febiger, 1968.
2. Axhausen, G.: Das Kiefergelenkknacken und seine Behandlung. Deutsche. Ztschr. Chir., *232*:238, ·1931.
3. Bauerle, J. E., and Archer, W. H.: Incidence of subluxation of the temporomandibular joint. J. Am. Dent. A., *43*:434, 1951.
4. Bayles, T. B., and Russell, L. A.: The temporomandibular joint in rheumatoid arthritis. J. Am. Dent. A., *28*:533, 1941.
5. Berlin, R., and Dessner, L.: Bruxism and chronic headache. Odont. Tskr., *68*:261, 1960.
6. Berry, D. C.: The relationship between some anatomical features of the human mandibular condyle and its appearance on radiographs. Arch. Oral Biol., *2*:203, 1960.
7. Blackwood, H. J. J.: Arthritis of the mandibular joint. Brit. Dent. J., *115*:317, 1963.
8. Blackwood, H. J. J.: Metastatic carcinoma of the mandibular condyle. Oral Surg., *9*:1318, 1956.
9. Block, L. S.: Tensions and intermaxillary relations. J. Prosth. Dent., *4*:204, 1954.
10. Boering, G.: Arthrosis of the temporomandibular joint. I. Clinical symptoms and radiological devices. Nederl. T. Tandheilk, *74*:79, 1967.
11. Boman, K. A.: Temporomandibular joint arthrosis and its treatment by extirpation of the disk; a clinical study. Acta chir. scandinav., Suppl. 118, 1947.
12. Brussell, I. J.: Temporomandibular joint diseases: Differential diagnosis and treatment. J. Am. Dent. A., *39*:532, 1949.

13. Bundgaard-Jörgensen, F.: Afslapningsövelser som led i behandlingen af habituelle dysfunktioner i mastikationsapparatet. Odont. Tskr., *58*:448, 1950.
14. Campbell, J.: Distribution and treatment of pain in temporomandibular arthrosis. Brit. Dent. J., *105*:393, 1958.
15. Carlson, S. D.: A possible explanation of dizziness in Costen's syndrome. Am. J. Orthodont., *41*:470, 1955.
16. Carraro, J. J., Caffesse, R. G., and Albano, E. A.: Temporomandibular joint syndrome. Oral Surg., *28*:54, 1969.
17. Cohen (Lord of Birkenhead): Facial neuralgias. Brit. Dent. J., *107*:9, 1959.
18. Cohn, L. A.: Factors of dental occlusion pertinent to the restorative and prosthetic problem. J. Prosth. Dent., *9*:256, 1959.
19. Coleman, R. D.: Temporomandibular joint: Relation of the retrodiskal zone to Meckel's cartilage and lateral pterygoid muscle. J. Dent. Res., *49*:626, 1970.
20. Cooper, A. P.: Treatise on Dislocations and Fractures of the Joints. London, J. & A. Churchill, Ltd., 1842, p. 393.
21. Copland, J.: Diagnosis of mandibular joint dysfunction. Oral Surg., *13*:1106, 1960.
22. Costen, J. B.: Classification and treatment of temporomandibular joint problems. Ann. Otol. Rhin. & Laryng., *65*:35, 1956.
23. Costen, J. B.: Syndrome of ear and sinus symptoms dependent upon disturbed function of the temporomandibular joint. Ann. Otol. Rhin. & Laryng., *43*:1, 1934.
24. Craddock, F. W.: Radiography of the temporomandibular joint. J. Dent. Res., *32*:302, 1953.
25. Decker, J. C.: Traumatic deafness as a result of retrusion of condyles of the mandible. Ann. Otol. Rhin. & Laryng., *34*:519, 1925.
26. Dessner, L.: Hyaluronidasbehandling av käkledsarthroses. Svensk. Tand. Tidskr., *49*:187, 1956.
27. Dixon, A. D.: Structure and functional significance of the intraarticular disc of the human temporomandibular joint. Oral Surg., *15*:48, 1962.
28. Ekensten, B.: Jamförande undersökningar av 400 St. käkleder i klinisket, röntgenologiskt och fonogram—metriskthänseende. Odont. Tidskr., *63*:18, 1955.
29. Engler, G. L.: Primary atypical facial neuralgias: An hysterical conversion symptom. Psychosom. Med., *13*:375, 1951.
30. Ericson, S., and Lundberg, M.: Structural changes in the finger, wrist, and temporomandibular joints. A comparative radiologic study. Acta. odont. Scand., *26*:111, 1968.
31. Eschler, J.: Elektrophysiologische und pathologische Untersuchungen des Kausystems. Deutsche Zahnärztl. Ztschr., *14*:39, 1959.
32. Findlay, I. A., and Kilpatrick, S. J.: An analysis of the sounds produced by the mandibular joint. J. Dent. Res., *39*:1163, 1960.
33. Foged, J.: Temporomandibular arthrosis. Lancet, *2*:1209, 1949.
34. Freese, A. S.: Costen's syndrome. A reinterpretation. A. M. A. Arch. Otolaryng., *67*:410, 1958.
35. Freese, A. S., and Scheman, P.: Management of Temporomandibular Joint Problems. St. Louis, The C. V. Mosby Co., 1962.
36. Freese, A. S.: The temporomandibular joint and myofascial trigger areas in the dental diagnosis of pain. J. Am. Dent. A., *59*:448, 1959.
37. Frenkel, G.: Untersuchungen mit der Kombination arthrographie und tomographie zur Darstellung des Discus articularis des menschen. D. Z. Z., *20*:1261, 1965.
38. Friedman, A. P., and Merrit, H. H.: Headache: Diagnosis and Treatment. Philadelphia, F. A. Davis Co., 1959.
39. Gärtner, F., and Preis, H.: Die Intra-artikuläre Hydrocortisontherapie bei Erkrankungen des Kiefergelenkes. Deutsche Zahnärztl. Ztschr., *11*:953, 1956.
40. Gelb, H., and Arnold, G. E.: Syndromes of the head and neck of dental origin: I. Pain caused by mandibular dysfunction. J. Dent. Med., *14*:201, 1959.
41. Goodfriend, D. J.: Dysarthrosis and subarthrosis of the mandibular articulation. Dent. Cosmos, *74*:523, 1932.
42. Goodfriend, D. J.: Symptomatology and treatment of abnormalities of the mandibular articulation (normal). Dent. Cosmos, *75*:844; 947; 1106; 1933.
43. Götte, H.: Zur Frage des intermediären Kiefergelenkknackens. Deutsche Zahnärztl. Ztschr., *15*:1629, 1960.

44. Hankey, G. T.: Temporomandibular arthrosis. An analysis of 150 cases. Brit. Dent. J., *97*: 249, 1954.
45. Harris, W.: The Facial Neuralgias. London, Humphrey Milford, Oxford University Press, 1937.
46. Hausser, E.: Der Aufban des Kiefergelenkes bei den verschiedenen Gebissanomalien. Deutsche Zahn-, Mund- und Kieferh'k., *16*:177; 266; 1953.
47. Henkel, G. H.: The role and applicability of hyaluronidase in clinical dentistry. Oral Surg., *9*:463, 1956.
48. Henny, F. A.: Intra-articular injection of hydrocortisone into the temporomandibular joint. J. Oral Surg., *12*:314, 1954.
49. Heuser, H.: Röntgenologische Untersuchungen über die Erkrankungen im Bereich des Kiefergelenkes. Deutsche Zahn-, Mund- und Kieferh'k., *14*:97, 1951.
50. Ireland, V. E.: The problem of the "clicking jaw." Roy. Soc. Med. Sect. Odont. Proc., *44*: 363, 1951.
51. Jarabak, J. R.: Electromyographic analysis of muscular and temporomandibular joint disturbances due to imbalances in occlusion. Angle Orthodont., *24*:170, 1956.
52. Kelly, H. T., and Goodfriend, D. J.: Medical significance of equilibration of the masticating mechanism. J. Prosth. Dent., *10*:496, 1960.
53. Kelly, H. T., and Goodfriend, D. J.: Vertigo attributable to dental and temporomandibular joint causes. J. Prosth. Dent., *14*:159, 1964.
54. Kleinman, H. Z., and Ewbank, R. L.: Gout of the temporomandibular joint. Report of three cases. Oral Surg., *27*:281, 1969.
55. Kyes, F. M.: Temporomandibular joint disorders. J. Am. Dent. A., *59*:1137, 1959.
56. Lindblom, G.: Disorders of the temporomandibular joint. Causal factors and the value of temporomandibular joint radiographs in their diagnosis and therapy. Acta odont. scandinav., *11*:61, 1953.
57. Lindblom, G.: Anatomy and function of the temporomandibular joint. Acta odont. scandinav., *17*:7, Suppl. 18, 1960.
58. Markowitz, H. A., and Gerry, R. G.: Temporomandibular joint disease. Oral Surg., *2*:1309, 1949.
59. Miller, S. C.: The practical solution to the prevention and cure of temporomandibular joint disturbances. J. Dent. Med., *8*:43, 1953.
60. Monson, G. S.: Impaired function as a result of closed bite. Nat. Dent. A. J., *8*:833, 1921.
61. Moulton, R.: Psychiatric considerations in maxillofacial pain. J. Am. Dent. A., *51*:408, 1955.
62. Myrhaug, H.: A new method of operation for habitual dislocation of the mandible. Acta odont. scandinav., *9*:246, 1951.
63. Myrhaug, H.: Etterundersökelse av opererte kjeveledd for arthrose-Kasuistikk. Norsk. Tandl. Tidsk., *63*:313, 1953.
64. Myrhaug, H.: Funksjonelle kjevelidelser med öresymptomer. Norsk. Tandl. Tidsk., *64*:61, 1954.
65. Myrhaug, H.: Parafunctions in gingival mucosa as cause of an otodental syndrome. Quint. Int., *1*:81, 1970.
66. Neuner, O.: Eine Behandlungsmethode der habituellen Luxation und Subluxation des Kiefergelenkes. Deutsche Zahn-, Mund- und Kieferh'k., *28*:215, 1958.
67. Nørgaard, F.: Temporomandibular Arthrography. Copenhagen, Einar Munksgaard, 1947.
68. Oshrain, H. I., and Sackler, A.: Involvement of the temporomandibular joint in a case of rheumatoid arthritis. Oral Surg., *8*:1039, 1955.
69. Perry, H. T., Jr.: Facial, cranial and cervical pain associated with dysfunction of the occlusion and articulations of the teeth. Angle Orthodont., *26*:121, 1956.
70. Perry, H. T., Jr.: Muscular changes associated with temporomandibular joint dysfunction. J. Am. Dent. A., *54*:644, 1957.
71. Pinto, O. F.: A new structure related to the temporomandibular joint and middle ear. J. Prosth. Dent., *12*:95, 1962.
72. Posselt, U.: Physiology of Occlusion and Rehabilitation. Philadelphia, F. A. Davis Co., 1962.
73. Prentiss, H. J.: A preliminary report upon the temporo-mandibular articulation in the human type. Dent. Cosmos, *60*:505, 1918.
74. Pringle, J. H.: Displacement of the mandibular meniscus and its treatment. Brit. J. Surg., *6*:375, 1918.

75. Ramfjord, S. P.: Diagnosis of traumatic temporomandibular joint arthritis. Calif. Dent. A. J. and Nev. Dent. Soc. J., *32*:300, 1956.
76. Ramfjord, S. P.: Dysfunctional temporomandibular joint and muscle pain. J. Prosth. Dent., *11*:353, 1961.
77. Redell, G.: Om intraartikulära kroppar i käkled. Sv. Tandl. Tidsk., *52*:301, 1959.
78. Rees, L. A.: Structure and function of the mandibular joint. Brit. Dent. J., *96*:125, 1954.
79. Ricketts, R. M.: Abnormal function of the temporomandibular joint. Am. J. Orthodont., *41*: 435, 1955.
80. Ross, I. F.: Effects of tensional clenching upon the structures of the neck. J. Periodont., *25*: 46, 1954.
81. Rushton, M. A.: Unilateral hyperplasia of the jaws in the young. Internat. Dent. J., *2*:41, 1951.
82. Schüle, H.: Elektromyographische Untersuchungen über die Wirkung von Myotonalytika auf die Kaumuskulatur. Deutsche Zahnärztl. Ztschr., *19*:495, 1964.
83. Schulte, W.: Zur funktionellen Behandlung des myo-Arthropathien des Kanorganes: Eine diagnostische und physio-therapeutisches program. D. Z. Z., *25*:422, 1970.
84. Schultz, L.: A curative treatment for subluxation of the temporomandibular joint or of any joint. J. Am. Dent. A., *24*:1947, 1937.
85. Schuyler, C. H.: Problems associated with opening the bite which would contraindicate it as a common procedure. J. Am. Dent. A., *26*:734, 1939.
86. Schwartz, L.: Disorders of the Temporomandibular Joint. Philadelphia, W. B. Saunders Co., 1959.
87. Schwartz, L.: Ethyl chloride treatment of limited, painful mandibular movements. J. Am. Dent. A., *48*:497, 1954.
88. Schwartz, L., and Tausig, D. P.: Temporomandibular joint pain—treatment with intramuscular infiltration of tetracaine hydrochloride: A preliminary report. New York Dent. J., *20*:219, 1954.
89. Sears, V. H.: Occlusal pivots. J. Prosth. Dent., *6*:332, 1956.
90. Seyffarth, H., and Steen-Johnsen, S.: Belastningsykkdommer i tyggeapparatet hos barn. Norsk. Tandl. Tidsk., *66*:295, 1956.
91. Siemssen, S. O.: Arteritis temporalis. Odont. Tidsk., *60*:314, 1952.
92. Shapiro, H. H.: Differential diagnosis of dental pain. Oral Surg., *4*:1353, 1951.
93. Sheppard, I. M.: The relation of occlusion and temporomandibular joint morphology to temporomandibular joint symptoms. J. Prosth. Dent., *6*:339, 1956.
94. Shohet, H.: The treatment of ear, facial, head, and other pains associated with pathologic temporomandibular joint. J. Prosth. Dent., *9*:80, 1959.
95. Sicher, H.: Structural and functional basis for disorders of the temporomandibular articulation. J. Oral Surg., *13*:275, 1955.
96. Sicher, H.: Temporomandibular articulation in mandibular overclosure. J. Am. Dent. A., *36*:131, 1948.
97. Sicher, H.: Problems of pain in dentistry. Oral Surg., *7*:149, 1954.
98. Shore, N. A.: Occlusal equilibration and temporomandibular joint dysfunction. Philadelphia, J. B. Lippincott Co., 1959.
99. Snawdon, J. W. E.: Fibrositis in the muscles of mastication. Roy. Soc. Med. Sect. Odont. Proc., *42*:153, 1949.
100. Summa, R.: The importance of the inter-articular fibro-cartilage of the temporo-mandibular articulation. Dent. Cosmos, *60*:512, 1918.
101. Thiemann, A.: Über nicht odontogene Kieferklemmen. Deutsche Zahnärztl. Ztschr., *5*:1052, 1950.
102. Thoma, K. H., and Goldman, H. M.: Oral Pathology. 5th ed. St. Louis, The C. V. Mosby Co., 1960.
103. Thomson, H.: Mandibular joint pain. Dent. Pract. & Dent. Rec., *13*:477, 1963.
104. Thonner, K.-E.: Aural symptoms in relation to the temporomandibular joint. Acta odont. scandinav., *10*:180, 1953.
105. Travell, J.: Ethyl chloride spray for painful muscle spasms. Arch. Physical Med., *33*:291, 1952.
106. Travell, J.: Temporomandibular joint pain referred from muscles of the head and neck. J. Prosth. Dent., *10*:745, 1960.

107. Vaughan, H. C.: Temporomandibular joint pain. A new diagnostic approach. J. Prosth. Dent., *4*:694, 1954.
108. Weeks, V., and Travell, J.: Postural vertigo due to trigger areas in the sternocleidomastoid muscle. J. Pediatrics, *47*:315, 1955.
109. Williams, H. L.: Meniere's disease. Springfield, Ill., Charles C Thomas, 1952.
110. Winters, S. E.: Staphylococcus infection of the temporomandibular joint. Oral Surg., *8*:148, 1955.
111. Wolff, H. G.: The nature and causation of headache. J. Dent. Med., *14*:3, 1959.
112. Wright, W. H.: Deafness as influenced by malposition of the jaws. Nat. Dent. A. J., *7*:979, 1920.
113. Zimmermann, A. A.: An evaluation of Costen's syndrome from an anatomic point of view. *In* Sarnat, B. G. (ed.): The Temporomandibular Joint. Springfield, Ill., Charles C Thomas, 1951, pp. 82–107.

Index